D0370385

STRESS AND THE HEART:
Interactions of the Cardiovascular System, Behavioral State, and Psychotropic Drugs

Second Edition

Stress and the Heart:
Interactions of the Cardiovascular System, Behavioral State, and Psychotropic Drugs

Second Edition

Editor

David Wheatley, M.A., M.D., M.R.C.Psych.
Head, General Practitioner Research Group
Twickenham, England

Raven Press ▪ New York

Raven Press, 1140 Avenue of the Americas, New York, New York 10036

© 1981 by Raven Press Books, Ltd. Previous edition © 1977 by Raven Press Books, Ltd. All rights reserved. This book is protected by copyright. No part of it may be reproduced, stored in a retrieval system, or transmitted, in any form or by any means, electronic, mechanical, photocopying, recording, or otherwise, without the prior written permission of the publisher.

Made in the United States of America

Library of Congress Cataloging in Publication Data

Main entry under title:

Stress and the heart.

Includes index.
1. Cardiovascular system—Diseases—Psychosomatic aspects. 2. Stress (Physiology) 3. Psychopharmacology. I. Wheatley, David, 1919–   . [DNLM: 1. Cardio-vascular diseases—Drug therapy. 2. Cardiovascular diseases—Etiology. 3. Psychotropic drugs—Pharma-codynamics. 4. Stress, Psychological. QV 77 S915]
RC669.S82   1981   616.1   80–28999
ISBN 0–89004–520–8

Great care has been taken to maintain the accuracy of the information contained in the volume. However, Raven Press cannot be held responsible for errors or for any consequences arising from the use of the information contained herein.

Second Printing, August 1981

616.1
S915
1981

Preface

In no system of the body are the manifestations of organic and psychiatric disease so intriguingly correlated as in the circulation of the blood. Thus, there are many similarities between symptoms of cardiovascular disease and the affective disorders, particularly when anxiety is predominant.

This is an uncharted ocean waiting to be explored. On the one hand, it is concerned with the influence of psychiatric symptomatology upon circulatory disorders, and, on the other hand, with the effects of the circulation upon psychiatric illness. The first edition of this book described the beginnings of this exploration into a field that covers the use of psychotropic drugs in circulatory disorders and, conversely, the use of cardiac drugs in psychiatric illnesses. Since then, further advances have occurred in these areas and promising and innovative pathways have been made into new areas, thus necessitating the second edition of this work.

The contributions to this volume encompass the five main fields of therapeutic practice associated with stress and cardiovascular function: coronary heart disease, cardiotoxic effects of psychotropic drugs, hypertension, cerebrovascular disease in the elderly, and beta-adrenergic blockade. In addition, much of the experimental work currently underway in the uses of drugs is presented. From its inception, this edition has been concerned with the working relationship between the clinician and the researcher. The average clinician is often unaware of much of the basic pharmacological research that forms the foundation of his subsequent therapeutic practice; conversely, many of those who are engaged in basic research do not always appreciate the clinical implications of their experimental work. It is the dual aim of this book to bridge these two gaps: the one between circulatory and psychiatric disorders, and the other between the laboratory and the clinician's consulting room.

An important additional section is concerned with the sociological aspects of the subject, which constitutes the epilogue to the book. Although the experimenter and the physician may consider the effects of stress and the methods of combating them pharmacologically, it is important as well to consider the nature of the stresses themselves, for this may also affect the heart and its workings. The nature, origin, and character of stress have changed considerably over the last 30 years and are important factors to consider when determining the best methods of managing the patient who is suffering from its effects. This applies particularly to the aged, who are the most vulnerable to the prolific stresses of present day life and in whom underlying cardiac abnormalities are most common.

In this second edition we have a number of new contributors who are pioneers in such uncharted and exciting areas as anti-anxiety drugs in coronary heart disease, beta-adrenergic blocking drugs in stressful situations and in schizophrenia, cardiotoxicity of antidepressants, yoga and bio-feedback in hypertension, nootropic drugs, and psychopharmacology in the elderly. Several of these contributions are appearing for the first time in published form, and others have been expanded and diversified for their initial presentation outside of their specialized fields.

The twin worlds of science and medicine owe an eternal debt to the genius of Hans Selye, whose original concept that stress—both physical and emotional— produces a set pattern of physical responses in the body, revolutionized scientific thinking and therapeutic practice. The contributors to this book are indeed honored that Dr. Selye has written the Introduction to their individual efforts to augment, each in his own way, the grand concept of stress and the heart, embracing as it does emotion, circulation, and stress.

David Wheatley

Contents

Contributors

Carl Burgess, M.B., M.R.C.P.
Lecturer
Department of Clinical Pharmacology
University of Southampton
Portsmouth, Hants, United Kingdom

Graham Burrows, M.D.
First Assistant and Reader
Department of Psychiatry
University of Melbourne
Royal Melbourne Hospital
Victoria 3050, Australia

**Malcolm Carruthers, M.D.,
M.R.C.G.P., M.R.C.Path.**
Senior Lecturer in Chemical Pathology
St. Mary's Hospital
London, United Kingdom

William J. Davidson, M.D.
*Department of Pharmacology and
Therapeutics*
Faculty of Medicine
University of Manitoba
Winnipeg R3E OW3, Canada

Richard Friedman, Ph.D.
Research Scientist and Assistant Professor
Long Island Research Institute
Department of Psychiatry
State University of New York
Stony Brook, New York 11794

David Griffith, M.R.C.P.
Assistant Lecturer in Medicine
The Royal Free Hospital
Hampstead, London, United Kingdom

John Gruzelier, M.D., Ph.D.
Senior Lecturer in Psychology
Charing Cross Hospital
Medical School
London, United Kingdom

**Anthony Hordern, M.D.,
F.R.C.P.Ed., F.R.C.P.,
F.R.C.Psych., FRANZCP,
D.P.M.**
Honorary Psychiatrist
Sydney Hospital
Sydney, Australia

Ian Hughes, B.Sc., Ph.D.
Senior Lecturer
Department of Pharmacology
University of Leeds
Leeds LS2 9JT, United Kingdom

**Ian M. James, Ph.D., M.B.B.S.,
F.R.C.P.**
*Senior Lecturer in Medicine and
Therapeutics*
Royal Free Hospital
Hampstead, London, United Kingdom

Hans Kopera, M.D.
Head, Clinical Pharmacology Unit
*Department of Experimental and Clinical
Pharmacology*
University of Graz
Graz, Austria

Mary F. Lockett, M.D., Ph.D.
Professor of Pharmacology
University of Western Australia
Nedlands, Australia

John F. Marwood, Ph.D.
Roche Research Institute
4–10 Inman Road
DEE DHY
New South Wales, 2099, Australia

Trevor Norman
Research Fellow
Department of Psychiatry
University of Melbourne
Royal Melbourne Hospital
Victoria 3050, Australia

Chandra H. Patel, M.D., M.R.C.G.P.
General Practitioner
Croydon, United Kingdom
and Senior Research Fellow
Department of Epidemiology
London School of Hygiene and Tropical
Medicine
London, United Kingdom

Richard Pearson, M.A., M.B., M.R.C.P.
Senior Medical Registrar
The Royal Free Hospital
Hampstead, London, United Kingdom

Henry I. Russek, M.D., F.A.C.C.
Research Professor in Cardiovascular
Disease
Clinical Professor of Medicine
New York Medical College
New York, New York 10029

Linda G. Russek, M.A.
Psychologist
The Russek Foundation
Staten Island, New York 10301

Bernd Saletu, M.D.
Section of Pharmacopsychiatry
Psychiatric University Clinic of Vienna
Vienna, Austria

Hans Selye, C.C., M.D., Ph.D., D.Sc.
Director
Institute of Experimental Medicine and
Surgery
University of Montreal
Montreal, Quebec, Canada

Leif Sourander, M.D.
Assistant Professor of Geriatric Medicine
University of Turku and Chief Physician
Department of Internal Medicine
City Hospital of Turku
Turku, Finland

Patrick Sourander, M.D.
Associate Professor of Pathology
University of Gothenburg
Gothenburg, Sweden

Peter Taggart, M.D., M.R.C.P., M.R.C.P.E.
Consultant Physician
Cavendish Medical Center and Senior
Lecturer in Cardiology
Middlesex Hospital
London, United Kingdom

Paul Turner, B.Sc., M.D., F.R.C.P.
Professor of Clinical Pharmacology
and Honorary Physician
St. Bartholomew's Hospital
London, United Kingdom
and Editor
British Journal of Clinical Pharmacology
London, United Kingdom

David Wheatley, M.A., M.D., M.R.C.Psych.
Head, General Practitioner Research
Group
Editor, Journal of Pharmacotherapy
and Clinical Assistant in Cardiology
St. John's Hospital
Twickenham, United Kingdom

Neil Yorkston, M.B., F.R.A.C.P., M.R.C.Psych., D.P.M., D.T.M.&H.
Consultant Physician
Bethlem Royal and Maudsley Hospitals
and Consultant Psychiatrist
Friern Hospital
London, United Kingdom

Saniha A. Zaki, M.B., Ch.B., M.S.C., D.P.M.
Senior Registrar
Friern Hospital
London, United Kingdom

Stress and the Heart, edited by D. Wheatley,
Raven Press, New York © 1981.

Introduction

Hans Selye

It is a pleasure to introduce this excellent volume on the effects of stress on the heart and circulatory system and the further interaction between pharmacological agents and the cardiovascular system under stress.

The historic background and general policy of this volume have been concisely outlined in the Preface by Dr. Wheatley. We need only to remind the reader, therefore, that the chief aim of the book is to bridge the gaps between circulatory and psychiatric disorders, on the one hand, and laboratory investigations, as well as clinical applications, on the other.

Since the volume focuses on the stress concept, it would be best to present the concept in general, as we understand it today, with major emphasis on its psychological and psychiatric implications. I shall pay special attention to those points considered most frequently in virtually every chapter. Much of this review is based on an article which I prepared for the Canadian Medical Association Journal (1), because the same fundamental problems seem to come up again in this present work, written as it is by clinicians and laboratory scientists who deal with stress, often from entirely unrelated points of view.

THE STRESS CONCEPT

More than four decades ago, we published a letter to the editor of *Nature,* entitled, "A syndrome produced by diverse nocuous agents" (2). Since that time, we have collected more than 150,000 publications (among them several hundred books) dealing with the different aspects of what is now known as the "stress concept," not only in virtually all fields of medicine, pathology, biochemistry, and medical jurisprudence but also in the behavioral sciences and philosophy. An encyclopedia quoting 7,518 key references is available under the title *Stress in Health and Disease* (3) and is meant to serve as a detailed guide to the pertinent literature. This voluminous and highly technical treatise appeared almost simultaneously with an entirely updated edition of *The Stress of Life* (4), first published about 24 years ago as a simple introduction to this field for general practitioners and medical students but formulated in a language understandable to educated lay persons.

The panoramic overview of the subject provided by the reexamination of all aspects of stress research was necessary for the presentation of the above-mentioned updated synoptic volumes. The compilation of these surveys, as well as many personal communications, made it opportune to present, as well, the simplest possible synopsis of those main points likely to cause difficulties in comprehension. It must be kept in mind that this introduction is not written for lay persons but for those who already have considerable understanding of the mechanism of stress reactions.

In retrospect, it is interesting to note that, irrespective of the specialties in which the stress concept has been used, the same 10 problems (some partly overlapping) have confused its application.

1. The definitions of stress, stressors, and the general adaptation syndrome (GAS).
2. Nonspecificity versus specificity.
3. Conditioning of stress responses by diverse endogenous and exogenous factors.
4. The GAS versus the local adaptation syndrome (LAS).
5. Direct versus indirect pathogens.
6. The definition of the "diseases of adaptation" (or stress-induced maladies).
7. Genetics versus self-control.
8. Syntoxic versus catatoxic agents.
9. The first mediator of the stress response.
10. Prophylaxis and treatment (the basic principles according to which the diseases of adaptation, or even feelings of distress in daily life, should be prevented or treated).

STRESS, STRESSORS, AND THE GAS

We have defined stress as "the nonspecific response of the body to any demand." A stressor is an agent which produces stress at any time. The GAS represents the chronological development of the response to stressors when their action is prolonged. It consists of three phases: (a) the alarm reaction, (b) the stage of resistance, and (c) the stage of exhaustion.

NONSPECIFICITY VERSUS SPECIFICITY

These terms may be applied to both the eliciting agent and the response. By nonspecific, we mean agents or responses characteristic of many effects or stimuli (e.g., the manifestations of the alarm reaction with the discharge of ACTH, corticoids, catecholamines, thymicolymphatic involution, eosinopenia, peptic ulcers). All these are nonspecific effects, since they can be elicited by innumerable agents that make an intense demand on the adaptability of the organism. On the other hand, the perception of green light is a highly specific response; it can be elicited only by the light of a given wavelength and only if this stimulus is applied to the retina. However, as we shall see when comparing the GAS and the LAS, even a highly specific local stimulus, such as intense light or sound, although acting specifically upon the eye or ear, respectively, can also cause a nonspecific, systemic (that is, general) stress reaction. It will do this if it is of sufficient magnitude to mobilize the general adaptive system of the entire body, e.g., by causing intense nervous arousal, with consequent stimulation of the hypothalamus-hypophysis-adrenocortical axis and generalized adrenergic responses.

Stereotyped nonspecific stress responses are highly specific in their manifestations but nonspecific in their causation, whereas generalized tissue catabolism, for example, is a nonspecific manifestation that may be evoked by many highly specific pathogens.

Thus specificity is always a relative phenomenon. Each agent that affects us (light, bacteria, hemorrhage, pain) has its own characteristics and, in addition, can cause stress, which is by definition a nonspecific demand for adaptation. Of course, certain agents and responses (e.g., long periods of excessive mental and physical work with consequent generalized fatigue) are predominantly nonspecific. Conversely, the perception of a certain light or sound wave and the production of Koplik's spots by the measles virus are highly specific in relation to both the evocative agents and the responses.

In this transition from the ideal, totally nonspecific, pure stress response to greater specificity, the first subdivision is the distinction between *eustress* and *distress,* the former being agreeable or healthy, the latter disagreeable or pathogenic. The way in which a certain stimulus will be received depends on its intensity and the particular receptiveness of the affected person. From these two main branches there can arise a virtually infinite number of ramifications in relation to the agents and the effects that are experienced during eustress and distress, respectively. This diversity depends primarily on conditioning.

CONDITIONING

The term conditioning is used in stress research not only in the Pavlovian sense but also to designate any factor that can influence the body's receptivity to a stressor (or stress-induced hormone).

As we have just seen, every agent posseses both stressor and specific effects; the latter can influence the stereotyped stress pattern by suppressing or enhancing some of its manifestations. It is precisely because all stressors must necessarily have some specific effects of their own that they cannot always elicit exactly the same response. In fact, even the same stimulus will act differently in different individuals, depending on endogenous conditioning factors (genetic predisposition, age, sex) or exogenous ones (treatment with hormones, drugs, exposure to environmental factors, including air pollution, social influences).

It is a lack of understanding of the role of conditioning that has so often prompted questions concerning two types of observations: (a) Qualitatively different stimuli of equal stressor potency (judged by their ability to elicit typical stress manifestations, e.g., ACTH, corticoid, or catecholamine production) do not necessarily cause the same stress syndrome in different individuals. (b) Even the same degree of stress induced by the same stimulus may provoke different lesions in different individuals.

GAS VERSUS LAS

We haved coined the term "systemic stress" to emphasize that a GAS is only elicited by stressors which directly or indirectly affect the whole body. On the other hand, a local adaptation syndrome, or LAS, is the response to nonspecific demands made on only one part of the body. Such demands may be made on a circumscribed, physically or chemically traumatized skin or connective tissue region; its manifestations then will be essentially those of inflammation, necrosis, or cell degeneration with regeneration. However, as we have said before, an intense LAS (in a limited muscle group, a sense organ, a brain region, etc.) may reach such proportions as to affect the body as a whole and produce a GAS through its secondary systemic stressor effects.

DIRECT VERSUS INDIRECT PATHOGENS

By direct pathogens, we mean those that act directly. Thus mechanical trauma, intense heat, or strong acids or alkalies will cause tissue damage, regardless of the body's response and, more particularly, irrespective of the defensive reactions characteristic of stress. That these pathogens are really direct and independent of any vital activity is best demonstrated by the fact that they will influence even a cadaver, which obviously cannot develop morbid lesions as a consequence of its own vital reactions.

Some other direct pathogens are endotoxins, spinal cord transection, and X-irradiation. Their effects (fever, paralysis, radiation syndrome) are not evident after death, yet they do act directly to a great extent. It is true that the body's defensive reactions (particularly the stress response) can be elicited by direct pathogens in the living organisms as a secondary consequence of their direct effects; however, their specific actions are not, or are only very slightly, influenced by the stress they produce.

Conversely, indirect pathogens act only, or predominantly, through the excessive or inappropriate defensive reactions which they elicit. For instance, emotional, immunological, and inflammatory reactions are primarily dependent on such indirect mechanisms.

DEFINITION OF DISEASES OF ADAPTATION OR STRESS-INDUCED MALADIES

Diseases of adaptation are primarily dependent on an excessive or inappropriate response to indirect pathogens. To this group belong all psychosomatic diseases, allergies, and other immunological responses, as well as excessive inflammatory reactions to agents which, in themselves, are harmless. In many of these maladies, it can readily be proven that the evocative agent itself is often not the cause of the trouble. For example, if emotional responses are prevented by suitable counseling or by psychopharmacological measures, or if immunological or inflammatory reactions are suppressed by glucocorticoids, it becomes clear that the evocative agent is not inherently pathogenic. Here we are dealing with the curious phenomenon that an essentially useful defensive reaction, developed in the course of evolution for protection (e.g., emotional arousal in preparation for fight, immunological and inflammatory responses to foreign intruders), can be the major cause of disease if the defense is inappropriate under the circumstances. It is true that, in the course of evolution, most of the inappropriate defense reactions have gradually been eliminated, whereas the fittest have survived. Evolution, however, is still in progess and is not yet perfect.

It should be remembered at this point that the platitude, "Nature knows best" is just as false as "Mother knows best." Nature may know best over millennia of further evolution, but meanwhile this is true only insofar as our brains have learned to correct false, automatic, adaptive defenses, using physical means (e.g., pharmacological, surgical) or mental ones (e.g., psychotherapeutic techniques, codes of behavior).

Even now there are many physicians who, in particular cases, have difficulty grasping the nonspecific aspect of the diseases of adaptation. Again and again, when faced with the interpretation of a peptic ulcer produced by a burn, they will quite justly emphasize that a peptic ulcer is a specific disease and a skin burn is a specific type of injury affecting a particular region of the body surface. Similarly, if a cardiac accident occurs in a patient after a violent marital dispute, these physicians will point out that both the result and the cause were specific; so why speak of a nonspecific stereotyped "stress" element?

Since this problem is so often misunderstood, it may be helpful to describe it in terms of well-known inanimate machines, all of which require energy to satisfy demands at an appropriate receptor. In patients, this is comparable to various highly specific morbid lesions produced by equally specific causative agents, but only if the latter generate a stress response.

Conditioning factors (innate or acquired) determine specifically which pathways and which receptors will be most sensitive to the common stimulus in any one case. Only a few responses are virtually always evident: massive acute energy liberation produces heat; massive acute stress stimulates the hypothalamus-pituitary-adrenocortical axis, as well as the catecholaminergic system, and causes catabolism.

If we compare this situation to energy utilization in inanimate machines, it is easy to see that an electric bulb, for example, placed directly in contact with a waterfall will not produce light, and an air conditioner will fail to perform properly if only soaked in its fuel. All the effects that can be produced by the inanimate receptors depend on energy derived from the diverse sources capable of furnishing it. Similarly, the diseases mentioned will not arise in patients exposed to the enumerated agents unless the latter do, in fact, produce stress.

Most of the apparent exceptions to the mediation of the diseases of adaptation by stress are readily explained. Thus some acute transient stressors (e.g., localized burns) are unlikely to cause hypertension because they do not act long enough; others (e.g., starvation, hemorrhage) will fail to raise blood pressure because they have a specific hypotensive effect.

GENETICS VERSUS SELF-CONTROL

We have already discussed in detail the various endogenous factors (to a large extent, inherited personality traits) and exogenous factors (environmental, including social) that determine the character of our response to stressors. In the last section, dealing with prophylaxis and treatment, we elaborate a code of behavior based on the natural laws that I believe to be highly efficacious in our achievement of homeostasis and happiness, behavior largely subject to self-control.

I do not think it is possible to answer, in quantitative terms, the eternal question about the relative importance of genetic predisposition and rational conduct, namely, our ability to respond to the exigencies of life by disciplined voluntary reactions, motivated by the pursuit of a goal which we really can and wish to achieve.

At present, there is great emphasis in medicine on inherited personality traits in the development of various stress-induced psychosomatic diseases, particularly with reference to the probability of coronary heart attack at an early age. We once described people with this behavioral pattern as the "stress seekers" or the "race horse type," as opposed to the easygoing "turtle type." In their now-classic studies, Friedman and Rosenman (5) refer to these as "Type-A" and "Type-B" persons, the former being particularly prone and the latter resistant to untimely coronary accidents during early middle age. These important investigations have been surveyed at length in *Stress in Health and Disease* (3). Suffice it here to reproduce one of their best descriptions of the coronary-prone personality:

> A Type-A behavior pattern is an action-emotion complex, shown by persons in chronic excessive struggle to achieve an unlimited number of things in the shortest possible time, perhaps against obstruction by other things or persons. The Type-A individual does not despair of losing the struggle, but confidently grapples with an endless succession of challenges. Type-A persons attempt to think, perform, communicate, and in general live more rapidly than do their peers."

This describes me perfectly! From the time I became addicted to medical research, at the age of 20, to the present (age 74 and still actively directing our institute), I have been the very prototype of this personality. Yet I have never had a coronary heart attack or any other manifestation of stress-induced illness. Let me emphasize that I am a great admirer of the excellent investigations that have led to the characterization of what we now know as the Type-A personality, primarily determined by genetic predisposition. I wish to console those born with this stigma, as I was, that the situation is not hopeless. We must learn to follow a code of behavior that turns distress into eustress. In any event, that is what has kept me healthy and happy, and even if I should die of a coronary accident before this book appears in print, it will not be "untimely." Besides, if I could be assured of survival until the age of 150 by turning into a "Type-B," I would not do it!

SYNTOXIC VERSUS CATATOXIC AGENTS

Syntoxic refers to agents that carry the message of coexistence with a potential pathogen. The best known examples of such chemical agents are syntoxic hormones, such as glucocorticoids, which suppress many of the usually helpful, defensive, inflammatory, or immunological reactions. Catatoxic refers to impulses for fight and aggression. Some natural steroid hormones (e.g., those of the testes) have catatoxic effects, but more effective are certain synthetic steroid hormone derivatives, such as pregnenolone-16α-carbonitrile, which induce aggressive drug-metabolizing enzymes in the liver. The latter can destroy a large number of pathogens (e.g., barbiturates, certain carcinogens, and digitalis compounds).

Not only chemical substances but people, as well, can be syntoxic or catatoxic. When a person is facing a potential aggressor, he may assume a syntoxic or catatoxic attitude; he may choose to act syntoxically and ignore the aggressor, or he may act catatoxically and fight against the potential threat.

THE "FIRST MEDIATOR" OF THE STRESS RESPONSE

Ever since the original description of the stress syndrome appeared, we have been puzzled by the nature of the "first mediator," which carries the message of stress from the area directly affected (e.g., a burned hand, an excited cerebral cortex, a vascular system depleted of blood) to the centers (e.g., hypothalamus, adenohypophysis) that regulate homeostatic reactions. We have learned a great deal about the latter, which represent the output of the stress centers, but very little is known about the nature of the input.

First, we have had to consider afferent nervous impulses and blood-borne chemical mediators, which carry the information that a state of stress exists. Undoubtedly in man, with his highly developed central nervous system, psychological stressors and emotional arousal, particularly, are of primary importance. This is especially true of the most common stressors of daily life (frustration, anger, fear, hate). Contrary to the opinion of some psychiatrists and psychologists, however, nervous arousal, particularly in the form of a conscious affect or emotion, cannot always be the common pathway. For example, typical activation of the hypothalamus-pituitary-adrenocortical axis and the adrenergic system can be accomplished by decortication, by surgical interventions under deep anesthesia, or by anesthesia itself.

Furthermore, stress occurs in lower animals and plants which have no central nervous system, and even in isolated cell colonies growing in tissue cultures. In addition, the entire hypophysiotropic area can be surgically isolated from the rest of the brain by a tubular knife (generally known as the Halász knife), pushed down from the cortex to the base of the skull. With this instrument, we can accomplish a complete "deafferentation" of the hypophysiotropic area, which then remains in contact with the hypophysis only through the stalk vessels. This operation causes no reduction in basal ACTH secretion (which, in fact, is usually above normal), and the adenohypophysis continues to respond to various stressors (ether, restraint, tourniquet shock, formaldehyde) by a rise in plasma ACTH and corticoid levels. In animals with such a completely isolated hypophysiotropic area, even the compensatory hypertrophy of the remaining adrenal is demonstrable after ablation of the contralateral gland. On the other hand, all these stress responses are abolished if the median eminence of the hypophysiotropic area is destroyed.

Hence it may be accepted, as well established today, that blood-borne stimuli can initiate the stress response even if emotional arousal (or any other cortical stimulus) is prevented from reaching the centers that produce corticotropin-releasing factor (CRF), the substance which induces the pituitary to produce ACTH.

As I said many years ago and repeated recently in an article on some persisting sources of "Confusion and controversy in the stress field" (6),

> As yet, nothing is known about the chemical nature of this first mediator; so far as we know, it may be a chemical by-product of activity or the lack of some important blood constituent that cells use up whenever they function. The identification of this first mediator appears to be one of the most fundamental tasks of future stress research.

Of course, a common feature of the body's response to any demand is energy consumption. Our analogy of inanimate machines raises the possibility that increased fuel consumption may be the common mediator in living machines also. In fact, an increase in the basal metabolic rate (BMR) often accompanies stress responses, but the two do not necessarily run parallel. Severe shock may be associated with a decrease in the BMR, whereas the administration of small doses of thyroid hormone can raise the BMR considerably with negligible manifestations of stress. The situation is somewhat comparable to that of an automobile which may use up large amounts of fuel and produce much energy without performing any work (locomotion) or causing any physical stress or strain in the machine outside of the motor itself. Conversely, running at full speed downhill over an extremely bumpy road with the engine completely cut off will expose the tires, springs, and other parts of the automobile to considerable stress, although there is no fuel consumption.

PROPHYLAXIS AND TREATMENT

A good deal of confusion has arisen in the literature with the recommendation of various drugs (tranquilizers, antiadrenergic agents, or even psychedelics and vitamins) to "eliminate stress." Some are undoubtedly useful in diminishing distress caused by excessive emotional lability; others are totally ineffective or even harmful in any kind of stress situation.

However, the first thing to keep in mind is that we must not suppress stress in all its forms but rather diminish distress and facilitate eustress, the satisfactory feeling that comes from the accomplishment of tasks that we consider worthwhile.

As I have said often, stress is the salt of life; few people would like to live an existence of no runs, no hits, no errors. Yet it is undoubtedly useful, from time to time, for the human machine to take a rest, and various techniques (transcendental meditation, the "relaxation response," Zen, Yoga, biofeedback, autohypnosis) have been devised to diminish all forms of biological stress temporarily to a level close to the minimum compatible with survival. Total elimination of stress is impossible, even during short periods, because that would involve the cessation of demands made upon any part of the body, including the cardiovascular, respiratory, and nervous systems. This would be equivalent to death.

Furthermore, it is undoubtedly of general value in certain situations, for the mobilization of useful adaptive reactions and an increase in general resistance, to use strong stressors [e.g., physical exercise, hydrotherapy, electroshock, insulin shock, pentylenetetrazol (Metrazol®) shock, nonspecific fever therapy]. The mechanism by which such stressors improve fitness and help the body's efforts to overcome diseases of adaptation is still unknown, yet the efficacy of these stressors has received ample empirical proof.

Experience has shown that often a change in activity (sometimes technically described as "deviation" or "diversion" of efforts) is more useful and more relaxing than complete rest. A person suffering extreme distress because of the continued use of his brain for a long time (e.g., in solving mathematical problems) will profit more from jogging, swimming, or fishing than from doing nothing; this is probably because his subconscious mind, if not otherwise engaged, continues to be preoccupied with the problems that caused his distress.

Little is known about why one or another type of stress treatment (shock therapy, relaxation, exercise) is more efficacious in special cases. Presumably, the conditioning factors associated with diverse prophylactic and therapeutic procedures, as well as those that accompany the harmful stressors that cause distress, so modify the stereotyped response that a certain degree of specificity becomes evident. For example, the various types of shock therapy are most useful in the treatment of certain psychoses. On the other hand, exercise, sauna, cold showers, and the many psychological relaxation techniques are more efficient in helping us to master the stress situations of everyday life; they turn the distress of fatigue and failure into the eustress of success and fulfillment.

To these time-honored procedures for the mastery of stress we have recently added a code of behavior described as "altruistic egoism." It is independent of, but compatible with, all religions and political doctrines, being based exclusively on biological laws regulating stress resistance on the cellular level. This code could not be outlined meaningfully here, but it has been described at length in *Stress Without Distress* (7). In essence, it accepts the reality that all living creatures are, and must be, primarily selfish; big fish must eat little fish or they will perish. None of us can expect others to look after us more than after themselves. However, we must meticulously avoid reckless selfishness, the kind that would induce a hooligan to kill a poor old widow for the few dollars in her piggy bank as long as he is sure that nobody can catch him. I object to this type of egoism not merely on moral grounds, for moralizing is not the domain of the physician, but also because reckless egoism is biologically unsound; it creates so many enemies and such feelings of uncertainty that it could never act as a satisfactory, permanent guideline through life.

However, we can rid ourselves of guilt feelings and inferiority complexes caused by our inability to be ideal altruists once we admit that egoism is an inescapable feature of all living beings. It is indispensable to the maintenance of both the individual and the species.

We must have a definite aim in life worth pursuing in order to satisfy our innate desire for accomplishment, self-expression, and creativity in our chosen occupation. It is biologically impossible to take literally the command, "Love thy neighbor as thyself." Man can die on command on the battlefield (as did the kamikaze pilots in the service of their Emperor); he can die on command as a martyr in the service of whatever God he accepts; but he cannot love on command. It is up to our neighbors to make themselves lovable. This code of behavior, based on altruistic egoism, tries to satisfy the natural egoistic tendencies of hoarding a capital for security. Most animals hoard food or building materials to assure their homeostasis in future time of need. In the case of man, however, this capital need not necessarily be stocked in the form of dollars, social position, or powerful weaponry, all of which may be taken away or become obsolete. It may be in the form of love and good will, achieved by learning to be useful to others.

I believe this can be done while still preserving the time-honored wisdom of the "Golden Rule." The ancient Hebrew version of "Love thy neighbor as thyself" may be translated, without loss of content, into modern language understandable to all contemporary people. The essence of this unassailable law of behavior can be retained and even enlarged into a motivating guideline if we rephrase it in terms of the scientifically oriented thinking of our times: "*Earn thy neighbor's love.*"

This will best assure homeostasis and resistance to stressors throughout life and give a satisfactory purpose to our activities. It will remove the need for destructive outlets or refuges from distasteful activities provided by violence, alcohol, or psychedelic drugs, which are at the root of "the crisis of our time."

We must recognize that man must work, that he must be selfish and hoard capital to assure his security; but who would blame the person whose egoistic and capitalistic tendencies express themselves in the unsatiable desire to accumulate the good will, esteem, and love of others by helping them, even if he is motivated by altruistic egoism?

Those who are interested in a code of behavior based on stress research may wish to know that this was the topic of my presidential address at the tremendously successful Second International Symposium on the Management of Stress (November 18–22, Monte Carlo, Monaco), the largest such meeting ever held. (Among the main speakers were several Nobel laureates: Sir Hans Krebs, Christian de Duve, Linus Pauling, and my former student, Roger Guillemin—as well as Jonas Salk, Mauricio Rocha e Silva, and William R. Barclay, Chief Editor of *JAMA*.) Future annual conventions are now being planned for the cities of Marakesh, Cairo, Tokyo, and Montreal, among others. The proceedings of all these congresses are to be published in the newly formed *Stress: The Official Journal of the Hans Selye Foundation and Its Affiliates,* to each issue of which I will be contributing a brief editorial.

In this introduction, I wanted to summarize the principal somatic and mental aspects of the stress syndrome as we see it today, after more than 40 years of experimental and clinical research on this and related subjects. I hope that this résumé will furnish a suitable framework for the special topics discussed by many distinguished authors in this anthology on stress.

REFERENCES

1. Selye, H. Forty years of stress research: The principal remaining problems and misconceptions. *Can. Med. Assoc. J.,* 1976, 115, 53.
2. Selye, H. A syndrome produced by diverse nocuous agents. *Nature (Lond.).* 1936, 138, 32.
3. Selye, H. *Stress in Health and Disease.* Butterworths, Reading, Massachusetts, 1976.
4. Selye, H. *The Stress of Life.* McGraw-Hill, New York, 1976.
5. Friedman, M., and Rosenman, R. H. Association of specific overt behavior pattern with blood and cardiovascular findings. *JAMA,* 1959, 169, 1268.
6. Selye, H. Confusion and controversy in the stress field. *J. Human Stress,* 1975, 1, 37.
7. Selye, H. *Stress Without Distress.* Lippincott, New York, 1974.

Prologue: Stress Factors in Coronary Heart Disease

It is obvious that the phenomenon of increasing morbidity due to coronary heart disease (CHD) and that of increasing stresses of everyday life are intimately related. The scientist, however, works with facts, and these are not always easy to acquire, particularly when emotional changes are involved.

In the opening chapter of this section, Henry Russek describes his extensive research into the sociological and occupational factors that contribute to the incidence of CHD and provides data collected from different types of individuals who are subject to varying degrees of emotional stress, both at work and in the home. His figures clearly illustrate the multicausal nature of CHD and the important of emotional stress in its etiology, whether deliberately endured by the patient or inflicted on him by genetic susceptibility.

This theme is carried a step further by Peter Taggart in the succeeding chapter, wherein he describes his research, undertaken in conjunction with Malcolm Carruthers, into a number of physical parameters associated with CHD and notes the influence on them of various stressful occupations. Not content with recording these associations, Taggart and Carruthers proceeded to study the effects of pharmacological "stress-blocking" (1).

The final chapter of the section, surveying the multietiological background of CHD, considers psychogenic factors, which play a part in many of the known causal factors of the condition. The impact of emotional stresses of various kinds on the cardiovascular system, and in particular on the sufferer from CHD, has been fully confirmed in many studies covering different aspects of the subject. The possibilities for treatment of the anxiety factor are then considered and the results of preliminary studies described to assess the use of antianxiety drugs in comparison to placebo. The therapeutic possibilities provided by such an approach may involve not only the amelioration of the symptoms of CHD (and particularly angina) but also prevention of myocardial infarction and the attainment of a more tranquil state in those who suffer from the condition.

In the first chapter of this section, the problem is defined as a result of research by survey; in the second, the theme is continued through the collection of physical data; finally, a therapeutic procedure is presented.

REFERENCE

1. Carruthers, M. *The Western Way of Death.* David-Poynter, London, 1974.

Stress and the Heart, edited by D. Wheatley,
Raven Press, New York © 1981.

Behavior Patterns and Emotional Stress in the Etiology of Coronary Heart Disease: Sociological and Occupational Aspects

Henry I. Russek and Linda G. Russek

THE MASTERY OF STRESS

While these observations emphasize that the magnitude of the stressors in our environment influences group susceptibility to coronary heart disease, they also reveal that the adaptive capacity of each person may be a major determinant of individual susceptibility. Thus there is mounting evidence to support the belief that vulnerability to coronary heart disease, mental and emotional disorders, and other psychosomatic syndromes may be correlated with the ability or inability of the individual to handle stress in continuum. All individuals have a characteristic manner of responding to an acute threat in keeping with the basic disposition of the personality, but it is only in those who fail to adapt to repetitive or continued stress that sustained reactions may predispose to subsequent disease. Cannon (46) was among the first to show the relationship of behavioral and emotional changes to physiologic responses. With the term "fight or flight reaction," he characterized a set of responses attributed to the adrenal medulla. Later studies by Selye (47) and Thorn (48) placed more emphasis on the sustained nature of the stress reaction, which they considered to be mediated through the action of the adrenal cortex. Since the ability or inability of individuals to master a continuing emergency situation is the major determinant of whether or not a sustained reaction takes place, methods have been devised to record responses which may shed light on the predisposition to subsequent disease.

Funkenstein and associates (49) have clearly shown in studies of young college students that many individuals fail to adapt to recurrent exposure to stressful stimuli. In experiments with laboratory-induced frustration at three weekly testing sessions, the authors were able to identify those subjects who exhibited a significant physiologic response initially, which either did not diminish or actually became accentuated in subsequent tests. In contrast, others were found in whom the degree of response was either minimal throughout or of diminishing intensity with repetitive exposures. Prospective studies would be valuable to confirm the validity of such methods for identifying future candidates for coronary heart disease. For the present, the hypothesis is most attractive and consistent with clinical and experimental observations.

Stress, Adaptation, and Evolution

If man is subject to the same evolutionary forces that Darwin observed in the lower animals a century ago, then he is participating in a process of natural selection which is determining who shall survive in the complex society which he has created. Since his appearance on this planet, homo sapiens have spent some 3.75 million years in the forest, 10,000 years on the farm, and only 300 years in the factory. Because adaptation to changing environment is a process that may require hundreds of thousands of years, modern man may have long to go in his continuing evolutionary development before acquiring the capacity to cope adequately with the relatively unfamiliar problems which now confront him. In this new environment of industrialized and mechanized society, many individuals appear to be responding to the symbolic and real challenges of daily living in the same manner as primitive man once reacted to the far greater threat to survival itself while inhabiting the forest and the cave. Moreover, while the fight or flight mechanism was apparently designed for short-term emergency needs, it appears that coronary-prone subjects often possess homeostatic mechanisms, which remain chronically mobilized in response to the demands of a rapidly changing environment. By sustained general autonomic arousal, such persons manifest a failure to master stress in continuum. From the resulting chronic activation of the defense center in the hypothalamus, cholesterol levels in the blood are maintained at a higher range, circulating catecholamines are present in increased concentrations, and clotting mechanisms are adversely affected. A high fat diet, cigarette smoking, lack of exercise, and diabetes could readily exert a harmful influence by exaggerating certain components of these physiologic expressions of fight or flight. Similarly, prolonged emotional stress, sociocultural mobility, or stressful life events could also bridge the gap between subclinical genetic predisposition and premature maturation of coronary artery disease.

Augmented Sympathetic Arousal and Ischemic Heart Disease

Although designed to be beneficial when danger threatens, catecholamines can also be detrimental. Their effect may lead to sudden rises in blood pressure, dangerous arrhythmias, and increased oxygen requirements for the heart. Aggregation of platelets in the microcirculation and diffuse myocardial necrosis are also well-known consequences of stress or prolonged catecholamine infusions (43). Of even greater interest is the role of augmented sympathetic arousal in the etiology of ischemic heart disease.

Reference has been made to laboratory studies which have shown significant differences in the capacity of normal individuals to mount a physiologic response to recurrent challenge (49). These observations take on added importance when considering the evidence that the pattern of reaction to stress may be a major determinant of susceptibility to future disease. There are now abundant data to indicate that patients with coronary disease respond to a variety of stresses with augmented catecholamine release when compared with normal subjects. Nestel (50) demonstrated a statistically higher vanilmandelic acid excretion in such patients after mildly painful stimuli or after the stress of doing arithmetic problems. Similarly, one of the major characteristics of the Type A coronary-prone individual is his excessive secretion of norepinephrine in response to a nonphysical competitive task (7). Even more conclusive is the finding in prospective studies that those in whom clinical coronary disease develops tend to produce twice as much epinephrine in a 24-hour period than the less coronary prone (45,51).

The possible importance of the sympathetic nervous system in the pathogenesis of clinical coronary disease is also suggested by the finding that a rise in diastolic pressure in the cold pressor test was the single most important variable for coronary heart disease prediction in a 23-year longitudinal prospective investigation conducted by Keys et al. (52). The relative risk ratio for coronary heart disease, death, or myocardial infarction of the hyperreactor group was 2.4 times that of the men who showed a rise of less than 20 mm. Type A behavior is associated with a heightened response to psychologic stimuli, whereas hyperreaction to cold represents an augmented response to physical challenge; one of us (LGR), however, has found no significant relationship between hyperreactivity to cold and Type A behavior pattern (53). If significant at all, therefore, hyperreactivity to cold must be an independent variable completely divorced from the psychosocial TypeA/B paradigm.

While considerable data attest to the significance of stress and augmented sympathetic activity in the etiology of coronary heart disease, certain conclusions concerning the extent of their influence can be drawn from natural experiments within the framework of human history. For example, the rarity of coronary episodes in German concentration camps and in the occupied Scandinavian countries during World War II indicates that morbidity and mortality are determined by the nature of the nutritional substrate upon which the psychologic and physiologic responses operate. In other words, stress and cholesterol appear to be dependent on each other for pathogenetic significance (6,16,17). In this connection, we have repeatedly emphasized that high fat diet and stressful living represent an exceptionally lethal combination; this is undoubtedly true for those without the genetic endowment to master stress.

Indirect confirmation of the importance of excessive and disproportionate sympathetic responses in the causation and progression of coronary heart disease has recently been obtained from long-term studies employing beta-adrenergic blocking agents. In one controlled trial of approximately 3,000 postinfarction patients in the United Kingdom, cardiac deaths were reduced by more than one-third in patients receiving the cardioselective beta-adrenergic blocker practolol. Although serious consideration is now being given to the use of such drugs after anterior myocardial infarction, there may also be good rationale for their use in selected coronary-prone subjects and those with known disease as prophylactic therapy before the advent of infarction.

The Stress of Modern Life

According to the data of statisticians, people in the United States enjoy more leisure than any civilization in history. Theoretically, at least, there can be no disagreement with this finding. In reality, however, this era of less work and more play is a tormenting illusion. It has been pointed out that the majority of the population work harder—at something—than we have ever done before (54). More than one in every 20 workers, according to the United States Census Bureau, is holding down two jobs, and some are managing three. Store owners work more than 50 hr per week, and physicians commonly work more. Despite mechanization, farmers are still engaged in their occupation for at least 50 hr per week, while top corporation executives spend 60 hr per week at their jobs, including the work they take home. More than one-third of married women are now employed outside the home, thus adding a job to the one they already have, and many men whose wives work also take on the extra job of helping to run the house. It is not until the average American arrives home at the end of the day, however, that the pressures of society start to close in (54). Far from being free from the demands of work or duty, much leisure time is regimented by participation in adult classes at night school, bowling, volunteer work, dancing lessons, bridge, community drives for funds, club meetings, and the like. Such obligatory use of leisure is not satisfying and may represent a poor antidote for the emotional stresses of daily business competition.

Atherosclerosis as a Pediatric Problem

In underdeveloped areas of the world, atherosclerosis is seen as an aging process in the latter decades of life; in Western society, it arises as a pediatric disorder. This is clearly demonstrated by the results of studies performed on soldiers killed during the Korean and Vietnamese wars (55). Although the dangers inherent in the typical American diet have frequently been emphasized in relation to the growing child, it seems incredible that the "stresses" to which a student is exposed during his 16 to 20 years in educational institutions have not been scanned for possible detriments to health (32–34). Quality education has become a scarce commodity and dedicated teachers an endangered species, necessitating more and more self-instruction at home. At the same time, demanding schedules and assignments no longer permit books to be read leisurely for pleasure or profit, but only superficially for grades. Frustrating assignments during holiday vacations or the scheduling of tests immediately thereafter destroy both the opportunity and the inclination for wholesome recreation and beneficial exercise. Other antidotes for stress in the form of hobbies, art, music, recreation, rest, and sleep are being sacrificed for the "benefits" of modern education. In the regimented setting at school, prescribed physical training is often neither enjoyable nor relaxing and may actually discourage continuation of athletic pursuits later in life. The once-popular ball games on city streets after school have largely vanished as a consequence of demanding homework assignments or easy access to television. Through activities such as science fairs, educators and parents alike seek to create scientists out of youngsters who scarcely have had time to be children. Compounding the effect of these pressures, unrelenting competition for high scholastic standing and college placement makes formalized education in the United States a highly traumatic experience for most students. Confirming this view, a recent study by the Carnegie Corporation has characterized most public schools as "aggressive," "grim," and "joyless."

With these considerations in mind, it would be difficult to conceive of a group of candidates more prone to ischemic heart disease than the graduating class of any medical school in the United States—unless they were the same individuals after the completion of their internship or residency. Little wonder that even 75 years ago Osler (14) called it the "doctors' disease."

PRIMARY AND SECONDARY PREVENTION IN ISCHEMIC HEART DISEASE

What Has Been Accomplished?

In the past two decades, we have witnessed a significant change in the saturated fat content of the American diet, along with the introduction of effective hypocholesterolemic agents. There has been a growing awareness of the need for exercise and normal body weight and the avoidance of tobacco. Diabetes and hypertension have been more effectively managed through better understanding and new drugs. Nonetheless, despite these apparent gains, there has been at best only questionable improvement in the mortality risk from coronary heart disease among the general population. Even among physicians, who are obviously the most knowledgeable in this area of prevention, no favorable alteration in longevity has occurred over the past 20 years (32–24). One must conclude, therefore, either that the "advances" thus far have been ineffective in dealing with the plague that now confronts us, or that inroads of progress are being counterbalanced by the growth of etiologic influences about which we have done or can do little. A new orientation is long overdue.

Preventive Medicine

Treatment today is largely focused on the end result of a disease process rather than on its prophylaxis. Therapeutic interventions may someday block the atherogenicity of a high fat diet, hypercholesterolemia, and emotional stress; until then, however, hygienic measures and preventive medicine must begin in childhood and continue throughout life if any real impact is to be made on the mortality risk from coronary heart disease. It has long been evident that the mental, emotional, physical, recreational, and spiritual needs of the young are being increasingly unfulfilled in both the academic and the home environments, despite unprecedented affluence. The resultant stresses may be responsible for the precocious atherosclerosis observed in our young people. American educational institutions certainly can play a crucial role in preventive cardiology. By teaching and encouraging the practice of sound prophylactic measures both at school and at home, we may finally curb the black plague of the 20th century. To accomplish this goal, however, education must be made an integral part of living, not a substitute for it.

Theoretical Considerations: Approaches to Stress Management

Stress research has clearly shown that every person inherits a genetically determined pattern of response to both emotional and physical demands. In some, the physiologic consequences of exposure to challenge reflects an augmented alarm reaction indicative of the inability of the individual to master stress. This genetic weakness may lie dormant or may be brought to clinical recognition by the struggle to survive in a competitive environment, by stressful life events, or by social and cultural mobility. Sustained arousal for fight or flight may be further aggravated by acquired behavioral characteristics, which create the atmosphere for repetitive crises in confronting life situations (Type A behavior pattern). Ideal therapy would allow an alarm reaction proportionate to the challenge, with rapid return to a state of relaxation when the threat has passed; it would confer diminishing responses to repetitive crises as an indication of the mastery of stress.

At present, a determined effort is being made by the medical and psychotherapeutic communities to mobilize a holistic treatment approach to stress management and to promote a new model of well-being called "wellness." This concept of wellness, different from the disease model, which states that one is well if he or she is without physical signs and symptoms, goes beyond the classic concept. Wellness includes higher levels of health derived from spiritual, mental, and emotional growth, education, and self-actualization. It encompasses an integration and complex combination of mind, body, and spirit, in contrast with the disease model, which relates to only one part, the body. Our increasing understanding of the interaction between mind and body and its role in the causation and exacerbation of psychosomatic diseases has engendered mounting interest in the wellness model. In our own program as in others across the country, a multidimensional approach is followed in an effort to provide, through experience and education, new and appropriate channels by which each individual can responsibly choose what proves most effective for him. The ability to make self-informed and responsible choices is considered the keynote of any desired outcome. The most notable therapeutic modalities and educational skills in use for this purpose are the following: (a) assertiveness training, (b) prescribed exercise, (c) cognitive restructuring therapies, (d) biofeedback with visual imagery, (e) meditation (relaxation response), (f) progressive Jacobsonian relaxation, (g) autogenic hypnosis, (h) individual and group psychotherapy, (i) body awareness training, and (j) dietary regulation.

The failure to master stress has been attributed to the rigidity of the response repertoire when evoked by challenges of varying magnitude. It is manifested by the inability to create, choose, and adapt expectations and beliefs, coping skills, and problem-solving techniques to meet the demands of the situation.

Cognitive restructuring therapies are concerned primarily with the psychologic aspects of language and communication. Whereas some cognitive restructuring therapists emphasize problem-solving, others are more concerned with coping skills. The problem-solving approach teaches the individual to stand back and systematically analyze a problem situation in the absence of any acute stress; the coping skills approach concentrates on what the individual must do when immediately confronted with an acute stressful situation. The problem-solving treatment is designed to teach the person how to identify problems, generate alternative solutions, tentatively select a solution, and then test and verify the efficacy of that solution. In contrast, Ellis's rational emotive therapy (RET) attempts to make the individual aware of negative self-statements and images and of the anxiety-engendering, self-defeating, and self-fulfilling prophecy aspects of such thinking.

Assertiveness training has proved to be most effective in providing a process and structure for thinking, feeling, and behaving which still allows for individualism in its use. Based on the theory of reciprocal inhibition, anxiety or anger cannot be present when assertive behavior is being utilized. We believe that assertiveness may be a civilized means of defusing the fight or flight mechanism, while still allowing the individual to defend himself in a manner appropriate to the perceived degree of threat.

Exercise is another valuable technique for neutralizing the cumulative effects of stress. Since the original purpose of the fight or flight mechanism was to activate the musculoskeletal system, regular exercise by recoupling the muscular component of the stress response may serve to neutralize the alarm reaction. Exercise may also divert attention from higher psychologic processing to more primitive bodily functions, thereby alleviating anxiety and tension.

The simplicity and potential of methods for obtaining the relaxation response, which is the reverse of the fight or flight phenomenon and which also appears to have a center of control within the hypothalamus, have stimulated wide public interest in this approach (see Chapter 14). The many techniques of meditation seem to have a common basis, namely, "restriction of attention to an unchanging source of stimulation." The result is essentially the same: predominance of alpha EEGs and a physiologic pattern of relaxation. Autogenic hypnosis, progressive Jacobsonian relaxation, and biofeedback with visual imagery are also effective modalities for redirecting attention to the internal environment by cognitive mediation, using pictures and internal auditory dialogue. Individual and group therapy are also valuable treatment modalities for both supporting and directing the course of emotional and behavioral change.

While behavior modification and cognitive restructuring therapies may reduce the build-up of stress, and meditation and exercise may encourage its discharge, there are also pharmacologic agents which are valuable in blunting its final expression. Thus the use of propranolol may prevent some of the important pathophysiologic consequences of the stress reaction by blocking chronotropic and inotropic effects, the aggregation of platelets in the microcirculation of the heart, the development of diffuse cardiac necrosis, and other responses, while sedatives and tranquilizers are useful in diminishing central autonomic hyperactivity.

CONCLUSIONS

Despite the application of primary and secondary preventive measures and significant advances in the treatment of angina pectoris and myocardial infarction, the overall morbidity and mortality from ischemic heart disease has not been appreciably altered in the past two decades in the United States. To date, it is evident that efforts have failed dismally in preventing the inexorable progression of coronary atherosclerosis and its disabling and fatal complications.

Abundant evidence now exists to indicate not only that high fat diet and stressful living form a most lethal combination, but also that each is dependent on the other for pathologic significance. It is therefore probable that dietary alteration, physical training, and environmental relaxation could prove effective prophylactically only if instituted early in childhood and maintained as a lifetime practice.

The simplicity and potential of methods for obtaining the relaxation response, which is the reverse of the fight or flight phenomenon, have stimulated many techniques of meditation. Thus behavior modification and cognitive restructuring therapies may reduce the build-up of stress, and meditation and exercise may encourage its discharge. There are also pharmacologic agents which are valuable in blunting its final expression.

ACKNOWLEDGMENT

This study was supported by The Russek Foundation, Inc., Staten Island, New York.

REFERENCES

1. Osler, W. Lectures on angina pectoris and allied states. *NY Med. J.*, 1896, 4, 224.
2. Arlow, J. A. Identification mechanisms in coronary occlusion. *Psychosom. Med.*, 1945, 7, 195.
3. Kemple, C. Rorschach method and psychosomatic diagnosis: Personality traits of patients with

rheumatic disease, hypertensive cardiovascular disease, coronary occlusion and fracture. *Psychosom. Med.,* 1945, 7, 85.

4. Wolf, S. G. Cardiovascular reactions to symbolic stimuli. *Circulation,* 1958, 18, 287.

5. Friedman, M., and Rosenman, R. H. Association of specific overt behaviour pattern with blood and cardiovascular findings: Blood cholesterol level, blood clotting time, incidence of arcus senilis, and clinical coronary artery disease. *JAMA,* 1959, 169, 1286.

6. Russek, H. I., and Zohman, B. L. Relative significance of heredity, diet, and occupational stress in coronary heart disease in young adults. *Am. J. Med. Sci.,* 1958, 235, 266.

7. Roseman, R. H., Friedman, M., Straus, R., Wurm, M., Jenkins, C. D., and Messinger, H. B. Coronary heart disease in the Western collaborative group study. *JAMA,* 1966, 195, 86.

8. Weiss, E. et al. Emotional factors in coronary occlusion. *AMA Arch. Int. Med.,* April 1957, 99, 628.

9. Buell, T., and Breslow, L. Mortality from coronary heart disease in California men who work long hours. *J. Chronic Dis.,* 1960, 2, 615.

10. Gertler, M. M. et al. *Coronary Heart Disease in Young Adults: Multidisciplinary Study.* Published for Commonwealth Fund by Harvard University Press, Cambridge, Mass., 1954, p. 65.

11. Yater, W. M. et al. Coronary artery disease in men 18 to 39 years of age: Report of 866 cases, 450 with necropsy examinations. *Am. Heart J.,* 1948, 36, 344 (Sept.), 481 (Oct.), 683 (Nov.).

12. Russek, H. I. Emotional stress and coronary heart disease in American physicians. *Am. J. Med. Sci.,* 1960, 240, 711.

13. Morris, J. N., Heady, J. A., and Barley, R. G. Coronary heart disease in medical practitioners. *Br. Med. J.,* 1952, 1, 503.

14. Osler, W. Angina pectoris, *Lancet,* 1910, 1, 697.

15. Smith, H. L. Incidence of coronary sclerosis among physicians, *JAMA,* 1937, 108, 1327.

16. Russek, H. I. Emotional stress and coronary heart disease in American physicians, dentists and lawyers. *Am. J. Med. Sci.,* 1962, 243, 716.

17. Russek, H. I. Stress, tobacco and coronary disease in North American professional groups; survey of 12,000 men in 14 occupational groups. *JAMA,* 1965, 192, 189.

17a. Russek, H. I. *Unpublished data.*

18. Snapper, L. *Chinese Lessons to Western Medicine: A Contribution to Geographical Medicine from the Clinics of Peiping Union Medical College.* Interscience, New York, 1941, p. 29.

19. Lown, B., and Stare, F. J. Atherosclerosis, infarction and nutrition. *Circulation,* 1959, 20, 161.

20. Ratcliffe, H. L., Yerasmides, T. H., and Elliott, G. A. Changes in the character and location of arterial lesions in mammals and birds in the Philadelphia Zoological Garden. *Circulation,* 1960, 21, 730.

21. Rikli, A. E. et al. U.S. Public Health Survey. Public Health Reports, Washington D.C., August, 1960.

22. Myasnikov, A. L. Influence of some factors on development of experimental cholesterol atherosclerosis. *Circulation,* 1958, 17, 99.

23. Uhley, H. N., and Friedman, M. Blood lipids, clotting and coronary atherosclerosis in rats exposed to a particular form of stress. *Am. J. Physiol.,* 1959, 197, 396.

24. Vlodaver, Z., Medalie, J., and Neufeld, H. N. Coronary arteries in immature monkeys, preliminary report of the relationships to activity and diet. *J. Atheroscler. Res.,* 1968, 8, 923.

25. Gunn, C. G., Friedman, M., and Buers, S. O. Effect of chronic hypothalamic stimulation upon cholesterol induced atherosclerosis in the rabbit. *J. Clin. Invest.,* 1960, 39, 1963.

26. Groen, J. J., Tijong, B. K., Willebrant, A. F., and Kamminga, C. J. Influence of nutrition, individuality and different forms of stress on blood cholesterol: Results of an experiment of 9 months duration in 60 normal volunteers. *Proc. Int. Cong. Diet,* Voeding, 1959, 19.

27. Lapiccirella, V., Lapiccirella, R., Abboni, F., and Liotta, S. Enquete clinique, biologique et cardiographique parmi les tribus nomades de le Somalie qui se nourrissent seulement de lait. *Bull. WHO,* 1962, 27, 681.

28. Mann, G. V., Schaffer, R. D., and Rich, A. Physical fitness and immunity to heart diseases in Masai. *J. Atheroscler. Res.,* 1965, 2, 1308.

29. Stout, C., Morrow, J., Brandt, E. N., Jr., and Wolf, S. Unusually low incidence of death from myocardial infarction: Study of an Italian-American community in Pennsylvania. *JAMA,* 1964, 188, 845.

30. Russek, H. I. Tobacco consumption and emotional stress in the etiology of coronary heart disease. *Geriatrics,* June 1964, 19, 425.
31. U.S. Public Health Service Report, Washington, D.C., 1968.
32. Russek, H. I., and Russek, L. G. Etiologic factors in ischaemic heart disease: The elusive role of emotional stress. In: *Myocardiology,* edited by E. Bajusz and G. Rona. University Park Press, Baltimore, 1972.
33. Russek, H. I. Emotional stress as a cause of coronary heart disease. *J. Am. Coll. Health Assoc.,* 1973, 22, 120.
34. Russek, H. I. Behaviour patterns, stress and coronary heart disease. *Am. Family Physician,* April 1974, 9, 117.
35. Bogdonoff, M. D., Estes, E. H., Jr., and Harlan, W. Psychophysiologic studies of fat metabolism. Read before the American College of Physicians, Chicago, April 21, 1959.
36. Steinberg, D., and Shafrir, E. Cortisone held "vital" to lipid rise in stress. *Med. News,* 1960, 6, 1.
37. Page, I. H. Atherosclerosis—a commentary. *Fed. Proc.,* 1959, 18, 47.
38. Raab, W., and Humphreys, R. J. Drug action upon myocardial epinephrine-sympathin concentration and heart rate: (Nitroglycerine, papaverine, priscol, dibenamine hydrochloride). *J. Pharmacol. Exp. Ther.,* 1947, 89, 64.
39. Raab, W., Chaplin, J. P., and Bajusz, E. Myocardial necroses produced in domesticated rats and in wild rats by sensory and emotional stresses. *Proc. Soc. Exp. Biol.,* 1964, 116, 665.
40. Groover, M. R., Jr., Seljeskog, E. L., Haglin, J. J., and Hitchcock, C. R. Myocardial infarction in the Kenya baboon without demonstrable atherosclerosis. *J. Angiol.,* 1963, 14, 409.
41. Dreyfuss, F., and Czaczkes, J. W. Blood cholesterol and uric acid of healthy medical students under stress of an examination. *Arch. Int. Med.,* 1959, 103, 708.
42. Still, J. W., and Heiffer, M. H. Blood viscosity in response to various stimuli. *Exp. Biol.,* April 26, 1958.
43. Haft, J. I, Microcirculatory platelet aggregation in the heart with epinephrine infusion. In: *Cardiovascular Problems: Perspectives and Progress,* edited by H. I. Russek. University Park Press, Baltimore.
44. Sharnoff, J. G. Stress-caused platelet rise called key to post-op. clots. Reported in *Med. News* from meeting of Am. Soc. Clin. Pathol.
45. Hames, C. "Most likely to succeed" as a candidate for a coronary attack. In: *New Horizons in Cardiovascular Practice,* edited by H. I. Russek. University Park Press, Baltimore, 1975, p. 129.
46. Cannon, W. B. *The Wisdom of the Body.* Norton, New York, 1932.
47. Selye, H. Stress. *Acta Montreal,* 1950.
48. Thorn, G. W. Diagnosis and treatment of adrenal insufficiency. Charles C Thomas, Springfield, Ill., 1952.
49. Funkenstein, D. H., King, S. H., and Drolette, M. *Mastery of Stress.* Harvard University Press, Cambridge, 1957.
50. Nestel, P. G. Stress and excretion of vanilmandelic acid. *Am. Heart J.,* 1967, 73, 227.
51. Kaplan, B. H. et al. Occupational mobility and coronary heart disease. *Arch. Int. Med.,* 1971, 122, 938.
52. Keys, A. et al. Mortality and coronary heart disease among men studied for 23 years, *Arch. Int. Med.,* 1971, 128, 201.
53. Russek, L. G. Relationship between two major risk factors in coronary heart disease. Dissertation, School of Human Behavior, U.S. International University, San Diego, 1977
54. Dempsey, D. Myth of the new leisure class. *The New York Times Magazine,* January 26, 1958.
55. Enas, W. F., Holmes, R. H., and Beyer, J. Coronary artery sclerosis in American soldiers killed during the Korean War. *JAMA,* 1953, 152, 1090.

Stress and the Heart, edited by D. Wheatley, Raven Press, New York © 1981.

Behaviour Patterns and Emotional Stress in the Etiology of Coronary Heart Disease: Cardiological and Biochemical Correlates*

P. Taggart and M. Carruthers

Emotion has long been known to be relevant to the cardiovascular system. In 1628 William Harvey included in his book on the cardiovascular system a report of "a strong man who, having received an injury and affront from one more powerful than himself, and upon whom he could not have his revenge, was so overcome with hatred and spite and passion, which he yet communicated to no-one, that at last he fell into a strange distemper, suffering from extreme oppression and pain of the heart and breast," from which the patient shortly died (1).

Many years later the celebrated English surgeon John Hunter, who suffered from angina which was readily induced by emotion, commented, "My life is at the mercy of any fool who shall put me in a passion." He died during a heated discussion at a hospital board meeting.

The English language abounds with colloquialisms such as "worked himself to death," "worried himself to death," "died of fright," and "I think you should take a few weeks off from work and relax," all of which testify to the belief held by lay persons and the medical profession alike that emotion is an important factor in both the etiology of coronary heart disease and the precipitation of acute cardiac events.

In the previous chapter, Henry and Linda Russek have amply demonstrated the association between sociological stress factors and the incidence of coronary heart disease. And yet emotional factors are not included on any list of so-called risk factors for coronary heart disease. There are three possible reasons for this lack of recognition of emotional factors in the etiology of the condition. First, the development and increased application of histochemical and biochemical techniques have tended to divert attention to those factors which are readily demonstrable and measurable. Second, emotional stress is difficult to quantify in terms that are universally acceptable, so that correlation between emotion and coronary heart disease is difficult. Finally, until relatively recently there has been no logical hypothesis to explain the physiological and biochemical mechanisms for such an association.

---

*Reprinted from Stress and The Heart, edited by D. Wheatley, first edition.

THE HYPOTHESIS

In 1969, one of us (MC) proposed a hypothesis (2) suggesting that emotion, acting via the intermediary of enhanced sympathetic activity, resulted in increased mobilization of free fatty acids (FFA) from adipose tissue. In the absence of metabolic demand, these were converted to triglycerides and were then available to be incorporated into atheroma.

This hypothesis, called the "chain of events," has substantial data to support each one of its links. Numerous, very elegant studies from the Karolinska Institute in Stockholm have demonstrated increased excretion of catecholamines in various emotional stress situations (3). Both epinephrine (adrenaline) and norepinephrine (noradrenaline) cause a rise in circulating FFA by lipolysis of triglycerides. Norepinephrine is very much more potent than epinephrine in this respect, and the increased FFA concentration tends to be more prolonged (4). Obese persons who have a higher resting FFA concentration exhibit particularly sustained increases (5), as do the physically less fit (6).

In the absence of immediate metabolic requirements, circulating FFAs are converted to triglycerides by the liver. These are not usually stored, but are recirculated as prebeta-lipoprotein; hypertriglyceridemia is statistically correlated with an increased tendency to develop clinically overt coronary heart disease (7). Furthermore, its deposition into vessel walls has been shown to be enhanced by high FFA concentrations (8).

Although the individual links in the hypothetical "chain of events" each receive substantial experimental support, it must be remembered that the demonstration of a possible mechanism does not imply a cause-and-effect relationship. In order to test this hypothesis further, we undertook a study designed to demonstrate four of these links simultaneously.

RACING CAR DRIVING

Racing car driving was selected because we considered it to exemplify an extreme emotional and aggressive situation associated with minimal

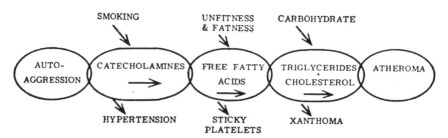

FIG. 3-1. The "Carruthers Hypothesis": a possible chain of events in the etiology of atheroma. (Figs. 3-1–3-6 reproduced by kind permission of the respective editors of the *Lancet* and *British Medical Journal*.)

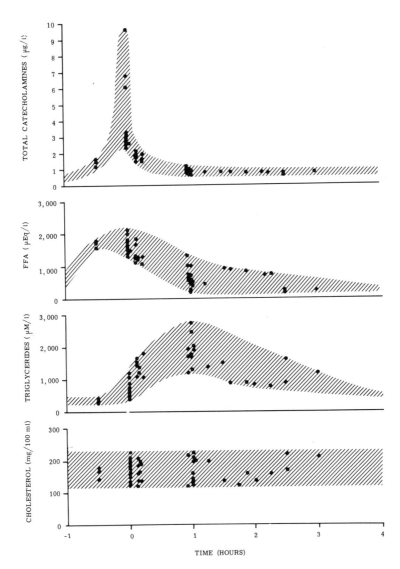

FIG. 3-2. Plasma catecholamine, free fatty acid, triglyceride, and cholesterol concentrations in racing car drivers. Time 0 indicates the end of their event.

physical effort. Thus, it might be expected to demonstrate magnification of certain biochemical changes that may occur in everyday life. Furthermore, changes in plasma concentration might be sufficiently great, we hoped, to be outside the error of the methods used.

Plasma samples were taken from racing drivers at various times within the 3-hr period following a race (9). The investigations involved 16 drivers,

2 of whom were studied repeatedly during the racing season, which consisted mostly of international events. The age range of these drivers was 22 to 39 years, and all were in apparent good health and of average build.

Figure 3-2 shows the effects of racing on the various plasma parameters measured in these subjects.

From these data it may be seen that the increase of plasma catecholamine and FFA concentrations roughly coincided in time. The delayed rise in plasma triglyceride concentration supports the contention of interconversion from FFA to triglyceride. In fact, there was a strong positive correlation between the total catecholamine levels below 2 μg/liter (32 estimations) and the FFA levels ($p < 0.01$). Including the further cases where the plasma total catecholamine levels were above this figure (43 estimations), the correlation was not nearly so strong, although it was still present ($p < 0.05$). In addition, there was a strong negative correlation between the FFA level and the triglyceride levels ($p < 0.001$).

These results suggest a linear relationship between the rapid rise in FFA and catecholamine levels until a FFA plateau is reached, with catecholamine levels of about 2 μg/liter. Above that level, no consistent rise occurs. The endogenous origin of triglyceride was demonstrated by electrophoretic patterns, and this study shows that maximal lipid response can be triggered by relatively low plasma catecholamine levels. However, it is of interest that in these racing drivers the resting levels were nevertheless relatively low. Although no far-reaching conclusions should be drawn from these observations, they may bear on the thesis that the development of atheroma may be promoted by recurrent elevations of blood lipids, induced by certain everyday emotional stresses.

EMOTION AND BLOOD BIOCHEMISTRY

If emotion is important in this context, it is appropriate to consider the possible interrelationships of different qualities of emotion and personality.

Friedman and his colleagues interviewed, by questionnaire, executives of a wide range of companies, as well as physicians, on their views concerning the cause of coronary heart disease (10). In both groups, 70% thought that the major causal factor was "a particular and rather specific type of emotional activity, namely that concerned with excessive drive, competition, meeting 'deadlines' and economic frustration." Less than 5% in either group considered worry or fear to be important.

Reference has already been made in Chapter 2 to the classic, and sometimes hotly disputed, delineation of coronary-prone and coronary-immune types of personalities (11). To enlarge upon these, the Type-A personality who is most likely to provoke coronary disease is characterized by:

1. an intense sustained drive to achieve self-selected but usually poorly defined goals,

2. profound inclination and eagerness to compete,
3. persistent desire for recognition and advancement,
4. continuous involvement in multiple and diverse functions constantly subject to time restrictions,
5. habitual propensity to accelerate the rate of execution of many physical and mental functions, and
6. extraordinary mental and physical alertness.

Type-B was formulated as the opposite of these.

The subjects were selected by lay associates and subsequently were subdivided by research interviewers into complete or incomplete patterns.

However, this classification has been subject to criticism. Mordkoff and Parsons (12) surveyed all the literature concerned with the search for a unique configuration of personality traits associated with coronary artery disease (CAD) or a "coronary personality." They observed that all the studies, with one exception, were retrospective in nature, and that inferences about CAD-predisposed personality traits made on this basis can be grossly misleading. They comment: "If proper attention is given to variables such as age, sex, socioeconomic status, criterial attributes, nature of comparison groups and, most importantly, the impact of the CAD upon the individual, then the personality configurations of CAD patients are more similar to the population strata from which they are drawn, than to other CAD patients from different population strata." In the one prospective study the authors found essentially no differences in pre-CAD personality between individuals who subsequently experienced myocardial infarction and those who did not (13). Furthermore, they used one of the most reliable and generally useful personality tests, the Minnesota Multiphasic Personality Inventory (MMPI).

Mai undertook a similar survey (14), pointing out that the predicted pattern may follow rather than precede the infarction, and that the published results do illustrate the importance of psychological response to an infarct, which can influence the interpretation given to retrospective surveys. Weiss et al. (15) studied the personality and life situation of 41 patients who had sustained a myocardial infarction during the previous 12 days, comparing these with 43 controls. They concluded that gradually mounting stress prior to the illness occurred significantly more often in the infarct patients than in the controls. They also noted the frequency with which the attack occurred on or near the anniversary of a significant event in their lives.

However valid Friedman and Rosenman's criteria for assessing behavior pattern, clinical pathological and biochemical differences were striking. In one study (11), Type-A persons showed much higher serum cholesterol concentrations although total calorie and fat intake, physical activity, height, weight, and age were comparable. The incidence of clinical coronary heart disease and arcus senilis was seven and three times more frequent, respectively, in Type-A than in Type-B persons. In a prospective study of over 3,500 men, known as the Western Collaborative Group Study, Friedman and Rosenman confirmed the association of well-recognized risk factors, such as cigarette smoking, family history, hypertension, and cholesterol beta-lipoprotein, with triglyceride concentrations. However, they noted that Type-A persons had higher serum lipids and greater daytime excretion of catecholamines. Of the subjects who died during a 5-year period, 22 of the 25 deaths due to coronary heart disease occurred in the Type-A group. Regardless of the cause of death, postmortem assessment showed coronary atherosclerosis to be six times more prevalent in the Type-A persons.

How, then, may personality differences be incorporated into the hypothetical model of Carruthers? Evidence is accumulating to suggest that different emotions are associated with different relative proportions of norepinephrine (4), so that the Carruthers model may be modified accordingly to place the major emphasis on norepinephrine as the lethal amine.

The Funkenstein hypothesis (16) proposed that norepinephrine release was associated with aggressive emotion, whereas epinephrine release was associated with anxiety. This agreed with the observations of Ax (17), who showed that subjects stimulated to fear and anger separately showed physiological responses resembling those of injections of epinephrine and a combination of epinephrine with norepinephrine, respectively. Although in broad agreement, Funkenstein, et al. considered that the pattern was more precise,

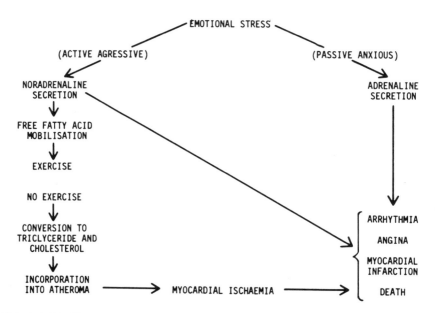

FIG. 3-3. Modification of the "Carruthers Hypothesis" to incorporate the possible influence of differential secretion of norepinephrine (noradrenaline) and epinephrine (adrenaline) in response to different emotional situations.

if the direction of anger was taken into account, i.e., by differentiating between anger with self and outward anger with, for example, the experimenter. Von Euler (18), who reviewed the available evidence, considered that fear and anger equated more closely with epinephrine and norepinephrine, respectively. Frankenhauser and Rissler (19) felt that epinephrine secretion was dictated largely by the presence of a high degree of arousal, and norepinephrine prevailed in situations where the outcome was inevitable.

PUBLIC SPEAKING

Increases in both plasma epinephrine and norepinephrine concentrations can be demonstrated under conditions of emotional stress, such as are experienced by speakers at public meetings. Common symptoms in such situations are: palpitations, dryness of the mouth, voice changes, hoarseness, and fear of failure or "drying up."

We studied a group of 30 subjects (23 with normal hearts and 7 with coronary heart disease) while they were speaking before an audience (20). Electrocardiographic tracings taken before and after exercise showed depression of the "J point" in 20 of the 23 normal subjects, but in only 1 of the 7 subjects with coronary heart disease. However, ischemic ST depression appeared or increased in 6 of the 7 coronary subjects. Ectopic beats at a rate of more than 6/min were recorded in 6 of the 23 normal subjects while they were speaking; 5 of the 7 coronary subjects had multiple and often multifocal ventricular ectopic beats. Furthermore, each of the 30 subjects studied while speaking developed some degree of tachycardia, the fastest heart rates reaching 180 beats/min. There was a mean maximum heart rate of 151 (range 125–180/min) in the 23 subjects with normal hearts, and in the 7 subjects with coronary heart disease, a mean maximum heart rate of 133/min (range 115–160/min) developed.

Since it is tempting to infer that the emotional responses in public speakers are mediated through the autonomic nervous system, we also studied the effect of the beta-adrenergic blocking drug, oxprenolol, administering either a single oral dose of 40 mg or a placebo to 15 subjects, 8 with normal hearts and 7 with coronary heart disease. These patients were studied while speaking on two occasions, once after taking placebo and again on a separate occasion after taking oxprenolol, these being administered on a double-blind basis. Figure 3-4 shows the changes in plasma catecholamines and FFA concentrations.

The total plasma catecholamine concentration was higher in the samples taken after speaking without medication than in those taken before speaking ($p < 0.05$). This was due entirely to the norepinephrine component ($p < 0.01$), no change being apparent in the plasma epinephrine. However, when the 15 subjects were studied while speaking after oxprenolol, there was

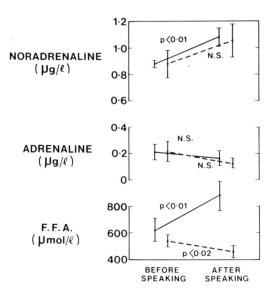

FIG. 3-4. Elevation of circulating free fatty acids (FFA) in response to the emotional challenge of speaking before an audience. —— Placebo; – – – – oxprenolol.

no increase in plasma catecholamine concentration in the samples taken immediately after the speech. After placebo, there was a highly significant increase in plasma concentrations of FFA, from a mean value of 622 (SD ± 376) meq/liter before speaking, to 822 (SD ± 499) meq/liter after speaking ($p < 0.01$).

The increase in plasma FFA concentrations occurring in association with raised norepinephrine levels accords with the theory that high levels of emotional activity, when accompanied by physical inactivity, can cause transient adverse changes in plasma-lipid patterns (20). Although the norepinephrine response to this situation is not as great as with the stress of racing driving, it is nevertheless still sufficient to trigger a pronounced lipid reaction.

Our data on plasma catecholamine concentrations are somewhat at variance with Frankenhauser and Rissler (19) and more in line with the original Funkenstein hypothesis (16). We would equate the increased plasma epinephrine concentrations observed in novice subjects about to experience their first descent by parachute (21), not simply with arousal but with fear; by either subjective or objective criteria they were terrified. We would equate the norepinephrine response that we observed among racing car drivers (9) with their sense of competition and aggression, not unlike the Type-A personality of Friedman and his colleagues. It could hardly be said that the outcome of a motor race was inevitable! (11.)

It is also of interest that experienced parachute jumpers showed far less

TABLE 3-1. *Parachute jumping. Plasma catecholamine concentrations on landing*[a]

	Norepinephrine (µg/liter)	Epinephrine (µg/liter)
Normal values	p (0.66 < 0.70 M < 0.82) = 99.36	p (0.06 < 0.10 M < 0.16) = 99.36
6 Experienced subjects n = 12	p (0.88 < 0.94 M < 1.22) = 99.36	p (0.29 < 0.53 M < 0.98) = 99.36
5 Beginners	p (0.93 < 1.08 M < 1.71) = 99.22	p (0.71 < 1.63 M < 2.72) = 99.22

[a] Predominant increase in epinephrine, particularly among the beginners. (Median values with confidence limits.) (Reproduced by kind permission of the respective editors of the *Lancet* and *British Medical Journal*.)

increase in plasma epinephrine concentrations, following a parachute descent, than did novices.

On the other hand, we have noted no obvious difference in the norepinephrine response between highly experienced and relatively inexperienced racing drivers. A possible implication of this is that experience and conditioning may be effective in reducing some of the metabolic responses to fear situations, but much less so in aggressive or "Type-A life style" situations.

ACUTE CARDIAC EVENTS

Another aspect of the association of emotion and coronary heart disease is the precipitation of acute cardiac events. For example, there is suggestive evidence that emotion may be relevant to the development of cardiac failure (22).

We have studied electrocardiogram (EKG) tracings taken from experienced drivers in busy city traffic, albeit following routes familiar to them (23). This investigation involved 32 normal individuals, and 24 with coronary heart disease. In the majority of both normals and coronary heart disease individuals, there were increased heart rates, including brief periods when the rate exceeded 140/min. S-T changes not due to tachycardia developed in 3 of the 32 normal individuals, and in no less than 13 of the 24 coronary heart disease patients. In addition, there were T-wave changes in the latter, and the S-T and T changes were gross in 6 of these patients. These were of such degree that if the circumstances had been an exercise test for the diagnosis of coronary heart disease, the results would have been classed as positive.

Plasma catecholamine levels were measured in 3 of the subjects with coronary heart disease immediately after driving, but there was little or no change compared to the resting levels (i.e., in contradistinction to the racing drivers). As a result of this investigation, we concluded that persons in whom angina is easily provoked or who are in borderline left ventricular failure should be advised not to drive.

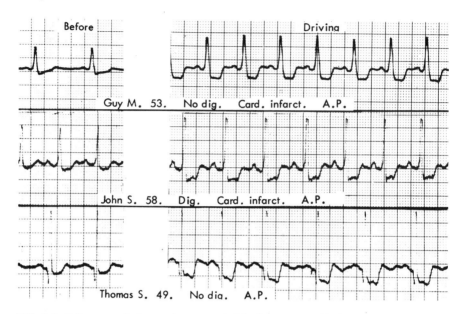

FIG. 3-5. S-T segment depression recorded in 3 persons with known coronary heart disease while driving their car in London traffic (**right**). Control tracings at the time of starting the test drive are included (**left**).

These changes are similar to those that occurred in 6 of the 7 persons with coronary heart disease monitored while speaking to an audience (20). In all instances these effects could be prevented by a single oral dose of 40 mg oxprenolol. This drug was also effective in preventing the emotionally induced tachycardia and the palpitation which, at times, may be distracting, unpleasant, and, in certain instances, possibly dangerous. Coronary heart disease is the major cause of death in men over 40 in Great Britain and the United States. Arrhythmia is probably the major determinant. Important ventricular arrhythmias were observed in 5 of the 24 coronary heart disease subjects driving in London traffic, and in 5 of the 7 similar persons speaking before an audience. No such ectopic activity was observed in the latter group when they were monitored on a separate occasion following the administration of oxprenolol.

We do not yet have sufficient data to assess the relative potency of endogenous epinephrine and norepinephrine on the S-T segment and arrhythmias in response to emotion. Such a relationship is likely to be complicated by the participation of parasympathetic activity which, in response to certain situations, may even be dominant (24,25). Thus, in a study of the effects of violent television programs and movies (24) vagal overactivity was demonstrated, in spite of increased epinephrine secretion, and slowing of the heart occurred. Further evidence of increased vagal overactivity was pro-

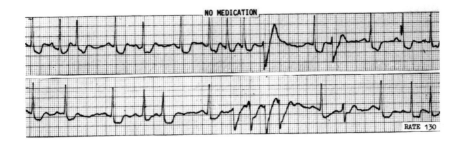

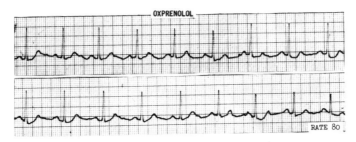

FIG. 3-6. S-T segment depression and ectopic activity, including a short run of ventricular tachycardia in a person with coronary heart disease monitored while speaking before an audience **(top)**. A normal electrocardiogram recorded from the same person on a separate but similar occasion prior to which he had taken an oral dose of 40 mg oxprenolol showing a normal heart rate, no ST-T changes, and no ectopic activity **(bottom)**.

vided by a sinus arrhythmia effect. This vagal inhibition of the heart was supported by changes in the levels of hormones such as growth hormone and glucagon. A neurohumeral aspect is thus added to the signs of parasympathetic activity. These appear to override the increase in sympathetic tone, indicated by a rise in urinary epinephrine secretion.

Levi (26) also has demonstrated increased urinary excretion of norepinephrine and epinephrine in subjects viewing almost any type of film, whether humorous, aggressive, or pornographic. Only bland, natural scenery films decreased the secretion of both amines. In our study, despite the evidence of vagal overactivity, the familiar plasma changes occurred, consisting of increases in FFAs and decreases in triglycerides.

We do not have sufficient data to draw useful conclusions about the period immediately following emotional arousal of different types. Since it is in the period immediately following exercise that ectopic activity is most prolific, rather than during exercise (27), it would be of interest to examine this period following emotion. It may be that both the extent and rate of change between the relative activity of the sympathetic and parasympathetic systems are important.

CONCLUSIONS

1. Emotion has long been thought to be relevant to the etiology of coronary heart disease and to the precipitation of acute cardiac events, although scientific proof of this has been lacking. Possible explanations for this lack include the difficulty in quantifying emotional stress, the advancement of techniques for histochemical and biochemical analysis which facilitate theories of dietary and other possible causes, and the absence of any obvious physiological and biochemical mechanisms by which the association of emotion and coronary heart disease may be effected.

2. An hypothesis is considered which relates emotion to coronary heart disease via the intermediary of enhanced sympathetic activity, leading to mobilization of free fatty acids and, in the absence of metabolic requirements, conversion of the latter to triglycerides. As norepinephrine is more powerful in its lipid mobilizing properties than epinephrine, this hypothesis is further examined in light of the different secretion of these two hormones in response to different emotions and personality types.

3. Tachycardia, EKG changes (including ST segment depression and arrhythmias), and even florid pulmonary edema can be emotionally induced. These are illustrated by our studies of racing drivers, public speakers, parachute jumpers, and automobile drivers in heavy traffic conditions.

4. The beta-adrenergic blocking agent oxprenolol has been shown to be effective in abolishing (a) the lipid response to emotion and the unpleasant symptoms sometimes associated with it, (b) tachycardia, (c) ST segment abnormalities, and (d) arrhythmias.

REFERENCES

1. Harvey, W. *Exercitatio Anatomica De Motu Cordis et Sanguinis in Animabilus.* Frankfurt-am-Main, 1628.
2. Carruthers, M. A. Aggression and atheroma. *Lancet,* 1969, 11, 1170.
3. Levi, L., ed. *Society, Stress and Disease.* Oxford University Press, Oxford, 1971.
4. Wenke, M. In: *Advances in Lipid Research,* Vol. 4, edited by R. Paolette and D. Kritchevsky. Academic Press, London, 1966.
5. Dole, V. P. A relation between non-esterified fatty acids in plasma and the metabolism of glucose. *J. Clin. Invest.,* 1956, 35, 150.
6. Johnson, R. H., Walton, J. L., Krebs, H. A., and Williamson, D. H. Post-exercise ketosis. *Lancet,* 1969, 2, 1383.
7. Lewis, B., Chait, A., Oakley, C. M. O., Wooton, I. D. P., Krickler, D. M., Onitin, A., Sigurdsson, G., and February, A. Serum lipoprotein abnormalities in patients with ischaemic heart disease: Comparisons with a control population. *Br. Med. J.,* 1974, 3, 489.
8. Rutstein, D. D., Castelli, W. P., and Nickerson, R. J. Heparin and human lipid metabolism. *Lancet,* 1969, 1, 1003.
9. Taggart, P., and Carruthers, M. Endogenous hyperlipidaemia induced by emotional stress of racing driving. *Lancet,* 1971, 1, 363.
10. Friedman, M., Rosenman, R. H., and Caroll, V. Changes in the serum cholesterol and blood clotting time in man subjected to cyclic variation of occupational stress. *Circulation,* 1958, 17, 852.
11. Friedman, M., and Rosenman, R. H. Association of a specific overt behaviour pattern with

increases in blood cholesterol, blood clotting time, incidence of arcus senilis and clinical coronary artery disease. *J.A.M.A.,* 1959, 169, 1286.

12. Mordkoff, A. M., and Parsons, O. A. The coronary personality—a critique. *Psychosom. Med.,* 1967, 29, 1.

13. Ostfeld, A. M., Lebovits, B. A., Shekelle, R. B., and Paul, O. A prospective study of the relationship between personality and coronary heart disease. *J. Chron. Dis.,* 1964, 17, 265.

14. Mai, F. M. M. Personality and stress in coronary disease. *J. Psychom. Res.,* 1968, 12, 275.

15. Weiss, E., Dlin, B., Rollin, H., Fischer, H., and Bepler, C. Emotional factors in coronary occlusion. *Arch. Intern. Med.,* 1957, 99, 628.

16. Funkenstein, D. H., King, S. H., and Drolette, M. The direction of anger during a laboratory stress-inducing situation. *Psychosom. Med.,* 1954, 16, 404.

17. Ax, A. F. The physiological differentiation between fear and anger in humans. *Psychosom. Med.,* 1953, 15, 433.

18. Von Euler, U. S. Quantitation of stress by catecholamine analysis. *Clin. Pharmacol. Ther.,* 1964, 5, 398.

19. Frankenhauser, M., and Rissler, A. Catecholamine output during relaxation and anticipation. *Percept. Mot. Skills,* 1970, 30, 745.

20. Taggart, P., Carruthers, M., and Somerville, W. Electrocardiogram, plasma catecholamines and lipids, and their modification by oxprenolol when speaking before an audience. *Lancet,* 1973, 2, 341.

21. Taggart, P., Carruthers, M., and Somerville, W. Emotions, Catecholamines, and the Electrocardiogram. In: *Progress in Cardiology,* vol. 7, p. 103, edited by P. N. Yu and J. F. Goodwin. Lea and Febiger, Philadelphia, 1978.

22. Perlman, L. V., Ferguson, S., Bergum, K., Isenberg, E. L., and Hammarsten, J. F. Precipitation of congestive heart failure: Social and emotional factors. *Ann. Intern. Med.,* 1971, 75, 1.

23. Taggart, P., Gibbons, D., and Somerville, W. Some effects of motor car driving on the normal and abnormal heart. *Br. Med. J.,* 1969, iv, 130.

24. Carruthers, M., and Taggart, P. Vagotonicity of violence. *Br. Med. J.,* 1973, 3, 384.

25. Taggart, P., Hedworth-Whitty, R.-B., Carruthers, M., and Gordon, P. Observation on the electrocardiogram and plasma catecholamines during dental procedures: The forgotten vagus. *Br. Med. J.,* 1976, 4, 787.

26. Levi, L. Stress and distress in response to psychosocial stimuli. *Acta Med. Scand.,* 1972, Suppl. 528.

27. Jelinek, M. V., and Lown, B. Exercise stress testing for exposure of cardiac arrhythmia. *Prog. Cardiovasc. Dis.,* 1974, 16, 497.

Stress and the Heart, edited by D. Wheatley,
Raven Press, New York © 1981.

Treatment of the Anxiety Factor

David Wheatley

As seen in the two previous chapters, behavioral and emotional stresses of protean kinds may be involved in the etiology of coronary heart disease (CHD). Individually, such factors can be classified into two groups, namely, those that are preventable and those that are not. Preventable factors include alcohol consumption, smoking, obesity, diet, climate, water supply, sexual activity, and exercise; nonpreventable factors are heredity and race.

As outlined in the preceding chapters, psychic and physical stresses of numerous kinds are important etiologic factors in CHD. In some instances, these may be preventable and in others they may not. Stress, therefore, forms an intermediate group between the preventable and nonpreventable factors in the etiology of CHD.

ETIOLOGIC FACTORS IN CHD

Under the heading of preventable factors are included a number of life habits and situations, which are potentially capable of modification, although social, financial, and individual characteristics may make this possible in some cases and not in others. For example, the alcohol drinker may be able to reduce or modify his consumption, whereas the alcoholic may not; some individuals may be able to reduce or stop smoking, whereas compulsive smokers cannot; obesity can be overcome by diet or anorectic drugs in some patients but not in others; some individuals may be able to change their diet, but others not preparing their own food may not; some living in extremely cold climates may be able to move to warmer ones but others may not; the chemical constitution of water supplies varies in different areas, and a change of residence is possible for some but not for others; oral contraceptives, the main iatrogenic factor involved in CHD, can be changed for other methods by some patients, but this is esthetically unacceptable for others; finally, some individuals who are coronary prone may be able to reduce their sexual activity, but others may not.

Alcohol

It has always been assumed that a moderate amount of alcohol, because of its peripheral vasodilator action, is beneficial in CHD, while excessive consumption, because of its profound effects on many body systems, is not (1,2). Recent studies, however, have established a negative association between moderate alcohol consumption and CHD (3–9). Thus Klatsby et al. (3) investigated the alcohol consumption of 464 patients before myocardial infarction (MI), controlling the results for cigarette smoking and other established risk factors. They found a statistically significant negative association between alcohol consumption and the subsequent first MI. There were significantly larger proportions of patients with MI in those patients who were nondrinkers as compared to both moderate and heavy drinkers.

Similar findings were recorded by Hennekens et al. (4), who compared the reported drinking habits of 568 men who had died of CHD with an equal number of matched controls. In contrast to the previous study (although again they found that the nondrinkers had a significantly higher incidence of CHD deaths), this was only in relation to light drinkers (up to 2 oz. alcohol daily), and the incidence was similar between the nondrinkers and heavy drinkers. The authors concluded that "These data provide strong evidence against a causal role of daily alcohol consumption in fatal CHD and are consistent with a small preventive action of 'any' v. 'no' daily drinking, although this relationship applies to light drinkers only."

Yano et al. (5) studied 7,705 Japanese patients over a 6-year period in Hawaii, among whom there were 294 new cases of CHD. Other studies (6,7) have shown a similar negative association between alcohol consumption and CHD, although in the case of the study by Stason et al. (7), there was evidence of a lower rate of CHD in subjects consuming six or more drinks daily.

The effects of alcohol on various blood parameters have also been investigated by Myrhed et al. (8), who studied 34 noncirrhotic males after acute drinking bouts and found no effects on the platelet count. Castelli et al. (9), reporting on a five-population study in the United States, found a strong relationship between reported alcohol intake and blood lipids, with a positive association with high density lipoprotein (HDL) cholesterol levels in all populations. There was a less strong but consistent negative association with low density lipoprotein (LDL) cholesterol. The authors speculated that alcohol produces a shift from LDL to HDL as a metabolic effect.

Perhaps one of the most recent studies concerns the specific effect of wine. St. Leger et al. (10) demonstrated a strong and specific negative association between CHD deaths and alcohol consumption, which they showed to be wholly attributable to wine consumption. They surveyed the death rates for males and females separately in the 55 to 64 age group from hypertensive disease, ischemic heart disease (IHD), cerebrovascular disease, and bronchitis, emphysema, and asthma. The only significant negative correlation was between IHD and wine ($r = -0.7$ males, -0.6 females) in contrast to beer (+0.2 and 0.3, respectively) and spirits (-0.3 and 0.3, respectively). Correlations in all the other conditions studied were low and not statistically significant. The implications are that a change from beer and spirit drinking to wine drinking might prove beneficial and might result in a reduction in heavy drinking of the former two alcoholic beverages.

Smoking

As outlined in Chapter 2, the association between smoking and CHD is not clear, although most studies report an adverse association between heavy smoking and CHD. Thus expert committees in many countries have concluded that cigarette smoking is a major risk factor in CHD. In the United Kingdom, about one-quarter of the 40,000 deaths in men and women under 65 who die each year from CHD are considered to be closely associated with cigarette smoking (11–13). This is a clearly preventable factor in the etiology of CHD.

Obesity

There are a number of reports of an adverse association between obesity and CHD (14,15). In a more recent study from Finland, Pelkonen et al. (16) studied serum lipid concentrations, relative body weight, and smoking habits in 1,648 middle-aged Finnish men who were subsequently followed for 7 years. Using multivariate analysis, these workers showed that serum triglyceride and cholesterol concentrations and smoking were all independently associated with cardiovascular mortality. Obesity influenced the death rates only in men with raised serum lipid levels, while smoking was associated with increased mortality when any combination of the other factors was present. The authors concluded that men who had raised triglyceride concentrations combined with smoking or obesity had the highest risk of cardiovascular death.

Weight reduction in overweight patients suffering from CHD is clearly a desirable aim, although this may not directly influence the disease process but rather exert indirect beneficial effects on reduction in hypertension and glucose intolerance when present, and plasma lipid levels (17). It may be that this is a variable factor in different individuals, depending on associations with exercise and occupation, and differing effects on hemodynamics in different individuals.

Diet

Apart from the long-standing controversy over the proportions of unsaturated and saturated fats in the diet, several other dietary factors have been associated with CHD.

The role of dietary fiber has been recently surveyed (18). An association between a diet high in cereal fiber and a reduced incidence of CHD was recorded by Morris et al. (19) in their follow-up study of 337 middle-aged men who participated in a dietary survey from 1956 to 1966. When reviewed at the end of 1976, clinical CHD had developed in 45 of these individuals. This showed two main relationships with diet, namely, a reduced incidence of the disease in relation to both a high energy intake and a high intake of dietary fiber.

Although there is a positive correlation between the death rate from CHD and sugar consumption in many countries (20,21), the latter is strongly correlated with saturated fat consumption and also with cigarette smoking. On the other hand, it has also been emphasized that the incidence of CHD is fairly low in many countries with a high sugar consumption, such as the Caribbean, Venezuela, and Mauritius (22). The association between CHD and high sugar intake does not appear to be well substantiated; nevertheless, this may constitute a risk factor, which can be easily controlled by the patient.

Onions and garlic appear to be potentially important dietary factors, the increased consumption of which may help to prevent CHD. A comment to Menon from a patient that clots in the legs of horses in France were treated with a diet of onions and garlic (23) led him and his co-workers to study the effects of onions on blood fibrinolytic activity. Dewar (24), one of Menon's co-workers, has recently surveyed the subsequent research efforts to isolate the fibrinolytic compounds from onions and garlic, showing that cycloallinin is an odorless compound of this type and can be synthesized (25–27). Although promising (28,29), this line of research appears to have become a "forgotten idea." Nevertheless, most patients should not find it difficult to increase their consumption of onions and garlic, particularly now that Mediterranean cuisine is becoming generally popular, and the odor of garlic on the breath may no longer be as unacceptable as it once was in other countries.

Climate

Extremes of either cold or heat can precipitate myocardial ischemia and even infarction. Neill et al. (30) placed damp towels filled with ice chips on the foreheads of 19 patients with CHD and six controls who were undergoing left heart catheterization for diagnostic purposes. Five of the patients with CHD developed typical angina pectoris after 2 to 3 min of exposure. This was accompanied by a marked increase in both systolic and diastolic blood pressure and in coronary blood flow in both patients and controls. In seven of the CHD patients, however, exposure to cold resulted in evidence of myocardial hypoxia.

The actual manifestations of these experimental changes are recorded in a paper by Glass and Zack (31), who examined death certificates in eastern Massachusetts after six blizzards from 1974 to 1978. They found that the total number of deaths was significantly higher in a "blizzard week" than in the preceding or subsequent weeks, and that deaths from IHD accounted for 90% of the excess total deaths. An association with elevation of blood pressure in response to cold is again suggested by a study of the cardiovascular responses of 28 subjects who swam in ice-cold water in the winter (32). Systolic blood pressure increased significantly while these individuals were waiting undressed in cold air before swimming, although after swimming there was no further increase in the blood pressure level. That excessive heat also may produce ischemic changes is illustrated by a study by Taggart et al. (33), who observed the effects of the intense heat of a sauna on patients with CHD and normal controls.

They found that a high proportion of subjects in both groups developed ischemic-like ST-T patterns during exposure to heat.

Finally, altitude may be important from a protective point of view. Ramos et al. (34) found no cases of MI or of even moderate CHD in 300 necropsies carried out at 14,000 feet in the Andes. Furthermore, studies in South America have shown that both angina and EKG changes due to myocardial ischemia are less common at high altitudes than at sea level (35). A further study was undertaken by Mortimer et al. (36) in relation to altitude in New Mexico. The authors found that with increasing altitude, there was a declining age-adjusted mortality for arteriosclerotic heart disease in men but not in women. Therefore, extremes of climatic conditions may have an important influence on CHD, as Davidson's experiments suggest (see Chapter 8).

Water Supplies

Various mineral constituents of drinking water have been implicated in the etiology of CHD. The association between a high salt content and hypertension is well known, and once again this may have an adverse effect on CHD (37–39). Cadmium concentration in water supplies has been the subject of several investigations. Østergaard (40), in a necropsy study, found renal cadmium concentration to be higher in normotensives than in hypertensives. On the other hand, administration of cadmium to laboratory animals can cause hypertension (41). This led Glauser et al. (42) to study blood cadmium levels in untreated hypertensive patients and normal controls. They found that the mean level in hypertensives was 11.1 ng/ml, while in controls it was only 3.4 ng/ml. Beevers et al. (43) found no significant differences between blood cadmium levels in 70 hypertensive patients and 70 controls matched for age and sex.

Beevers et al. (44) also investigated blood levels of lead in 135 hypertensive patients and 135 age- and sex-matched normal controls in relation to the level of lead in tap water. They found a positive correlation between blood lead and tap water lead and concluded that "in the West of Scotland high blood-pressure is associated with high blood-lead levels, which might explain the high prevalence of cardiovascular disease in the area."

A number of studies have suggested that hard drinking water may exert a protective influence in CHD. This may be associated with the relative magnesium-potassium and potassium-sodium ratios in hard and soft drinking water. Nationwide studies in the United States and Great Britain have shown an inverse relationship between water hardness and cardiovascular mortality (45). In a survey of mineral content of hard and soft waters, Elwood et al. (46) produced evidence to suggest that it is only the calcium concentration in hard water that contributes significantly to the overall negative association between hardness and CHD. On the other hand, Chipperfield and Chipperfield (47) suggest that it is the ratios between magnesium and potassium and between sodium and potassium that are the important factors influencing the incidence of CHD. It appears that hard water does exert some protective effect in CHD, and sufferers from the condition might consider moving to a hard water area to take advantage of this protective influence.

Sex

Sexual activity may exert an adverse effect in CHD in two different ways between the sexes. The use of oral contraceptives by women may increase the risk of MI, particularly if associated with cigarette smoking (48). The findings of the study suggested that the rate of MI is increased approximately fourfold among women using oral contraceptives. Furthermore, in combination with 25 or more cigarettes per day, the rate increases at least 20-fold and more probably about 40-fold. Further confirmation for the increased risk of CHD due to oral contraceptive use is provided by a study undertaken by Wallace et al. (49) of women attending 10 North American lipid research clinics. They found that, compared with controls, oral contraceptive users showed increased cholesterol, triglyceride, and LDL and very low density lipoprotein (VLDL) levels, and that these levels were positively associated with the quantity of the estrogen components.

In both sexes, intercourse culminating in orgasm may cause transient tachycardia, hypertension, and hyperventilation (50). Heart rates of 180 beats/min and blood pressures of 230/130 mm Hg have been recorded at orgasm in normotensive individuals (51). EKG abnormalities have not been observed in normal men and women during intercourse (51). In patients suffering from CHD, angina commonly occurs during coitus (50,52).

Although women suffering from CHD might be well advised to use mechanical means of contraception in preference to hormonal methods, with respect to sexual intercourse, members of both sexes might prefer to take the risk involved rather than lead a life of abstinence.

Exercise

There is evidence that regular exercise may exert a protective effect in the prevention of CHD. Morris et al. (53) have shown a striking difference in the relative risk of CHD between middle-aged sedentary male civil servants undertaking different levels of leisure activities. Those who stated that they undertook vigorous exercise had about one-third the incidence of CHD than those who did not. Occupational exercise has been studied by Paffenberger and Hale (54) in the United States. These authors classified dock workers into high, medium, or low caloric output jobs in a follow-up study lasting 22 years. They found that the high-activity workers had CHD death rates almost one-half those found in the medium and low categories, although there was little difference between the latter two. The association was observed especially for sudden death, which was about three times as frequent in the moderate and light activity categories. Previous studies by Morris and colleagues on active bus conductors, as compared to sedentary bus drivers, and active postmen as compared to sedentary clerks, have recorded similar findings.

Physical fitness involving regular exercise is beneficial in the prevention of CHD; but it is debatable as to what dangers may be involved in patients with CHD who take up physical activities, such as jogging, for the first time when they are already suffering from the disease. This is a potentially dangerous procedure, and the sensible course might be to start gradually graded increases in exercise; one of the best forms for the CHD sufferer is walking.

Heredity

Of the nonpreventable factors (at least as far as the individual patient is concerned) in CHD, heredity is undoubtedly the most important (55). In a study from Finland, the probability of CHD developing before the age of 65 in a man whose brother has just suffered a heart attack was 52 to 65% (in different regions), as compared to 5 and 31% respectively, in brothers of healthy controls (56).

Although individuals may not be able to thwart nature's inheritance, a knowledge of the increased risk in those with a strong history of CHD can at least lead them to undertake other preventive and therapeutic measures. Such individuals may be able to lessen the risk to some extent by giving attention to the other etiologic factors, which have already been described, and by subjecting themselves to periodic cardiologic and blood pressure checks. Rissanen and Nikkila (56) showed that a man with a family history of CHD has no increased risk unless he has a raised blood pressure or serum cholesterol level. Herein lie possibilities for prevention in coronary-prone individuals.

Race

The often lauded association between CHD and the type of fat consumption receives a considerable measure of vindication when the rare incidence of death from cardiovascular disease in Eskimos is considered (57). It would seem logical to attribute this to the high consumption of polyunsaturated fatty acids by Eskimos and the finding of longer bleeding times and reduced platelet aggregations in their race (57). Dietary factors, however, cannot explain other differences that have been demonstrated between different races, such as those found in the study by Gordon et al. (58,59) comparing the United States, Honolulu, and Puerto Rico, and those in the study by Gordon and Marmot et al. in Japan, Hawaii, and the United States (58–60). (These studies are considered in more detail in Chapter 14.)

The effect of race and the incidence of CHD is by no means a simple matter and may consist of many factors. To what extent the adoption of a racial culture with an inherant low incidence of CHD might benefit the sufferer or potential sufferer from CHD coming from another country is a matter of intriguing conjecture.

EMOTIONAL STRESS AND ANXIETY

The importance of emotional stress and, in particular, anxiety, in CHD must be considered against the background of the multifactorial etiology of the condition, of which the most important known factors have been surveyed. The role of emotional stress may then be viewed in perspective, its importance assessed, and the possibilities for treatment considered.

Experimental Evidence

The etiologic role of emotional stress in human CHD has already been surveyed by Russek and Russek in Chapter 2 and the pioneering work of Selye in the laboratory in the Introduction to this volume. Animals may not provide a very good paradigm for the human situation in this context since, as Freeman (61) points out: "animals necessarily have the ability to adapt, albeit within certain limits, to environmental change." Thus stress and the response to it are normal components of the life of the majority of animals in the wild, as has been vividly illustrated by Folkow (62), describing a lion attack on a grazing antelope. Epinephrine release accomplishes an instantaneous shift of cardiac output from the gastrointestinal tract to the skeletal muscle, so that within a 2-sec interval, the animal turns to flee. Situations such as this are an everyday occurrence in the antelope's life, and its cardiovascular responses to them do not result in any adverse effects on that system. For the average human being, however, an acutely stressful situation is not an everyday event, and although his nervous and cardiovascular systems may be prepared for it, the psychologic effects of such a response may be profound.

The stresses that assault the individual in everyday life are ubiquitous although more likely constituted in a series of mild stressful events uneventful in themselves but possibly amalgamating in a susceptible individual to produce an appreciable stimulus to the body's stress mechanisms. The modification of these responses by mental inhibition might also be considered, as pointed out by Eliot and Forker (63).The simplistic "fight-or-flight" response to stressful situations may be substantially modified or completely nullified by man's social environment. Thus central mental control in the human may prevent the fulfillment of cardiovascular readiness to respond to stress, resulting in prolonged periods during which these cardiovascular changes are maintained.

Life events may play an important role in this context, these being characterized by various stressful events, such as death of a relative, family illness, marital problems, financial problems, overwork, or inability to reach prescribed standards. Even relatively minor events, such as a nonserious car accident, inability to obtain a prized object, or interpersonal relationships of a frustrating nature, may produce long-continued emotional stress and maintain changes in the cardiovascular system in response.

Schiffer et al. (64) investigated 43 subjects with and without IHD, subjecting them to a 12-min tape recorded "stress quiz." This consisted of 35 questions, becoming progressively more difficult and resembling everyday situations, in which people were asked to perform difficult mental tasks. For the entire group, during the quiz, the mean pulse rate rose from 76 to 87 per min and the mean blood pressure from 136/87 to 158/94 mm Hg, differences which were highly significant. Of the 43 subjects, 33 were classified as "executives." These were subdivided into three groups: (a) without angina, (b) with angina, and (c) with angina and hypertension. Both of the angina groups responded with significantly greater rises in blood pressure than either the executives without angina or the 10 patients who were classified as "nonexecutives." Furthermore, the pulse and blood pressure rises in response to the quiz were higher in the executives with angina than in the nonexecutives with angina. Finally, during the test, 10 of the 14 executives with angina pectoris experienced ST segment depression greater than 0.5 mm. There was a high correlation between these depressions and bicycle exercise testing.

The influence of personality is considered in Chapter 2. It is of interest that the studies of Friedman and Rosenman have received some confirmation in Great Britain (65). Behavioral research of this nature must also be confounded by the problem as to which came first, psychiatric or organic morbidity. Lloyd and Cawley (66) assessed psychiatric morbidity in 100 consecutive male patients under age 65 1 week after their first MI. Significant psychiatric morbidity was discovered in 35 of these patients. In 16, this had been evident before the infarct, and it was these patients who showed a wider range of psychopathology than those whose symptoms had been precipitated by the infarct. These workers concluded that psychiatric morbidity in cardiac patients is not necessarily a result of the disease process.

The psychologic effects of coronary heart disease on the patients' spouses must also be considered. A study by Mayou et al. (67) has shown substantial and persistent psychologic symptoms in 82 wives of men suffering their first infarction. The authors concluded that the attitudes and behavior of the wives (as well as the general quality of family life) were important determinants of the rate and extent of the patients' recovery.

To what extent are some of the important risk factors reviewed in the opening part of this chapter associated with psychiatric morbidity, as either cause or effect? If we briefly consider the factors outlined, such an association is credible in a number of instances. For instance, the consumption of alcohol whether, this be excessive or selective, is clearly influenced by psychogenic factors. The heavy drinker uses alcohol as a tranquilizer, while the social drinker uses it as a euphoriant. Similarly, nicotine may act as a tranquilizer, and many individuals smoke excessively in response to long-continued emotional stress. In this context, Horowitz et al. (68) used a life events questionnaire to determine presumptive stress in 575 middle-aged men in relation to smoking, blood pressure, and cholesterol levels. They found significant differences in stress levels only between smokers and nonsmokers.

The many and varied psychologic aspects of obesity are best indicated by the following quote from Craddock's (69) book on the subject:

> The majority of obese people probably have no obvious psychological factors affecting their tendency to obesity. Many of them are people who eat under the minor stresses of everyday life instead of, or as well as, smoking, drinking alcohol or tea, or biting their nails. They are often hypersensitive individuals whose reaction to life is passive rather than active, and they have been conditioned to eat as a reward since early childhood. They therefore eat when under stress, whereas most people are less hungry and lose weight when under stress, owing to increased adrenalin production which mobilises fat and glucose.

The composition of an individual's diet in relation to CHD is primarily a matter for education. Nevertheless, there may be a small psychologic component in that some patients may respond to and maintain dietary instructions, while others will not. The same remarks apply to the factors of climate and composition of water supplies.

Psychologic factors are heavily implicated in the effects of sex on CHD. It is well known that sudden deaths do occur during or shortly after sexual intercourse. It has been suggested, however, that these usually occur in clandestine circumstances, such as the bordello or the mistress's boudoir, or when the relationship has been between an older man and a younger woman (70). It is perhaps only in the placid ambiance of established marriage that sex may be safely indulged in by the sufferer from CHD. The physiologic effects of sexual intercourse are probably minimal since the oxygen cost to the heart is little more than that incurred by mild exertion (49). On the other hand, exercise itself may produce beneficial psychogenic effects for, as Hill (71) remarks referring to rehabilitation after MI, increasing exercise may help to liberate self-expression in physical activity.

With increasing knowledge of the risk factors involved in CHD by the general public, the psychologic effects of a family history of CHD may be of considerable importance. The public generally attributes familial involvement to a heterogeneous collection of ailments, and the phrase "it runs in the family" is well known to general practitioners. Fear of succumbing to the same ailment that killed one's forebears is a potent causal factor in CHD. Indeed, when also widely appreciated, the effects of race may also influence prognosis in this condition. Therefore, emotional stress and anxiety may play a part, either greater or lesser, in most of the known etiologic factors concerned with CHD.

THE ROLE OF PSYCHOTROPIC DRUGS

Little has been written on the use of psychotropic drugs to counteract the psychogenic factors involved in CHD, whether in a prophylactic or a therapeutic role. It is a widely established practice, however, perhaps more so in the United States than in the United Kingdom, to prescribe tranquilizing drugs immediately after MI and for various periods thereafter. This well-established therapeutic custom has not been systematically evaluated by the established method of the controlled clinical trial.

Our own report on the use of an antianxiety drug in comparison to placebo in patients who had suffered their first MI was published recently (72,73). This was followed by a report by Samet and Geller (74) of a double-blind comparison between a benzodiazepine and placebo. In our study, described below, patients who had suffered their first MI were treated for a period of 3 months with either clorazepate or placebo. In the study by Samet and Geller (74), lorazepam was compared to placebo over a 4-week period in 66 patients suffering from a variety of cardiovascular disorders, including disturbances of rhythm and hypertension. In both studies, significant advantages were demonstrated in those patients who received the active medications.

Stressful emotions may even produce effects on the blood-clotting mechanisms themselves. Schneider and Zangari (75) studied the plasma clotting time, relative viscosity, hematocrit, erythrocyte sedimentation rate, and prothrombin time in 16 normal volunteers, nine normotensive patients, and 12 hypertensive patients. They observed: "With anxiety, fear, anger or hostility, the clotting time was shortened, the relative viscosity increased, and blood pressure elevated." The authors speculated that these effects might be part of a protective reaction in response to stress, when offensive action may be needed. Such a pattern might protect against excessive blood loss in armed combat and result in increased oxygen transportation in the blood. Such a pattern, however, if chronic or inappropriate, might favor intravascular thrombosis.

A recent study on the effect of hematocrit on cerebral blood flow (CBF) in man supports these findings (76). It showed that CBF was significantly lower in patients with hematocrit values in the higher ranges. Furthermore, after reduction of hematocrit by venesection, CBF increased by a mean of 50%. This improvement in flow was largely due to a reduction in viscosity. The authors concluded that hematocrit values in the generally accepted upper limit of normal may be important in the production of occlusive vascular disease.

Etiologic receptor sites for drugs that relieve tension and anxiety would not appear to be lacking in CHD in both treatment and prevention.

CLORAZEPATE AFTER INFARCTION

Following MI, patients can be expected to feel anxiety as a reaction to their condition. We sought to determine whether or not an antianxiety drug might help in the management of such patients. We chose patients who had already suffered one MI because the diagnosis would not be in doubt in such cases. Also, it was assumed that such patients would be particularly apprehensive of a second (and probably fatal) infarction.

Clorazepate, a long-acting benzodiazepine, can be given as a single dose at night (77), making it convenient for long-term treatment of patients who are going about their daily life and continuing to work. Patient compliance is also likely to be better with a single daily dose than with multiple doses (78). In a double-blind trial, either clorazepate in a single nightly dose of 15 mg or a matching placebo was given for 3 months (72). Patients were assigned randomly to either the drug or placebo group.

Patient Data

Contrary to expectation, it was difficult to find patients who had experienced one MI and who were also exhibiting a sufficient level of anxiety (73). Of the 41 patients who met the entry criteria, 20 received clorazepate and 21 placebo.

Data were recorded on possible stressful events, diagnostic details, and clinical and investigational findings. Analysis showed that many of these factors did not differ from the findings in the general population, except with respect to family history of arteriosclerosis, economic factors, and occupational and recreational activities.

Family History

Nearly half the patients ($N = 19$) had a family history of arteriosclerotic disease. Interestingly, among 64 parents and siblings who had died, 29 of the deaths (45%) were from cardiovascular disease or its complications.

Besides the details concerning a family history of arteriosclerotic disease, other data were revealing. The majority of spouses and parents were engaged in relatively lowly occupations (presumably without much mental stress) and were nearly all classified as having been successful in life (again, presumably with no mental stress). There seemed to be a combination of extrovert father with introvert mother, and a preponderance of extrovert spouses.

Sociologic Data

Socioeconomic data were also recorded for 38 of the 41 patients. A patient was considered "self-made" if he was born into a low economic group but made his way despite that handicap, if he had a physical disability which he overcame, or if he became successful in any way due to his own efforts.

The patient was classified as having "appropriate achievements" if his occupation and lifestyle were what might have been expected from his upbringing and intellectual attainments. Any patient who in his formative years was afforded some considerable advantage over his peers (for example, wealthy parents, an inheritance, or chance fortune) was classified under "inherited advantage."

There was a relatively high proportion of self-made persons (19 cases, 45%), which might have been expected since such persons would be exposed to considerably more mental stress than those in other categories. (There was an equal number of patients in the "appropriate achievements" category, but no patients fell into the "inherited advantage" group.)

The proportion of patients with active occupations [79% (30 patients) compared with 21% (eight patients) with sedentary jobs] seems high in relation to the general population. On the other hand, there was only a slightly higher proportion of patients in competitive than in noncompetitive occupations. The statistics for active occupations might seem at variance with the idea that physical exercise is beneficial in preventing CHD.

A high proportion of the patients in this study were involved in aggressive/competitive recreations, but mainly as spectators. Of those participating in noncompetitive recreations, a higher proportion were in those classified as sedentary than in those involving physical exertion. These proportions are in keeping with the proposition that physical exercise is beneficial in the prevention of CHD and that a sedentary life is detrimental.

Comparability of Groups

While the sample was small, the two groups matched well, with only one exception: six patients in the placebo group had had severe infarcts, compared with only one in the clorazepate group.

The patients themselves made daily records of their anginal attacks, including number of attacks, whether they occurred at rest or exercise, precipitating cause if known, number of trinitrate tablets taken, other medicines and doses, general well-being, and exercise tolerance. Figure 4.1 shows the mean anginal attack rate per 2-week period in the two treatment groups.

The anginal attack rate is difficult to analyze because attacks tend to vary

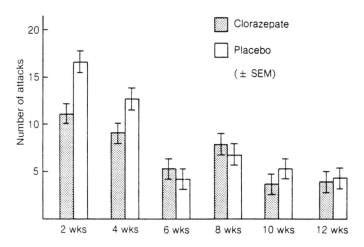

FIG. 4.1. Mean anginal attack rates per 2-week period.

greatly between patients and at different times in each patient. Thus during the first 2 weeks on clorazepate, the attack rate at rest varied from 0 to 39, while the attack rate on exercise varied from 0 to 21. Nevertheless, the figures did tend to even out over the 12 weeks of the trial, making comparisons possible.

For the first 2 weeks of treatment, patients given clorazepate had a mean anginal attack rate of 10.1 (SEM ± 2.4), which dropped progressively to 4.5 (SEM ± 1.2) by the end of the trial. In contrast, the patients given the placebo had a mean attack rate of 17.1 (SEM ± 2.8). Although the rate also fell progressively to 5.2 (SEM ± 1.5) by the end of the trial, the mean anginal attack rate was considerably higher during the first 4 weeks on placebo than on the antianxiety drug. None of the individual differences at any period of the trial is statistically significant, nor is the combined result of all assessment periods.

Nitroglycerin Requirements

A better measure of the frequency of anginal attacks is the requirement for nitroglycerin, provided that nitroglycerin tablets are taken only to relieve attacks, as in this trial (Fig. 4.2).

The mean nitroglycerin requirement was much higher in the patients on placebo than in those on clorazepate. In the patients given clorazepate, the mean nitroglycerin requirement was 7.7 (± 2.0) during the first 2 weeks and dropped progressively to 4.6 (± 1.6) at the end of the 12-week treatment period. In contrast, patients given the placebo had a mean nitroglycerin requirement during

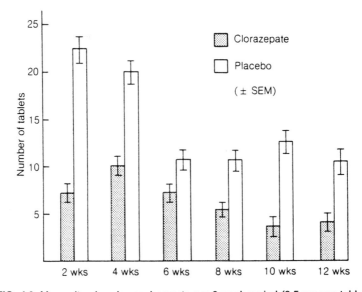

FIG. 4.2. Mean nitroglycerin requirements per 2-week period (0.5 mg per tablet).

the first 2 weeks that was three times that of the clorazepate group, namely, 22.5 ($\pm$ 7.9). As with the clorazepate-treated patients, the mean nitroglycerin requirement declined progressively during the trial but only to a rate of 11.3 ($\pm$ 6.7) by the end of the trial.

None of the between-group differences at any period of the trial is statistically significant, although the difference recorded in the first 2 weeks is nearly so ($p < 0.06$). If we combine all the figures for all six periods as representing the total nitroglycerin requirement over the full period of the trial, however, then the difference becomes highly significant ($p < 0.01$) in favor of the patients who received clorazepate.

Cardiovascular Measures

Blood pressure, pulse rate, and rhythm were recorded every 2 weeks throughout the trial. There was a greater reduction in both mean systolic and mean diastolic pressures in the patients treated with clorazepate than in those treated with placebo. The reduction in systolic pressure in the clorazepate series was statistically significant by the end of the trial ($p < 0.02$), but this was not so in the placebo group. None of the diastolic pre-post differences was statistically significant in either series. Analysis of covariance did not reveal any significant between-group differences at the last assessment.

Six patients in the clorazepate group and five in the placebo group had raised systolic blood pressures initially (150 mm Hg or more). Five of the six clorazepate patients were normotensive by the end of the trial. Only one placebo patient was normotensive. Four patients in the clorazepate series and two in the placebo group had a diastolic hypertension of 100 mm Hg or more. All four clorazepate patients and one of the two placebo patients became normotensive by the end of the trial. Clearly, no deduction can be drawn from these small numbers.

Although there was a slight reduction in mean pulse rate during the trial in both series of cases, there were no statistically significant differences; nor were there any significant differences between the two series of patients in relation to regularity of rhythm.

Psychiatric Symptoms

Psychiatric symptomatology was recorded using the General Practitioner Research Group nine-item anxiety rating scale (78) and the Hopkins Symptom Check List (79) recorded by the patients themselves. Figure 4.3 shows the mean changes recorded with these two scales.

There were statistically significant pre-post differences on the physicians' rating scale but not on the patients' scale starting at 4 weeks and thereafter in the case of clorazepate ($p < 0.01$) and at 8 weeks and thereafter in the case of placebo ($p < 0.05$). Analysis of covariance, however, did not show any between-drug differences on either of the scales.

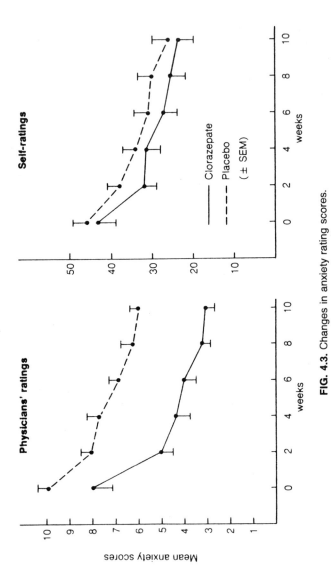

FIG. 4.3. Changes in anxiety rating scores.

Global Assessments

At the end of the trial, the investigators made an assessment of overall changes in the patients' condition. Assessments were made of 15 of the 18 patients remaining in the clorazepate group and 18 of the 20 in the placebo group. The results are shown in Table 4.1.

A significantly larger proportion of the patients treated with clorazepate were classified as "greatly improved" compared with those given placebo. Using a chi-square test, this difference is statistically significant in favor of clorazepate ($p < 0.05$).

Other Factors

Clorazepate was tolerated well by the patients; the proportion of patients experiencing no side effects was high for both the clorazepate and placebo groups. The most important possible side effect of a benzodiazepine drug of this type is drowsiness, but only three patients receiving clorazepate experienced drowsiness, compared with two patients receiving placebo.

If necessary on clinical grounds, physicians were permitted to add other drugs. Ten of the patients receiving placebo required additional medication, compared with five patients receiving clorazepate. This difference, however, is not statistically significant.

Beta-blocking drugs were those most frequently used. The addition of these drugs to placebo treatment resulted in a considerable reduction in nitroglycerin requirements (as compared with all cases), but this reduction was not as marked in the case of the clorazepate series. The overall between-group differences recorded in nitroglycerin requirements might have been even greater had beta-blocking drugs not been used in some cases.

Finally, six patients (29%) dropped out of the placebo series, compared with two (10%) in the clorazepate series, but this difference is not statistically significant. Further infarction occurred in three patients who were receiving placebo but in none receiving clorazepate. Again, this difference is not statistically significant.

TABLE 4.1. Physicians global assessments of improvement by the end of the trial

Global assessment	Clorazepate	Placebo
Greatly improved	11 (79%)[a]	5 (33%)[a]
Same	3	9
Worse	0	0
Much worse	0	1
Not applicable	1	3
Not recorded	3	2

[a]$p < 0.05$.

PREINFARCTION STUDIES

In the postinfarction study described, a number of design defects emerged, not least of which was the lack of a preliminary control period. This was not included because it had been originally intended to treat 200 cases, and with such large numbers the control period would not have been required. Nevertheless, the results showed a consistently lower anginal attack rate and nitroglycerin consumption in patients treated with clorazepate than in those treated with placebo. Furthermore, in the case of the nitroglycerin requirements, the differences were marked at all periods of the trial, being statistically significant in favor of clorazepate over placebo. Without an initial control period, however, it cannot be concluded that the two treatment groups were originally homogeneous in regard to frequency and severity of anginal attacks.

The main reason for the relatively small number of patients included in the trial was the difficulty in finding patients who had suffered one MI who also exhibited a sufficient level of anxiety symptoms. It may be that MI occurring for the first time, rather than being an anxiety-provoking event, may actually constitute an anxiety-relieving one. Thus many sufferers from CHD, as seen in Chapter 2, are leading highly stressful lives often manifested by an increasing burden of responsibility and activity, both at work and in the home. Such individuals are under constant pressure to increase their efforts, with subsequent increasing financial liability. When such an individual suffers an infarction, this may produce consternation not only in his home environment but also at his place of work. Neither spouse nor employer wishes to lose a person of ability upon whom both depend, and the exhortations to strive more greatly are immediately replaced by exhortations to relax. Gone suddenly are the long working hours, the pressures to succeed, and possibly even marital emotional frigidity. In fact, MI is a socially acceptable excuse for such individuals to totally reduce their levels of activity, both mental and physical.

We have therefore turned our attention to an earlier stage in the disease, namely, the study of patients suffering from angina pectoris, particularly with an increasing severity of attacks, who have not yet suffered an actual infarction. In this second trial, clorazepate was again compared to placebo. Although the study is still in progress, some preliminary results on the first 35 patients who completed the full trial period are available. The design of the trial was similar to the first study, patients being treated throughout with either clorazepate (15 mg daily) or placebo for a period of 12 weeks, according to random selection. In this trial, however, an initial 2-week control period was included, during which no treatment was given other than trinitrate tablets to relieve attacks.

Preliminary Results

On breaking the code, it was found that 20 patients had received clorazepate and 15 placebo. The results for the four clinical measures are summarized in Table 4.2. It is apparent from these mean figures that the variance was much

TABLE 4.2. Physical measures in angina patients treated with clorazepate and placebo

2-Week periods	Anginal attacks		GTN used		General well being		Exercise tolerance	
	Clorazepate	Placebo	Clorazepate	Placebo	Clorazepate	Placebo	Clorazepate	Placebo
Control 2 weeks	31.6 ($\pm$8.9)	29.4 ($\pm$6.5)	32.8 ($\pm$9.5)	28.7 ($\pm$6.4)	18.2 ($\pm$1.4)	17.7 ($\pm$1.6)	17.2 ($\pm$1.6)	15.5 ($\pm$1.6)
Third 2 weeks	24.1 ($\pm$10)	13.1 ($\pm$3.1)	20.5 ($\pm$9.4)	12.9 ($\pm$3.5)	23.4 ($\pm$2.6)	22.4 ($\pm$2.5)	21.5 ($\pm$2.2)	20.1 ($\pm$2.1)
Sixth 2 weeks	18.9 ($\pm$10.7)	14.5 ($\pm$3.1)	17.9 ($\pm$11)	14.2 ($\pm$3.3)	27.2 ($\pm$2.7)	20.7 ($\pm$2.5)	25.3 ($\pm$2.5)	18.7 ($\pm$2.5)

greater in these patients who had not suffered a MI than in the previous trial described. The mean number of anginal attacks in the clorazepate series during the 2-week control period was 31.6 (SEM ± 8.9), while in the placebo group it was 29.4 (± 6.5). In fact, during the control period, the number of anginal attacks varied from 1 to 124 in individual patients in the clorazepate group, and from 0 to 89 in the placebo group. Because of these large variances, it is difficult to make any statistical comparisons between the results recorded, and the numbers so far are too small to stratify the cases into groups according to the frequency of anginal attacks during the control period.

Considering the anginal attack rate, it is seen that in both series of patients, the mean rate was reduced by about 50%, comparing the last 2 weeks of the trial to the control 2 weeks. The results were similar for the number of nitroglycerin tablets used per 2-week period. The reduction in anginal attack rate and nitroglycerin tablets used was statistically significant at 8 and 10 weeks ($p <$ 0.02) but not at 12 weeks for the clorazepate group, and statistically significant at all periods of the trial for the placebo group ($p < 0.02$).

Considering general well being and exercise tolerance, in the clorazepate group, there was significant improvement in both measures by the last 2 weeks of the trial ($p < 0.005$ and < 0.02, respectively); but in the placebo group, there was no significant improvement on either measure. The Wilcoxon summed rank test was used to test for significant between-group differences, but in neither case was the difference statistically significant.

IMPLICATIONS FOR FUTURE RESEARCH

The preliminary results from this second study in preinfarction patients demonstrate once again the power of suggestion. The patients treated with placebo responded as well as those treated with the active drug. In view of the large variance in the assessment parameters during the control period, future studies may require more defined criteria with respect to severity in order to obtain more homogeneous active and placebo treatment groups.

A number of effective prophylactic drugs are now in clinical use in the treatment of CHD. Therefore, it is perhaps more realistic to assess the effectiveness of an antianxiety drug compared to placebo when added to prophylactic treatment of this nature. Such drugs are mainly beta-adrenergic blocking drugs or calcium ion antagonists and long-acting coronary vasodilators. With this in mind, our group has planned a study to compare diazepam to placebo randomly allocated to patients for an 8-week trial period, all of whom are also receiving verapamil (Cordilox®), an established calcium ion antagonist. The type of patient our investigators are seeking for inclusion in this study is the one with angina pectoris of moderate severity and relatively free of anginal attacks, but who also suffers from predominant complaints, such as emotional tension, restlessness, anxiety, and sleep disturbances. Otherwise, this study is being conducted on similar lines to those already described.

It is apparent that trying to assess the effectiveness of treatment of the anxiety factor in CHD is fraught with problems in view of the considerable variations in severity which occur in this condition, not only between individuals but at different periods of time in the same individuals. Nevertheless, our preliminary results suggest that the use of an antianxiety drug may be of benefit not only in improving the clinical state of the patients but also in the prevention of future MIs.

CONCLUSIONS

It is apparent that there is a diverse etiologic background to CHD, comprised of many factors, most of which are capable of modification by sociologic or pharmacologic means. Alcohol, smoking, obesity, diet, climate, water supply, sexual activity, and exercise can be listed. Associated with many of these factors is an inescapable psychic element.

The evidence for an adverse effect of emotional stress on CHD is compelling and provides a good case for the assessment of anxiety-relieving drugs in prophylaxis and treatment. By allaying the anxiety element by such means, not only may symptoms be relieved but prognosis improved by delaying or preventing MI.

Some substance for this proposition has been provided by a randomized double-blind comparison undertaken by the General Practitioner Research Group to compare the antianxiety drug clorazepate to placebo in patients who had suffered their first MI. The treatment period was 3 months, and the mean anginal attack rate and mean nitroglycerin requirements were significantly less in the patients treated with active drug than in those treated with placebo. There was also a greater reduction in mean blood pressure with clorazepate; and in both treatment groups, there was a significant reduction in anxiety symptoms.

The study was then extended to patients who had not as yet suffered MI but were experiencing increasing severity of anginal attacks. The preliminary results in this study, which was conducted on similar lines to the previous one, indicate that both active and placebo preparations produced highly significant relief of the symptoms of CHD, although with no significant differences between them. In this study, there was a much greater variance in the frequency of anginal attacks than in the patients who had suffered MI. It will be necessary to allow for this in the continuing research program of the group in this area.

REFERENCES

1. Paul, O., Lepper, M. H., Phelan, W. H., et al. A longitudinal study of coronary heart disease. *Circulation,* 1963, 28, 20–31.
2. Wilhelmsen, L., Wedel, H., and Tibblin, G. Multivariate analysis of risk factors for coronary heart disease. *Circulation,* 1973, 48, 950–958.
3. Klatsby, A. L., Friedman, G. D., and Sigelaub, A. B. Alcohol consumption before myocardial infarction. *Ann. Intern. Med.,* 1974, 81, 294–301.

4. Hennekens, C. H., Robner, B., and Cole, D. Daily alcohol consumption and coronary heart disease. *Am. J. Epidemiol.*, 1978, 107, 196–200.

5. Yano, K., Rhoads, G. G., and Kagan, A. Coffee, alcohol and risk of coronary heart disease in Japanese-Americans. *N. Engl. J. Med.*, 1977, 297, 405–409.

6. Berecochea, J. E. *Health Consequences of Drinking Practices: Kind of Beverage and Subsequent Mortality.* Prepared for the Wine Institute, Berkeley, California, 1978.

7. Stason, W. B., Neff, R. K., Miettinen, O. S., and Jick, H. Alcohol consumption and non-fatal myocardial infarction. *Am. J. Epidemiol.*, 1976, 104, 603–608.

8. Myrhed, M., Berglund, L., and Bottiger, L. E. Alcohol consumption and hematology. *Acta Med. Scand.*, 1977, 202, 11–14.

9. Castelli, W. P., Gordon, T., Hijortland, M. D., et al. Alcohol and blood lipids. *Lancet*, 1977, 2, 153–155.

10. St. Leger, A. S., Cochrane, A. L., and Moore, F. Factors associated with cardiac mortality in developed countries with particular reference to the consumption of wine. *Lancet*, 1979, 1, 1017.

11. Joint Working Party. Prevention of coronary heart disease. *J. R. Coll. Phys.*, 1976, 10(3), 21.

12. Kahn, H. A. The Dorn study of working and mortality among U.S. veterans. *Natl. Cancer Inst. Monogr.*, 1966, 19, 1.

13. Ball, K., and Turner, R. Smoking and the heart. The basis for action. *Lancet*, 1974, 2, 822.

14. Gordon, T., and Kannel, W. B. The effects of overweight on cardiovascular disease. *Geriatrics*, 1973, 28, 80.

15. Keys, A. et al. Coronary heart disease: Overweight and obesity as risk factors. *Ann. Intern. Med.*, 1972, 77, 15.

16. Pelkonen, R., Nikkila, E. A., Koskinen, S. et. al. Association of serum lips and obesity with cardiovascular mortality. *Br. Med. J.*, 1977, 2, 1185.

17. Leelarthaepin, B., Woodhill, J. M., Palmer, S. J., and Blacket, R. B. Obesity, diet and type II hyperlipidaemia. *Lancet*, 1974, 2, 1217.

18. Annotation. The heart and the bowel—what have they in common. *J. Pharmacother.*, 1978, 1, 4, 120.

19. Morris, J. N., Marr, J. W., and Clayton, D. G. Diet and heart: A postcript. *Br. Med. J.*, 1977, 2, 1307.

20. Keys, A. Sucrose in the diet and coronary heart disease. *Atherosclerosis*, 1971, 14, 193.

21. Yudkin, J. Sucrose and cardiovascular disease. *Proc. Nutr. Soc.*, 1972, 31, 331.

22. Joint Working Party. Prevention of coronary heart disease. *J. R. Coll. Phys.*, 1976, 10(3), 45.

23. Menon, I. S., Kendal, R. Y., Dewar, H. A., and Newall, D. J. Effects of onions on blood fibrinolytic activity. *Br. Med. J.*, 1968, 3, 351.

24. Dewar, H. A. Onion, garlic and the circulatory system. *J. Pharmacother.*, 1978, 2(2), 44.

25. Augusti, K. T., Benaim, M. E., Dewar, H. A., and Virden, R. Partial identification of the fibrinolytic activity in onion. *Atherosclerosis*, 1975, 21, 409.

26. Virtanen, A. I., and Matikkala, E. J. The structure and synthesis of cycoalliin isolated from alluim cepa. *Acta Chem. Scand.*, 1959, 3, 623.

27. Agarwal, R. K., Dewar, H. A., Newall, D. J., and Das, B. Controlled trial of the effect of cycoalliin on the fibrinolytic activity of venous blood. *Atherosclerosis*, 1977, 27, 347.

28. Jain, R. C., Vyas, C. R., and Mahotma, O. P. Hypoglycaemic action of onion and garlic. *Lancet*, 1973, 2, 1491.

29. Jain, R. C. Onion and garlic in experimental atherosclerosis. *Lancet*, 1975, 1, 1240.

30. Neill, W. A., Angus Duncan, D., Kloster, F., and Mahler, D. J. Response of coronary ciculation on cutaneous cold. *Am. J. Med.*, 1974, 56, 471.

31. Glass, R. I., and Zack, M. M. Increase in deaths from ischaemic heart disease after blizzards. *Lancet*, 1979, 1, 485.

32. Zenner, R. J., De Decker, D. E., and Clement, D. L. Blood-pressure response to swimming in ice-cold water. *Lancet*, 1980, 1, 120.

33. Taggart, P., Parkinson, P., and Carruthers, M. Cardiac responses to thermal, physical and emotional stress. *Br. Med. J.*, 1972, 3, 71–76.

34. Ramos, D. A., Kruger, H., Muro, M., and Arias-Stella, J. Patologia del hombre nativo de las grandes alturas: Investigacion de las causos de muerte en 300 autopsias. *Bol. San. Panam.*, 1967, 62, 497–501.

35. Ruiz, L., Figueroa, M., Horna, C., and Penaloza, D. Prevalencia de la hipertension arterial y

cardiopatia insquemica en las grandes alturas. *Arch. Inst. Cardiol. Mex.,* 1969, 39, 474–489.

36. Mortimer, E. A., Monson, R. R., and MacMahon, B. Reduction in mortality from coronary heart disease in men residing at high altitude. *N. Engl. J. Med.,* 1977, 296, 581–585.

37. Morgan, T., Adam, W., Gillies, A., et al. Hypertension treated by salt restriction. *Lancet,* 1978, 1, 227–230.

38. Annotation. Hypertension—Salt poisoning. *Lancet,* 1978, 1, 1136–1137.

39. Trowell, H. C. Hypertension and salt. *Lancet,* 1978, 2, 204.

40. Østergaard, K. Cadmium and hypertension. *Lancet,* 1977, 1, 677–678.

41. Fassett, D. W. In: *Metallic Contaminants and Human Health,* edited by D. H. K. Lee, Chapter 4, p. 97. New York, 1972.

42. Glauser, S. C., Bello, C. T., and Glauser, E. M. Blood-cadmium levels in normotensive and untreated hypertensive humans. *Lancet,* 1976, 1, 717–718.

43. Beevers, D. G., Campbell, B. C., Goldberg, A. et al. Blood-cadmium in hypertensives and normotensives. *Lancet,* 1976, 2, 1222–1224.

44. Beevers, D. G., Erskine, E., Robertson, M. et al. Blood-lead and hypertension. *Lancet,* 1976, 2, 1–3.

45. Annotation. Progress in the water story. *Br. Med. J.,* 1978, 1, 264.

46. Elwood, P. C., St. Leger, A. S., and Morton, M. Mortality and the concentration of elements in tap water in county boroughs in England and Wales. *Br. J. Prevent. Soc. Med.,* 1977, 31, 178–182.

47. Chipperfield, B., and Chipperfield, J. R. Relation of myocardial metal concentrations to water hardness and death-rates from ischaemic heart disease. *Lancet,* 1979, 2, 709–712.

48. Shapiro, S., Slone, D., Rosenberg, L. et al. Oral-contraceptive use in relation to myocardial infarction. *Lancet,* 1979, 1, 743–746.

49. Wallace, R. B., Hoover, J., Barrett-Connor, E. et al. Altered plasma lipid and lipoprotein levels associated with oral contraceptive and oestrogen use. *Lancet,* 1979, 2, 111–114.

50. Hellerstein, H. K., and Friedman, E. H. Sexual activity and the postcoronary patient. *Arch. Intern. Med.,* 1970, 125, 987–999.

51. Littler, W. A., Honour, A. J., and Sleight, P. Direct arterial pressure, heart rate and electrocardiogram during human coitus. *J. Reprod. Fertil.,* 1974, 40, 321–329.

52. Tuttle, W. B., Cook, W. L., and Fitch, E. Sexual activity in postmyocardial infarction patients. *Am. J. Cardiol.,* 1964, 13, 140.

53. Morris, J. N., Chave, S. P. W., Adam, C. et al. Vigorous exercise in leisure time and the incidence of coronary heart disease. *Lancet,* 1973, 1, 333.

54. Paffenberger, R. S., and Hale, W. E. Work activity and coronary heart mortality. *N. Engl. J. Med.,* 1975, 292, 545.

55. Slack, J., and Evans, K. A. The increased risk of death from ischaemic heart disease in first degree relatives of 121 men and 96 women with ischaemic heart disease. *J. Med. Genet.,* 1966, 3, 239–257.

56. Rissanen, A. M., and Nikkila, E. A. Coronary arterial disease and its risk factors in families of young men with angina pectoris and in controls. *Br. Heart J.,* 1977, 39, 875–883.

57. Dyerberg, J., and Bang, H. O. Haemostatic function and platelet polyunsaturated fatty acids in Eskimos. *Lancet,* 1979, 2, 433–435.

58. Gordon, T., Garcia-Palmieri, M. R., Kagan, A. et al. Differences in coronary heart disease in Framingham, Honolulu and Puerto Rico. *Am. J. Med.,* 1977, 62, 707.

59. Gordon, T. Mortality experience among the Japanese in the United States, Hawaii and Japan. *Public Health Report,* 1957, 72, 543–553.

60. Marmot, M. G., Syme, S. L., Kagan, A. et al. Epidemiologic studies of cornary heart disease and stroke in Japanese men living in Japan, Hawaii and California: Prevalence of coronary and hypertensive heart disease and associated risk factors. *Am. J. Epidemiol.,* 1975, 102, 514–525.

61. Freeman, B. M. Physiological basis of stress. *Proc. R. Soc. Med.,* 1975, 68, 427.

62. Folkow, B. Role of sympathetic nervous system. In: *Coronary Heart Disease and Physical Fitness,* edited by O. A. Latsen and R. O. Malmborg. University Press, Baltimore, 1971.

63. Eliot, R. S., and Forker, A. D. Emotional stress and cardiac disease. *JAMA,* 1976, 236, 20, 2325.

64. Schiffer, F., Hartley, L. H., Schulman, C. L. et al. The quiz electrocardiogram: A new diagnostic

and research technique for evaluating a relation between emotional stress and ischaemic heart disease. *Am. J. Cardiol.,* 1976, 37, 41–47.

65. Heller, R. F. Type A behaviour and coronary heart disease. *Br. Med. J.,* 1979, 2, 368.
66. Lloyd, G. G., and Cawley, R. H. Psychiatric morbidity in men one week after first acute myocardial infarction. *Br. Med. J.,* 1978, 2, 1453–1454.
67. Mayou, R., Foster, A., and Williamson, B. The psychological and social effects of myocardial infarction on wives. *Br. Med. J.,* 1978, 1, 699–701.
68. Horowitz, M. J., Benfari, R., Hulley, S. et al. Life events, risk factors and coronary disease. *Psychosomatics,* 1979, 20, 9, 586–592.
69. Craddock, D. *Obesity and its Management,* second edition. Churchill Livingstone, Edinburgh, 1973.
70. Annotation. Coitus and coronaries. *Br. Med. J.,* 1976, 1, 414.
71. Hill, O. The psychological management of psychosomatic diseases. *Br. J. Psychiatry,* 1977, 131, 113–126.
72. Wheatley, D. Clorazepate in the management of coronary disease. *Psychosomatics,* 1979, 20, 3, 195–205.
73. Wheatley, D. Coronary heart disease: Treating the anxiety component. In: *Progress in Neuropsychopharmacology (in press).*
74. Samet, C. M., and Geller, R. D. Anxiety associated with cardiovascular disorders: A study using lorazepam. *Psychosomatics,* 1979, 20, 10, 709–713.
75. Schneider, R. A., and Zangari, B. S. Variation in clotting time, relative viscosity and other physio-chemical properties of the blood accompanying physical and emotional stress in the normotensive and hypertensive subject. *Psychosom. Med.,* 1951, 13, 289.
76. Thomas, D. J., du Boulay, G. H., Marshall, J. et al. Effect of haematocrit on cerebral blood-flow in man. *Lancet,* 1977, 2, 941.
77. Wheatley, D. A single-dose anti-anxiety drug. *Practitioner,* 1975, 215, 98.
78. Wheatley, D. *Psychopharmacology in Family Practice.* Appleton-Century-Crofts, New York, 1973.
79. Derogatis, L. R., Rickels, K., and Rock, A. F. The SCL-90 and the MMPI: A step in the validation of a new self-report scale. *Br. J. Psychiatr.,* 1976, 128, 280.

Prologue: Beta-Adrenergic Blockade in Psychiatry

The first section of this book surveyed the impact of stress on the heart as manifested by coronary heart disease. The importance of behavior patterns and emotional stress in the etiology of this, perhaps the most dramatic manifestation of heart disease, was amply demonstrated by Taggart and Carruthers in their chapter, which provided an indication as to the pharmacologic means by which these factors may be combated. Chemical blockade of the beta-adrenergic receptors in the heart results in abolition of many of the adverse biochemical and behavioral responses to stressful situations. In this section of the book, this theme is carried further. The authors of the various chapters consider in detail the indications for the use of this pharmacologic approach in the treatment of various emotional and psychiatric situations.

In the opening chapter, Ian James and his colleagues describe how beta-adrenergic blocking drugs can be used with benefit to combat the effects of "stage fright," and neatly pose the question as to what extent this may be justified in normal life situations. A distinction must of course be made between individual variability that enables one person to meet a stressful situation with calm and confidence but yet another with so much apprehension that functional ability, otherwise normal, is impaired. As the authors point out, the effects of stage fright may be so calamitous as to deprive a gifted individual of his ability to make use of those gifts. It would be hard to justify withholding pharmacologic therapy under these circumstances, and indeed this might comprise a form of prophylaxis in the prevention of consequent psychiatric disorders, such as depression and anxiety states.

In the second chapter of the section, the theme moves from normal life situations to the abnormal situation of an anxiety state and the effects of the various forms of this psychiatric illness on those who suffer from it. To what extent beta-adrenergic blockade may constitute a specific remedy for this type of affective disorder remains to be seen, but this form of treatment does provide an alternative to the ubiquitous benzodiazepines that are, at present, being questioned by many clinicians as to their suitability, particularly for long-term use. The dangers of drug dependence and withdrawal symptoms are only now coming to be appreciated with these drugs, together with the problem of daytime drowsiness, particularly when they are used as hypnotics. The beta-blocking drugs would seem to provide a safe physiologic alternative for the treatment of this distressing condition in all its guises.

Finally, a much more important indication for beta-blockers is described by Neil Yorkston, who has pioneered the use of beta-blocking drugs in the treatment of schizophrenia. For this condition, however, much larger doses must be employed than in the treatment of stressful situations and anxiety states. Nevertheless, these appear to be relatively well tolerated by psychotic patients. In the long-term treatment of chronic schizophrenia, confirmation of these early results with beta-adrenergic blockade may provide a form of treatment that need not interfere quantitatively with the quality of the patient's life. As an alternative to the psycholeptic drugs, with their serious side-effects (such as parkinsonism and dyskinesia), drugs of the beta-blocker series may provide a new therapeutic dawn for the patient suffering from this, the most intractable form of psychotic disorder.

Stress and the Heart, edited by D. Wheatley,
Raven Press, New York © 1981.

Stressful Situations

D. Griffith, R. Pearson, and I. M. James

When man descended from the trees, there is little doubt that catecholamines
were an unqualified success. In most ways, this remains the case today. Not
only is their basal secretion essential for the maintenance of life, but the outpour-
ing that occurs in response to stressful stimuli and their ability to mobilize
the body for action are invaluable assets. In some ways, however, conditions
and desirable responses to these conditions have changed. In modern society,
there is a different set of demands on the human frame. This is reflected in a
narrower sense in differing patterns not only of life but of death and morbidity,
with an increasing prevalence of cardiovascular problems. While there is no
question that the enormous benefits bestowed by catecholamines still far outweigh
any drawbacks, it is now possible to see that some facets of their actions may
actually be disadvantageous in certain spheres of human activity.

PERFORMANCE OF SKILLED TASKS

One such case is the performance of skilled tasks in which physical control
rather than sheer physical exertion is paramount yet where maintenance of
mental alertness is essential. Today, such skilled behavior is often carried out
under adverse and stressful conditions. The relationship between apprehension
and the performance of such tasks has been described by the "Yerkes-Dodson"
law (1). Initially, performance improves as apprehension increases, largely due
to increased motivation of the subject. Further anxiety, however, is not associated
with additional improvement in performance, and if apprehension continues
to increase, performance rapidly deteriorates. A classic example of this is stage-
fright, which is the problem we chose to investigate.

Stage-Fright

The psychologic and physiologic mechanisms responsible for the complex
interaction that occurs in stage-fright are difficult to unravel but almost certainly
involve the sympathoadrenal system. Mental stress is often associated with activation of the sympathetic nervous system, resulting in the clinical manifestations
of palpitations, hyperventilation, sweating, and tremor. Such sensations may
not only in themselves interfere with the performance of skilled tasks, but they
often enhance the anxiety in susceptible individuals, with the result that the
very sensations are associated with feelings of fear. It has long been known

that the infusion of catecholamines or their release from a pheochromocytoma can cause anxiety and fear. There appears to be a positive feedback system of anxiety causing catecholamine release, which itself causes further anxiety.

Traditionally, centrally acting drugs have been used in an attempt to combat the adverse effects of anxiety on performance. Their administration, however, is associated with unwanted sedation, which in turn leads to a deterioration in performance. The pharmaceutical companies that manufacture these drugs usually advise that people should not work with machinery or drive when taking them. The correct aim should be to control anxiety without causing concomitant undesirable depressant effects on the central nervous system.

Apart from this aspect of the problem, catecholamine release may also result in other adverse changes, both biochemical and cardiovascular. Thus, as described in Chapter 3, the mobilization of free fatty acids from adipose tissue and their subsequent conversion to triglycerides may, if they are not utilized, play an important role in the genesis of atheroma (2). There is also evidence that the increasing morbidity of cardiovascular disease and the increasing stresses of everyday life are intimately related, as Russek and Russek demonstrated in Chapter 2. Furthermore, studies of racing drivers, public speakers, parachutists, and car drivers in heavy traffic have shown that tachycardia and ECG changes, such as ST segment depression and dysrhythmias, can be precipitated by stress (see Chapter 3).

As noted in Chapter 3, beta-adrenoceptor blocking drugs have been shown to be effective not only in abolishing the lipid response to emotion but also in attenuating or abolishing stress-induced tachycardia, ST segment abnormalities, and dysrhythmias (3). Thus there is a good argument for protecting the patient with coronary artery disease from the ravages of stress by the use of beta-adrenoceptor blocking drugs. Indeed, the use of such drugs in anyone over middle age subjected to stress might be indicated on cardiovascular grounds alone. First, however, it is essential that their effect on performance be fully assessed.

The use of beta-adrenoceptor blocking drugs in the treatment of anxiety was first suggested by Granville-Grossman and Turner (4). Their efficacy in this respect has been confirmed in a number of studies (5–8) which are fully described in the next chapter. Turner and Hedges (9) have shown that the beta-adrenoceptor blocking drug oxprenolol, given orally to normal volunteers, produces no adverse changes in tests of central nervous system function.

PUBLIC MUSICAL PERFORMANCES

The main purpose of our study was to determine the effect of oxprenolol on anxiety-induced disturbances engendered by giving a musical performance in public, rather than to assess disturbances caused by artificial stress. While some degree of apprehension on the part of the performer is often said to be essential for an optimal musical performance, it is nevertheless well recognized by professional musicians that excessive anxiety may have an incapacitating effect and may be truly catastrophic, as many performers—and audiences—will testify. We investigated string players exclusively because the effect of tremor in particular is more easily observed in this group of musicians.

Clinical Trial of Oxprenolol

Twenty four healthy string players between ages 18 and 47 years and comprising six men and 18 women were recruited from the London Colleges and Academies of Music. All were intent on making music a career, and none claimed to suffer from undue nervousness. A conventional two-way crossover double-blind clinical trial design was used. The subject was assessed on two separate days, once on 40 mg oxprenolol and once on identical placebo. Drugs, coffee, and alcohol were forbidden on the day of the study but a standard light lunch with soft drinks was provided each day. Each player took either the oxprenolol or the placebo 90 min before the recital. Those who received oxprenolol on the first day had the placebo on the second day, and vice versa, equal numbers taking drug and placebo on each day. The order of administration was randomly allocated and the code broken only after all the results had been obtained.

The Stress of a Solo Debut

A realistic degree of anxiety was engendered in the subjects by mounting the study under concert conditions at the Wigmore Hall, London, where a solo debut is widely regarded as a testing experience. Performances were tape-recorded using a battery of obvious microphones. Press, radio, and television access to the hall was allowed and controlled as far as possible to make both days equally stressful. Before performance, both the subjective sensations of the players and certain physiologic variables were assessed. Anxiety was scored by a graded scale from 1 ("nonchalant") to 6 ("panicky") and by a visual analog rating scale (VARS) from 0 mm ("I feel relaxed") to 100 mm ("I feel petrified"). Pallor, hand sweating, hand coldness, and tremor were graded, and blood pressure and pulse were recorded.

Musical assessment was carried out by two professors from the London College of Music, both experienced music competition adjudicators. They carried out the assessment blind to drug therapy, medical records, and to each other's scoring. Each recitalist played two pieces, the first with music and the second from memory. The pieces were marked from 0 to 10 with respect to each of the following important musical points: (a) accurate shifting (of hand position), vibrato, intonation, and musicianship with respect to the left hand, and (b) bowing, lack of tremor, and musicianship for the right hand. The maximum possible score for each piece was 70. Memory was separately scored 0 to 10.

Immediately after performing, subjects chose a word to describe their performance varying from terrible *(1)* to very good *(5)*. They also used a VARS to describe their emotional state from "I feel euphoric" (0 mm) to "I feel hopeless" (100 mm).

Effects of Beta-Blockade

Review of the results of the physiologic variables before performance (Table 5.1) showed that oxprenolol caused a significant fall in pulse rate from 99 to 75 per min and of systolic blood pressure from 125 to 110 mm Hg. Tremor was less with the drug but was not usually completely abolished. There was a tendency for the hands to become less sweaty and less cold, but this did not reach a statistically significant level. Surprisingly, oxprenolol appears to have slightly increased facial pallor. The performers' subjective sensations of nervousness were significantly decreased by oxprenolol as assessed either by the VARS or graded scales (Table 5.1).

Musical Assessments

Musical assessment showed that oxprenolol produced a highly significant improvement in the total scores ($p < 0.0001$ by analysis of variance) and seemed to be more effective when taken for the first session than when taken for the second (Table 5.2). The mean (pooled) scores were higher for the second session than for the first. Listed in Table 5.3 are the mean scores for the individual aspects of musicianship. Memory, which was separately scored, was not significantly affected by the drug.

The players themselves assessed their problems with tremor and stiffness as being significantly less on oxprenolol. There was a significant improvement in

TABLE 5.1. *Assessment before performance*

Parameter	Placebo	Oxprenolol	Significance
Heart rate (per min)	99.00 ± 2.6	75.00 ± 1.7	< 0.0001[a]
Systolic blood pressure (mm Hg)	125.00 ± 2.3	110.00 ± 2.5	< 0.0001[a]
(Scaling 0–3)			
Facial pallor	0.25 ± 0.09	0.63 ± 0.17	NS[b]
Sweaty hands	2.00 ± 0.22	1.83 ± 0.21	NS[b]
Cold hands	1.21 ± 0.21	0.83 ± 0.18	NS[b]
Tremor	2.12 ± 0.16	1.50 ± 0.16	< 0.02[b]
Nervousness (VARS) 57.	57.00 ± 4.0	46.00 ± 4.8	< 0.05[c]
0 (relaxed) to 100 (petrified)			
Nervousness (graded)	3.71 ± 0.23	2.92 ± 0.24	< 0.005[b]
1 (nonchalant) to 6 (panicky)			

Means $\pm$ standard error of means are shown.
[a] Paired *t*-test.
[b] Signs test.
[c] Wilcoxon's matched pairs signed ranks test.
NS, not significant.

TABLE 5.2. *Mean values for analysis of variance of total scores of musical assessors' record*

Session	Placebo	Oxprenolol	Pooled results
First	47.1	51.5	49.3
Second	50.3	51.1	50.7

how the musicians felt they had performed, and they were also happier after the performance.

In summary, the main point is that oxprenolol, a beta-adrenoceptor blocking agent, caused a significant improvement in musical performance. Although overall mean improvement was only about 5%, in some subjects there was a 30% improvement, and in one individual this figure reached 73%. The reasons for the overall improvement in the total musical scores are of some interest. An appreciable factor in the improvement was the effect on tremor, to which approximately 30% of the total improvement was attributable. Other components also improved significantly (Table 5.3), and although these may be difficult to interpret exactly in physiologic terms, it is apparent that skill, coordination, and judgment are all involved.

Another point of interest was that while there was a highly significant difference between drug and placebo on the first day, on the second this difference was not seen, the principal reason being the improved score on the second occasions (Table 5.2). The fact that the greater effect was seen on the first performance when stress and anxiety were greatest raises the possibility that the need for the drug would lessen with time. Once a performer has coped successfully with a situation, he or she has greater confidence for subsequent occasions.

TABLE 5.3. *Mean scores for the musical assessors' record of individual aspects of musicianship*

Variable	Placebo	Oxprenolol minus placebo	p^a
Left hand			
Accurate shifting	6.74	+0.22	NS[b]
Vibrato	6.69	+0.21	NS
Intonation	6.48	+0.34	<0.02
Musicianship	6.53	+0.26	<0.05
Right hand			
Bowing	6.86	+0.44	NS
Tremor	8.64	+0.79	<0.02
Musicianship	6.79	+0.31	<0.05
Total	48.72	+2.57	<0.01
Memory	6.29	+0.56	NS

[a] Paired *t*-test. NS, not significant.

USE OF BETA-BLOCKERS IN NORMAL INDIVIDUALS

As mentioned previously, a role for beta-adrenoceptor blocking drugs in acutely stressful situations has been suggested by other workers for various reasons. Evidence is accumulating to support the contention that emotion may exert important untoward effects on the cardiovascular system, not only in patients with coronary artery disease but also in normal subjects. The evidence for this is both biochemical and electrophysiologic.

These facts, taken with the beneficial effect on anxiety-induced disturbances of performance, strengthen the case for using beta-adrenoceptor blocking drugs in normal individuals under acute emotional stress. Whether or not these drugs should be used by musicians, or indeed by others whose performance of a skilled task is adversely affected by stress, is a question for which there is at present no simple answer. Each case must be judged on its own merits. Although the decision must ultimately rest with the subject and his or her personal physician, there are several points that could influence that decision. If future career prospects or livelihood depend on the task, then the case for using the drug becomes strengthened. Beta-adrenoceptor blocking drugs used intermittantly in relatively small doses may enable people to adapt successfully to stressful occasions. Although the use of drugs in such situations is often deplored, the nonaddicting, peripherally acting beta-adrenoceptor blocking drugs may be more acceptable than the sedatives or alcohol so often used. Further studies are needed to confirm their efficacy in this and other similar situations. The results of this study give cause for limited optimism.

CONCLUSIONS

The catecholamine secretion that occurs in man as a response to stressful stimuli is an invaluable asset, but some facets of catecholamine actions may actually be disadvantageous in certain spheres of human activity. An example is in the performance of skilled tasks where physical control is paramount and the maintenance of mental alertness essential.

The psychologic and physiologic mechanisms occurring in stage-fright almost certainly involve the sympathoadrenal system. The symptoms resulting from stimulation of the system, such as palpitations, hyperventilation, sweating, and tremor, may not only interfere with the performance of skilled tasks but often continue to perpetuate anxiety in susceptible individuals.

Beta-blockade with oxprenolol proved highly effective, as compared to placebo, in 24 string musicians subjected to the stress of a solo debut. Not only were the performers' subjective sensations of nervousness significantly decreased, but their musical performances were significantly improved.

There is a strong case for using beta-adrenoceptor blocking drugs in normal individuals under acute emotional stress, particularly when future career prospects or livelihood may depend on the task being undertaken.

REFERENCES

1. Tyrer, P. Choice of treatment for anxiety. *Practitioner,* 1977, 219, 479.
2. Carruthers, M. Aggression and atheroma. *Lancet,* 1969, 11, 1170.
3. Taggart, P., Gibbons, D., and Somerville, W. Some effects of motor car driving on the normal and abnormal heart. *Br. Med. J.,* 1969, iv, 130.
4. Granville-Grossman, K., and Turner, P. The effect of propranolol on anxiety. *Lancet,* 1966, 1, 788.
5. Wheatley, D. Comparative effects of propranolol and chlordiazepoxide in anxiety states. *Br. J. Psychiatry,* 1969, 115, 1411.
6. Tyrer, P. J., and Lader, M. H. Response to propranolol and diazepam in somatic and psychic anxiety. *Br. Med. J.,* 1974, 2, 14.
7. McMillan, W. P. Oxprenolol in anxiety. *Lancet,* 1973, 1, 1193.
8. Burrows, G. D., Davies, B., Foil, L. et al. A placebo controlled trial of diazepam and oxprenolol for anxiety. *Psychopharmacology,* 1976, 50, 177.
9. Turner, P., and Hedges, A. In: *New Perspectives in Beta-Blockade,* edited by D. M. Burley, J. H. Fryer, R. K. Rondel, and S. H. Taylor. CIBA Laboratories, Horsham.

Stress and the Heart, edited by D. Wheatley,
Raven Press, New York © 1981.

Beta-Blocking Drugs in Anxiety

David Wheatley

Adrenergic blocking drugs are divided into two types: alpha-blocking and beta-blocking. Phentolamine, phenoxybenzamine, and tolazoline are examples of the former. They are rather esoteric compounds; because they are generally peripheral vasodilators and hypotensive agents, their main uses have been in the diagnosis and treatment of pheochromocytoma.

The beta-blocking drugs exert their main effects on the cardiovascular system and are established in clinical practice for the treatment of various disorders of cardiac function, such as the arrythmias (1), coronary heart disease (CHD) (2), and hypertension (3). Labetalol (Trandate®) is unique in combining both alpha- and beta-adrenergic blocking actions (4).

The potential importance of adrenergic beta-blockade as a therapeutic measure in CHD is demonstrated dramatically in the work of Taggart and Carruthers (see Chapter 3). The direct clinical application of such findings has been demonstrated by a number of workers. Wilhelmsson et al. (5) reported highly significant effects of alprenolol in reducing the incidence of sudden deaths after myocardial infarction (MI) over a period of 2 years. Norris et al. (6) demonstrated the protective effect of propranolol in patients with threatened MI. In a long-term study involving 3,053 patients with MI, subsequent treatment with practolol significantly reduced the eventual mortality due to reinfarction by 38% in comparison to placebo (7). Swedberg et al. (8) have reported prolongation of survival in congestive cardiomyopathy as a result of using beta-receptor blockade. Their finding that beta-blockade improved myocardial function is supported by the experimental work of Vaughan Williams et al. (9), who showed that long-term beta-adrenoceptor blockade produced an increase in the relative volume of vascular elements in the myocardium. The authors speculated that the relative increase in capillaries and shorter diffusion pathway for oxygen could raise oxygen availability, which would have direct application in clinical situations.

ANTIANXIETY EFFECTS

The beneficial cardiovascular effects of the beta-blocking drugs are not in doubt, but how have they come to be advocated for the treatment of anxiety? This use is based on their property of slowing the pulse, which is effective even in subjects with normal pulse rates. The beneficial effects of this pharmacologic maneuver in allaying anxiety under stressful situations is amply demonstrated in the previous chapter. Another striking example of reduction in stress-induced tachycardia by a beta-blocking drug has been recorded by Foster et al. (10), who monitored eight surgeons while operating, finding their mean heart rate to be 121 beats/min, with maximum rates in some cases of more than 150 beats/min. In contrast, the surgeons' heart rates during busy outpatient clinics lay within normal limits. The stress-induced tachycardia during operation was abolished by 40 mg oxprenolol taken 1 hr before; this reduced heart rates during operations to below those recorded during the outpatient clinics. The heart rates were recorded by a cassett tape-recorder worn on a belt around the surgeon's waist. The ECG signal was monitored by two chest electrodes. Thus continuous ambulatory monitoring was achieved.

Apart from this basic action of the beta-blocking drugs, many of the features of anxiety are those that characterize hyperactivity of the adrenergic system. Therefore, in addition to slowing the tachycardia that is a prominent feature of anxiety states, beta-blocking drugs should also help to control a number of the other symptoms of anxiety: tremor, sweating, restlessness, palpitations, and other psychosomatic manifestations. Indeed, so effective are the beta-blocking drugs in these contexts, that they have become part of the standard therapy for hyperthyroidism, which produces similar symptoms. Thus they have been used alone to control the symptoms of thyroid overactivity, to prepare patients for thyroid surgery, and in combination with antithyroid drugs and radioactive iodine (11).

Animal pharmacology has provided evidence for the antianxiety effect of propranolol, since Bainbridge and Greenwood (12) showed that both D- and L-propranolol reduced the reactivity to novel stimuli in rats made hyperactive by septal lesioning. Furthermore, Valzelli et al. (13) showed that propranolol reduces aggression in mice first kept in isolation and then placed in groups, whereas Richardson et al. (14) suggested that the antianxiety effects of the drug might be due to effects on the amygdala.

Clinical Trials

The use of propranolol to treat anxiety was first suggested by Granville-Grossman and Turner in 1966 (15). They undertook a double-blind comparison between propranolol and placebo and demonstrated significant antianxiety effects from the active compound. Subsequently, our own group undertook a trial comparing propranolol to chlordiazepoxide, which was conducted under the usual double-blind procedures on 105 patients suffering from anxiety (16). We found similar effects from the two drugs, with no statistically significant differences between them at any period of the trial. When considering specific items of the rating scale used, however, there was a significantly better response to chlordiazepoxide in depressive mood and sleep disturbance, although improvement in tachycardia and tremor was similar with both drugs.

The use of beta-blockers in anxiety has been reviewed by Kelly (17). Trials have been undertaken with the following drugs: propranolol (18,19), oxprenolol

(20–23), sotalol (24,25), and practolol (26). In these studies, comparisons were made to either placebo or standard benzodiazepine drugs, such as diazepam and chlordiazepoxide. Equivalent antianxiety effects were demonstrated for propranolol, oxprenolol, and practolol, although the studies with sotalol were not as convincing. Tyrer and Lader (24) compared it to placebo using a crossover design of 2 weeks of treatment with each (24). According to the patients' preferences, there were no differences between the two treatments. On the Hamilton Anxiety Scale, however, somatic symptoms were helped by the active drug. Salkind and Silverstone (25) undertook a double-blind comparison between sotalol (120 mg/day) and diazepam (15 mg/day) and placebo in 44 patients suffering from anxiety. Treatment was randomly assigned and was continued for 4 weeks. The authors found that both active drugs produced a statistically significant improvement in the first 2 weeks, but that by the end of 4 weeks, there were no differences between active drugs and placebo.

Oxprenolol has been the subject of three more recent studies. In a double-blind comparison, Johnson et al. (27) compared 11 cases treated with oxprenolol to 13 treated with diazepam and five treated with placebo (27). The investigators found that diazepam produced a more rapid effect, and that by the end of the trial, this differed significantly from placebo but not from oxprenolol. On the other hand, the relief of anxiety with oxprenolol by the end of the trial did not differ significantly from that recorded with placebo. In view of the small numbers of patients per treatment group, not much significance should be attached to these findings. It is of interest that the authors were unable to demonstrate any differences in response between somatic and psychic symptoms.

In contrast, Burrows et al. (28) undertook a similar study on 22 patients treated with oxprenolol, 20 with diazepam, and 20 with placebo. After 3 weeks of treatment, significantly better results were recorded with the two active drugs as compared to placebo, although there were no significant differences between the two drugs themselves. These authors also failed to demonstrate any differences in response between somatic and psychic symptoms. Finally, Becker (29) compared 23 patients treated with oxprenolol to 23 treated with propranolol under double-blind conditions for 2 weeks. He was not able to demonstrate any differences in response between these two different beta-blocking drugs.

General Practice Studies

Our own group recently completed a double-blind comparison between practolol and chlordiazepoxide in anxiety. Patients were treated for 4 weeks with one or the other drug according to random selection. The trial included all cases of anxiety, provided symptoms had been present for at least 1 week; cases with mild depressive symptoms were also included, provided anxiety was the predominant diagnosis.

The daily dosage of the drugs was: practolol, 300 mg, and chlordiazepoxide, 30 mg, both being administered t.d.s. A total of 63 patients received treatment,

34 with practolol and 29 with chlordiazepoxide. Results were assessed initially and at the end of 1, 2, and 4 weeks using defined global ratings, the GPRG nine-item physician rating scale, and the NIMH patient self-rating scale (30). On all three measures, slightly better results were recorded for chlordiazepoxide than for practolol, although there were no statistically significant differences except in the proportion of patients experiencing no effect at the end of the fourth week. This proportion was significantly higher with practolol than with chlordiazepoxide ($p < 0.05$). Relief of anxiety was similar with the two compounds, and there were no statistically significant differences at any period of the trial.

Side effects spontaneously volunteered by the patients and attributed to the medication were recorded; in addition, a specific question was asked concerning drowsiness, together with a control question concerning increased alertness. The incidence of side effects was similar with the two drugs (practolol, 14 cases, 41%; chlordiazepoxide, 11 cases, 38%), as were the relative severities (severe: practolol, two cases, 14%; chlordiazepoxide, one case, 9%). However, drowsiness occurred more frequently with chlordiazepoxide (nine cases, 31%) than with practolol (seven cases, 20%), although the difference was not statistically significant for the numbers involved. Increased alertness occurred in five cases on each medication (14 and 17%, respectively).

We have also studied the effects of two other beta-blockers, namely, acebutolol and tolamolol (subsequently withdrawn because of adverse effects in animals),

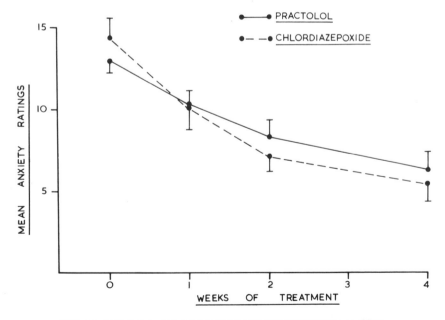

FIG. 6.1. Relief of anxiety by practolol and chlordiazepoxide (± SEM).

during clinical trials of these two drugs in hypertension and CHD, respectively (31). Although the initial mean level of anxiety in these patients was low, anxiety symptoms were significantly relieved in both studies. In the absence of any control group, however, no conclusions can be drawn concerning the possible effects of these two drugs in anxiety states.

Apart from the studies on propranolol, practolol (now withdrawn because of toxic effects), and oxprenolol, the evidence for antianxiety effects from the other beta-blockers described is not substantial. This does not imply that the drugs may be without antianxiety effects, but the studies generally were undertaken either on small numbers of patients or with a rather unsatisfactory crossover design, involving treatment for only short periods of 1 or 2 weeks.

THE BETA-BLOCKER FAMILY

A large number of drugs of this type have been introduced into clinical practice, although research on this type of compound has been aimed at producing drugs with a more highly selective cardiogenic action. In particular, attempts have been made to discover beta-blocking drugs that are highly specific in their effects in CHD and hypertension (beta$_1$ specificity), with as little effect as possible on the bronchi (beta$_2$ effects), since the use of these drugs is severely limited in asthmatic patients. A number of differences have emerged between the different beta-blocking drugs with respect to various pharmacologic actions. Some of these that may be relevant to psychotropic effects are listed in Table 6.1.

MODE OF ACTION IN ANXIETY

There are indications that the action of the beta-blocking drugs in anxiety may be a peripheral rather than a central one. Propranolol is marketed for therapeutic use as a racemic mixture of the dextro- and levo-forms; Bonn (32) conducted trials on this preparation, in comparison to D-propranolol and practolol. Both DL-propranolol and practolol are active peripheral beta-adrenergic blockers (33), but D-propranolol is not (34). Both D- and L-propranolol enter the brain, but practolol does not (35). Therefore, Bonn concluded that these results indicated that the peripheral beta-adrenergic blocking drugs, DL-propranolol and practolol, significantly improved anxiety states, but that the nonbeta-blocking drug D-propranolol had no such effect. As little practolol enters the brain, Bonn concluded that the antianxiety action of the beta-blocking drugs must be attributable to their peripheral action and not to a central one. Thus the antianxiety effect of these drugs is independent of their ability to penetrate to the central nervous system (CNS).

It has been suggested that, since the effectiveness of beta-blocking drugs in anxiety is due to their peripheral action, they are more effective against somatic than psychic symptoms. This suggestion is based on a study reported by Tyrer and Lader (36), who undertook a double-blind crossover trial in 12 chronically

TABLE 6.1. *Some pharmacologic properties of the beta-blocker family*

Property	Beta-blocker[a]											
	Prop	Pract	Ox	Met	Sot	Tim	Pind	Aceb	Aten	Nad	Al	Lab
Cardioselective	−	+	−	+	−	−	−	±	+	−	−	−
Intrinsic sympath. activity	−	+	+	−	−	−	++	±	−	−	+	−
Membrane stabilizing	+	−	±	+	−	−	±	+	−	−	++	+
Lipid solubility	+	−	+	±	−	−	−	+	−	−	+	−
Passes to CNS	+	−	+	±	±	−	+	−	−	(−)	+	−
Antianxiety	+	+	+	?	±	−	?	?	?	?	?	?

[a]Prop, propranolol; Pract, practolol; Ox, oxprenolol; Met, metoprolol; Sot, sotalol; Tim, timolol; Pind, pindolol; Aceb, acebutolol; Aten, atenolol; Nad, nadolol; Al, alprenolol; Lab, labetalol.

anxious patients, giving propranolol, diazepam, and placebo for 1 week each. The authors concluded that diazepam was, in general, more effective than propranolol or placebo in relieving anxiety, but that propranolol was more effective than placebo in patients with predominantly somatic symptoms. This was not the case in those with predominantly psychic symptoms. Tyrer and Lader suggested that propranolol should be reserved for patients whose anxiety symptoms are mainly somatic.

This conclusion is based on flimsy evidence. Patients were divided into two groups of six predominantly suffering from somatic anxiety and six predominantly from psychic anxiety. It was shown that in the former group there was an equivalent response to diazepam and propranolol, but that in the latter group there was a significant response to diazepam only. These significant responses were based on the total Hamilton Anxiety scores. These authors do not seem to have undertaken separate analyses on the psychic and somatic components of the Hamilton scale. Also, it seems doubtful whether significant clinical conclusions can be drawn from 1 week's treatment. Although it was stated that "order effects of treatment were allowed for," it is difficult to see how some carryover of effect could have been avoided with such short treatment periods and no intervening washout periods.

Subsequent studies undertaken on larger groups of patients with longer treatment periods have failed to differentiate any specific action of beta-blocking drugs in relation to benzodiazepines, in the relief of somatic and psychic symptoms, respectively (27–29).

The ideal antianxiety drug should combine effectiveness against both somatic and psychic symptoms. Beta-blocking drugs that enter the CNS in high concentrations might be relatively more effective as antianxiety agents, since they might exert both peripheral and central actions. That considerable differences exist between the different members of the beta-blocking family in this respect has been demonstrated by Day and Hemsworth (37).

Central CNS Effects

In animal studies, a number of beta-adrenoceptor antagonists have been shown to cross the blood-brain barrier following systemic administration (37–39). In a more recent study by Street et al. (40), the uptake of radioactively labeled propranolol, oxprenolol, metoprolol, acebutolol, practolol, and atenolol into brain, liver, and lung tissue was studied 5 min after intravenous administration in rats. All the beta-adrenoceptor antagonists, including the least lipophilic compounds atenolol and practolol, were detected in brain tissue 5 min after systemic administration. The level of propranolol in the brain, however, was 40 and 67 times greater than the levels found for atenolol and practolol, respectively. Furthermore, the drugs could be divided into groups with high brain concentrations (propranolol, oxprenolol, and metoprolol) and low concentrations (acebutolol, practolol, and atenolol).

The ability of these drugs to pass the blood-brain barrier is due at least in part to their relative lipophilicity (41). The findings of Street et al. (40) are in keeping with the properties of the compounds they investigated in this respect (see Table 6.1). On the grounds of high lipophilicity, alprenolol and pindolol could be added to the group of beta-blocking drugs that would be highly concentrated in the brain and nadolol to those that would only achieve low concentrations. Once again, this is in keeping with the known effects of these drugs (see Table 6.1).

There is evidence from animal pharmacology that concentrations of beta-blocking drugs in the brain may produce behavioral responses. Costain and Green (42) investigated the effects of various beta-blocking drugs on the 5-hydroxytryptamine (5-HT)-induced hyperactivity response in rats following administration of tranylcypromine followed by L-tryptophan. The authors found that alprenolol, sotalol, pindolol, oxprenolol, and timolol *(sic)* all inhibited the hyperactivity response to some degree, whereas atenolol, practolol, labetalol, and acebutolol, which only passed the blood-brain barrier poorly, did not inhibit the 5-HT-mediated behavior. On the other hand, metoprolol, which is well concentrated in the brain, did not inhibit this behavior. The authors attributed this to the fact that metoprolol is a highly cardioselective (B_1 selective) drug. In another test for effects on dopamine-mediated behavior, circling (behavior) was produced in unilateral nigrostriatal lesioned rats by methamphetamine. None of the drugs tested had a statistically significant effect on circling, although alprenolol did decrease the total number of turns in all animals tested. The workers concluded that nonselective (B_1 and B_2) adrenoceptor antagonists, which have a high brain/blood ratio following peripheral injection, block 5-HT-mediated behavioral responses in the rat.

In addition to lipophilicity, the degree of plasma protein binding of beta-blockers may affect their ability to pass the blood-brain barrier. Cruickshank et al. (43) investigated the CNS pharmacokinetics in man of three beta-blockers: atenolol (Tenormin®), which is highly water soluble and not highly plasma protein bound; propranolol (Inderal®), which is highly lipid soluble and highly plasma protein bound; and metoprolol (Lopressor®), which is moderately lipid soluble and not highly plasma protein bound. All patients were neurosurgical and required a routine lumbar puncture. The mean blood/cerebrospinal fluid (CSF) ratio for atenolol was $\simeq 10:1$, for propranolol $\simeq 19:1$, and for metoprolol $\simeq 1:1$. Despite the low CSF levels of propranolol, in two patients who came to ablative surgery, a high concentration of propranolol in brain tissue was seen, with a mean brain/CSF ratio of $\simeq 335:1$ and brain/blood ratio of $\simeq 33:1$. In another patient who also came to ablative surgery who had been treated with atenolol, the mean brain/CSF ratio was $\simeq 1:1$, with a brain/blood ratio of $\simeq 0.2:1$.

There are striking differences between different beta-blockers, both in their ability to pass the blood-brain barrier and in relation to their relative concentrations in brain and CSF. Of perhaps even more interest from the point of view of possible behavioral effects of these drugs is a consideration of the areas of brain in which they become concentrated, for these also vary considerably between different drugs of the series. In a study undertaken by Garvey and Ram (44), tissue distributions of propranolol, pindolol, and sotalol were investigated in rats, tissue distribution being determined after 14 days of treatment. Propranolol and a metabolite were concentrated in the hippocampus, whereas pindolol was concentrated in the septum. Significant central concentrations of sotalol were not demonstrable. The authors speculate that this uptake of propranolol may be responsible for the tranquilizing effect of the drug. A sedative effect was observed in their experiments in both normotensive and hypertensive animals. As well as being concentrated in the hippocampus, propranolol is also taken up by several other brain areas, such as the hypothalamus and septum.

It is possible that selective uptake in different areas of the brain may be a factor in determining whether or not a beta-blocking drug has antianxiety effects.

Membrane-Stabilizing Activity

A number of studies provide evidence for a central action by beta-blocking drugs, which may be associated with their membrane-stablizing action. Thus, in contradistinction to the studies undertaken by Bonn (32), Bainbridge and Greenwood (12) found in rats that D-propranolol was just as good a tranquilizer as DL-propranolol. Similar results were recorded by Speizer and Weinstock (45). As Koella (46) observes:

> These findings strongly suggest that the central damping effect of DL-propranolol, at least as observed in this particular animal model, is due not to the drug's beta-adrenergic blocking action but presumably to some other membrane-active influence which it exerts. Accessory properties of these beta-blocking drugs—e.g., their well-known local anaesthetic action (membrane "stabilisation")—could perhaps be responsible for such "non-beta" effects, although the local concentration at central sites might be too small for such mechanisms to become effective.

In this connection, it is of interest that the tricyclic antidepressants also possess local anesthetic activity (47). This effect has been suggested as an explanation for the cardiotoxicity exhibited by these drugs (see Chapter 10).

Hellenbrecht et al. (48) characterized the nonspecific membrane affinity of a number of beta-adrenergic blocking drugs by determining their hydrophobicity, surface activity, and local anesthetic activity. The authors found that the drugs investigated could be divided into three main groups, according to their physiochemical properties and their nonspecific pharmacologic effects. Among the most active were alprenolol and propranolol, while oxprenolol and pindolol were intermediate, and sotalol and practolol were the least active.

Combining Beta-Blocker and Benzodiazepine

Another possibility would be to combine a beta-blocking drug (peripheral action) with a benzodiazepine (central action). This has been the subject of a recent study undertaken by our research group on the combination of timolol with chlordiazepoxide.

Timolol is a noncardiospecific beta-blocking drug which differs from propranolol in not having membrane-stablizing properties (see Table 6.1). The indications for its use are similar to those for propranolol. In particular, it has been combined with a thiazide diuretic in the treatment of hypertension (49).

The trial was a double-blind comparison between timolol and chlordiazepoxide (hereafter referred to as the timolol group) and placebo and chlordiazepoxide (hereafter referred to as the placebo group). Patients were allocated to one or the other treatment by random selection, and the dose of timolol (10-mg tablets) (or placebo) was increased as necessary from one to four daily (10 to 40 mg timolol). Chlordiazepoxide was prescribed in a standard dose of 10 mg t.d.s. throughout (30 mg/day).

In total, 47 patients were treated. On breaking the code, it was found that 23 had received timolol and 24 placebo. Results were assessed using the Leeds Self-Rating Scale (50) completed by the patients and the Hamilton Anxiety Scale completed by the physicians. The trial period was 4 weeks. The results are shown diagramatically in Figure 6.2.

Significant pre-post differences were recorded in both treatment groups from the end of the first week onward, but analysis of covariance failed to show any between-group differences at any period of the trial. Similar results were recorded on the Leeds Self-Rating scale and on the Leeds Anxiety and Depression subscales. The somatic items on the Hamilton scale were also analyzed separately. This showed a mean reduction in somatic item score for the timolol group of 1.75 ($\pm$ 0.74) and a reduction of 3.59 ($\pm$ 0.56) for the placebo group. These two mean change scores were tested for significant differences using the t-test, which gave $t = -2.022$ (i.e., in favor of placebo), a difference which is virtually statistically significant ($p = 0.051$). On this analysis of the somatic items, better results were recorded for the group treated with placebo plus chlordiazepoxide than for the group treated with timolol plus chlordiazepoxide.

Apart from showing any enhanced antianxiety effects from the combination of the beta-blocking drug and benzodiazepine, the results, at least on the somatic items, were if anything better in the group receiving the benzodiazepine alone. It cannot be determined whether the combination offers no advantages over the single components in the treatment of anxiety or, alternatively, whether timolol is a beta-blocking drug without antianxiety effects.

Is There a Specific Compound for Anxiety?

In an attempt to determine why the combination of timolol and chlordiazepoxide proved relatively ineffective in the study described, the properties of timolol, recorded in Table 6.1, were reviewed. Timolol differs from propranolol in the lack of membrane-stablizing properties and in the fact that it does not pass in any appreciable concentration to the CNS. Practolol, an effective antianxiety

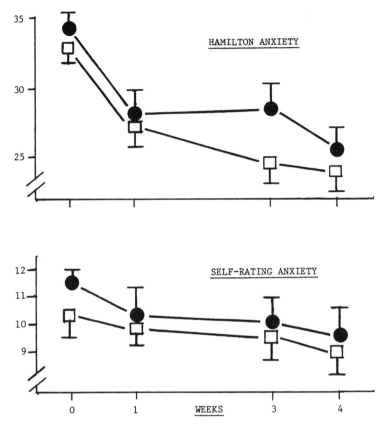

FIG. 6.2. Changes in mean scores of total Hamilton Anxiety Scale **(upper tracings)** and of Anxiety Sub-scale of Leeds Self-Rating Scale **(lower tracings).** Closed circles, timolol + chlordiaz; open squares, placebo + chlordiaz.

drug, also lacks both these properties. To determine if different beta-blocking drugs may have differing effects on anxiety symptoms as a result of varied combinations of pharmacologic effects, a series of trials, in comparison to both placebo and benzodiazepines, should be conducted. In this respect, pindolol might be of interest since it possesses membrane-stabilizing properties, appears in the CNS in high concentration (like propranolol), and has intrinsic sympathetic activity (like practolol). Such a trial is at present being planned by our group. In a small pilot study involving eight patients suffering from anxiety treated for 3 weeks with pindolol, there was a reduction in the mean Hamilton anxiety rating score from 28.9 (SEM $\pm$ 2.4) initially to 24.7 ($\pm$ 2.4) by the end of the trial period. Despite this modest result, the reduction in mean score is statistically significant ($p = 0.01$, Wilcoxon signed rank test).

Other compounds that may be of interest in this connection are acebutolol and metoprolol. Acebutolol has been shown to reduce tachycardia and improve symptoms of tension in individuals taking part in competition rifle shooting (51). There are no reports of the use of acebutolol in anxiety neurosis, but reference has been made to a study by our group to compare acebutolol to bendrofluazide and the combination of acebutolol with bendrofluazide in cases of hypertension. In this study, anxiety ratings were made before and after treatment; although anxiety symptoms were relieved, the differences were not statistically significant (52).

Metoprolol has been employed to investigate the preventive action of beta-blockade on the response to mental stress (53). In this study, mental stress was artificially induced by a so-called "speech-delayer," whereby an artificial speech disturbance is induced. By means of acoustic feedback from a tape-recorder, speech is disintegrated, severely disturbing the subject's intention to speak. Attempts to adjust to this state lead to a pronounced increase in heart rate and rise in blood pressure. Although metoprolol prevented the rise in heart rate, it had no effect on the raised blood pressure and no effects on reaction time, opticomotor coordination, or concentration ability. It is debatable, however, to what extent this artificial induction of a stress situation may be related to anxiety states occurring in patients.

There is both experimental and clinical evidence to suggest that different beta-blocking drugs may exert different effects on the CNS and in psychiatric disorders. It is unfortunate that a uniform series of tests in both experimental areas has not been undertaken with a number of beta-blocking drugs; it is difficult to make comparisons between results that are recorded with widely differing experimental and clinical procedures.

CLINICAL USEFULNESS

Although the beta-adrenergic blocking drugs may not exert any better antianxiety effect than the benzodiazepines, an advantage might be a reduced incidence of side effects, particularly drowsiness, in the treatment of ambulatory patients at home. This would have particular relevance to the driving of motor vehicles, since in the study by Taggart and Carruthers of oxprenolol in racing drivers, there was no impairment of performance as a result of taking the drug (see Chapter 3).

Freedom from Drowsiness

In the two studies by our group on propranolol and practolol, respectively, compared to chlordiazepoxide, the overall incidence of side effects did not differ significantly, although the incidence of drowsiness was less in both studies with the beta-blocking drug. Even on summating the figures for drowsiness from both trials, there was no significant difference between the incidence with the beta-blocking drugs and that with chlordiazepoxide.

In contrast to these two formal studies on anxiety, in two studies of tolamolol (not now marketed) and acebutolol in coronary disease and hypertension, respectively, the incidence of side effects in general and drowsiness in particular was low. Of 64 patients treated with tolamolol, only one complained of "listlessness" (2%); of 56 patients treated with acebutolol, only one complained of drowsiness (2%). The occurrence of drowsiness as a side effect may be related to the condition being treated. In the case of anxiety neurosis, the production of a tranquilizing effect may induce a sensation of relaxation or drowsiness, in contrast to previous feelings of tension occasioned by the illness. As we have seen in the two studies in the cardiovascular conditions, the levels of anxiety were not very high; this may have contributed to the very low level of drowsiness recorded in these two studies.

On the other hand, in a double-blind controlled trial between propranolol and methyldopa in hypertension (described in Chapter 15), drowsiness was specifically asked for, in contradistinction to the other studies described, in which side effects were recorded only if spontaneously volunteered by the patients. Inevitably, the incidence of all side effects is considerably higher when they are specifically elicited, and this study proved to be no exception. Nevertheless, the incidence of drowsiness with propranolol (six of 30 cases, 20%) was considerably less than with methyldopa (14 of 37 cases, 38%).

The recorded side effects, including drowsiness, in other published studies on the use of beta-blockers in anxiety are low. Becker (29) recorded two cases of drowsiness in 23 patients treated with propranolol and in one of 23 treated with oxprenolol. In a survey of adverse reactions associated with propranolol in 35 hypertension trials involving 1,435 patients, Conway (54) recorded a 4.18% incidence of fatigue and lack of energy, together with an incidence of drowsiness of only 0.49%. In the period from 1972 to 1977 in Australia, only two cases of drowsiness had been reported with propranolol as compared to one with practolol, four with pindolol, and none with either alprenolol or oxprenolol (55). The low incidence of CNS psychiatric side effects with beta-blocking drugs has been demonstrated in the United States in a number of double-blind trials of timolol compared to placebo in hypertension (56). No significant differences were demonstrated in the incidence of either type of side effect between 168 patients receiving placebo and 176 patients receiving timolol for 12 weeks.

Even more important are studies which have been undertaken using various psychomotor tests after beta-blocking drugs. In comparison to placebo, Turner and Hedges (57) found no significant changes in serial subtraction, disc dotting performance, or critical flicker frequency after single doses in healthy volunteers. Lader and Tyrer (58), using single oral doses of propranolol (120 mg), sotalol (240 mg), or placebo, could discern no evidence of central effects on reaction time, key tapping, card sorting, digit symbol substitution, and symbol copying, or on EEG recordings. Ogle and Turner (59) found no effects from single oral doses up to 160 mg propranolol on pursuit rotor and reaction time in eight subjects. As Turner (60) observes:

even where a statistically significant performance decrement has been found in normal subjects, it has been very small in comparison with the effects of a known sedative drug such as one of the benzodiazepines.

The recognition of serious side effects of practolol (61,62) has necessitated its withdrawal from general clinical use. It remains to be seen whether these serious complications (corneal damage, sclerosing peritonitis) occur also with any of the other beta-blocking drugs available, although this seems unlikely. For example, since propranolol has been in use much longer than practolol, in view of clinical awareness of the complications of the latter, it would be expected that any problems with propranolol would have been reported by now. However, an occasional report indicating one or other of the beta-blockers in use does appear in the correspondence columns of medical and scientific journals. Such isolated reports should not bar the continued use of these drugs in clinical practice.

CONCLUSIONS

There is sufficient evidence to demonstrate that the beta-adrenergic blocking drugs, or at least propranolol and practolol, exert antianxiety effects comparable to those of the benzodiazepines.

The results of our studies indicate that the level of side effects is lower with the beta-blocking drugs than with comparable antianxiety agents, such as the benzodiazepines. This may be of considerable importance when treating the ambulant patient, particularly if his or her daily life and work involves driving a motor vehicle. Although we were unable to demonstrate statistically significant differences in the incidence of drowsiness in our two studies on anxiety, the low incidence of this side effect in the two studies with tolamolol and acebutolol, respectively, may be of importance. It is also noteworthy that the reported incidence of drowsiness from the use of beta-blockers in treating cardiovascular disorders is low and in most cases no more than that which occurs with placebo medication.

Although there are notable contraindications to the use of beta-blocking drugs, particularly in patients with cardiac failure, other cardiac conditions, or asthma, the newer compounds of this type that are being introduced will probably prove to be considerably more cardiospecific than their predecessors. Therefore, with the exception of practolol, there is no reason not to use these drugs to treat anxiety. In the case of practolol, the severe toxic effects that can be produced preclude its use in the treatment of anxiety. These effects, however, are peculiar to practolol. Undoubtedly, rigid screening procedures will be undertaken with the new beta-blocking drugs to ensure that they are free of similar toxic actions.

There is no evidence that the beta-blocking drugs produce drug dependence, as can happen with the benzodiazepines. If this is confirmed in clinical practice, it may be an important advantage for this group of drugs and a strong argument for their use in preference to conventional antianxiety agents.

The suggested distinction between the response of somatic and psychic symptoms, respectively, to beta-blockers has not been confirmed by subsequent studies. The action of beta-blocking drugs in the treatment of anxiety states may be due to both a peripheral and a central action. In this context, considerable differences may exist between different members of the beta-blocker family. Further research is required to elucidate the antianxiety effects of the many different individual beta-blocking drugs that are now available for clinical use.

REFERENCES

1. Sloman, G., and Stannard, M. Beta-adrenergic blockade and cardiac arrhythmias. *Br. Med. J.,* 1967, 4, 508.
2. Prichard, B. N. C., and Gillam, B. M. S. Assessment of propranolol in angina pectoris: Clinical dose response curve and effect on electro-cardiogram at rest and at exercise. *Br. Heart J.,* 1971, 33, 473.
3. Prichard, B. N. C., and Gillam, B. M. S. Treatment of hypertension with propranolol. *Br. Med. J.,* 1969, 1, 7.
4. Phillips, L. A. Labetalol: A clinical review. *J. Pharmacother.,* 1977, 1, 1, 35.
5. Wilhelmsson, C., Vendin, J. A., Wilhelmsen, L. et al. Reduction of sudden deaths after myocardial infarction by treatment with alprenolol. *Lancet,* 1974, 2, 1157.
6. Norris, R. M., Sammel, N. L., Clarke, E. D. et al. Protective effect of propranolol in threatened myocardial infarction. *Lancet,* 1978, 2, 907.
7. Multi-Centre International Study: Supplementary Report. Reduction in mortality after myocardial infarction with long-term beta-adrenoceptor blockade. *Br. Med. J.,* 1977, 2, 419.
8. Swedberg, K., Waagstein, F., Hjalmarson, A., and Wallentin, I. Prolongation of survival in congestive cardiomyopathy by beta-receptor blockade, *Lancet,* 1979, 1, 1374.
9. Vaughan Williams, E. M., Tasgal, J., and Raine, A. E. G. Morphometric changes in rabbit ventricular myocardium produced by long-term beta-adrenoceptor blockade. *Lancet,* 1977, 2, 850.
10. Foster, G. E., Evans, D. F., and Hardcastle, J. D. Heart-rates of surgeons during operations and other clinical activities and their modification by oxprenolol. *Lancet,* 1978, 1, 1323.
11. Carroll, P., Woods, K. L., and Kendall, M. J. Hyperthyroidism and β-adrenoceptor blockade. *J. Pharmacother.,* 1980, Vol 3 (No. 2) p. 64.
12. Bainbridge, J. G., and Greenwood, D. T. Tranquillizing effects of propranolol in rats. *Int. J. Neuropharmacol.,* 1971, 10, 453.
13. Valzelli, L., Giacolone, E., and Garattini, S. Pharmacological control of aggressive behavior in mice. *Eur. J. Pharmacol.,* 1967, 2, 144.
14. Richardson, J. S., Stacey, P. D., Cerauskio, P. W., and Musty, R. E. Propranolol interferes with inhibitory behavior in rats. *J. Pharm. Pharmacol.,* 1971, 23, 457.
15. Granville-Grossman, K., and Turner, P. The effect of propranolol on anxiety. *Lancet,* 1966, 1, 788.
16. Wheatley, D. Comparative effects of propranolol and chlordiazepoxide in anxiety states. *Br. J. Psychiatry,* 1969, 115, 1411.
17. Kelly, D. Beta-blockers in anxiety. *J. Pharmacother.,* 1978. 1, 3, 91.
18. Tyrer, P. J., and Lader, M. H. Response to propranolol and diazepam in somatic and psychic anxiety. *Br. Med. J.,* 1974, 2, 14.
19. Tyrer, P. J., and Lader, M. H. Physiological and psychological effects of dl-propranolol, d-propranolol and diazepam in induced anxiety. *Br. J. Clin. Pharmacol.,* 1974, 1, 379.
20. Gaind, R., Suri, A. K., and Thompson, J. Use of beta blockers as an adjunct in behavioural techniques. *Scot. Med. J.,* 1975, 20, 284.
21. Krishnan, G. Oxprenolol in the treatment of examination nerves. *Scot. Med. J.,* 1975, 20, 288.
22. McMillin, W. P. Oxprenolol in anxiety. *Lancet,* 1973, 1, 1193.
23. Elsdon-Dew, R. S. Clinical trials of oxprenolol in anxiety. *Scot. Med. J.,* 1975, 20, 286.

24. Tyrer, P. J., and Lader, M. H. Effects of beta-adrenergic blockade with sotalol in chronic anxiety. *Clin. Parmacol. Ther.,* 1973, 14, 418.
25. Salkind, M. R., and Silverstone, J. T. The clinical and psychophysiological effects of a beta-adrenergic blocking agent (sotalol) in anxiety. *Psychopharmacologia,* 1972. 26 (Supplement) 72. Springer-Verlag, Berlin.
26. Bonn, J. A., Turner, P., and Hicks, D. C. Beta-adrenergic receptor blockade with practolol in the treatment of anxiety. *Lancet,* 1972, 1, 814.
27. Johnson, G., Singh, B., and Leeman, M. Controlled evaluation of the beta-adrenoceptor blocking drug, oxprenolol in anxiety. *Med. J. Aust.,* 1976, 1, 909.
28. Burrows, G. D., Davies, B., Foil, L., et al. A placebo controlled trial of diazepam and oxprenolol for anxiety. *Psychopharmacology,* 1976, 50, 177.
29. Becker, A. L. Oxprenolol and propranolol in anxiety states. A double-blind comparative study. *S. Afr. Med. J.,* 1976, 50, 16, 627.
30. Wheatley, D. *Psychopharmacology in Family Practice.* Heinemann, London, 1973.
31. Wheatley, D. (ed.) *Stress and the Heart,* first edition. Raven Press, New York, 1977.
32. Bonn, J. A. Beta-blocking drugs in anxiety. Paper read at symposium on Psychopharmacology of the Circulatory System, held at the 1st World Congress of Biological Psychiatry, Buenos Aires, 1974.
33. Dunlop, D., and Shanks, R. G. Selective blockade of adrenoceptive beta receptors in the heart. *Br. J. Pharmacol.,* 1968, 32, 201.
34. Barrett, A. M., and Cullum, V. The biological properties of the optical isomers of propranolol and their effects on cardiac arrhythmias. *Br. J. Pharmacol.,* 1968, 34, 53.
35. Scales, B., and Cosgrove, M. B. The metabolism and distribution of the selective adrenergic beta-blocking agent practolol. *J. Pharmacol. Exp. Ther.,* 1970, 175, 338.
36. Tyrer, P. J., and Lader, M. H. Response to propranolol and diazepam in somatic and psychic anxiety. *Br. Med. J.,* 1974, 2, 14.
37. Day, M. D., and Hemsworth, B. A. The central uptake of beta-adrenoceptor antagonists. *J. Pharm. Pharmacol. [Suppl.],* 1977, 29, 52.
38. Wong, K. K., and Schreiber, E. C. Recent developments in beta-adrenergic blocking drugs. *Drug Metab. Rev.,* 1972, 1, 101.
39. Garvey, H. L., and Ram, N. Centrally induced hypotensive effects of β-adrenergic blocking drugs. *Eur. J. Pharmacol.,* 1975, 33, 283.
40. Street, J. A., Hemsworth, B. A., Roach, A. G., and Day, M. D. Tissue levels of several radiolabelled β-adrenoceptor antagonists after intravenous administration in rats. *Arch. Pharmacodyn. Ther.,* 1979, 237, 2, 180.
41. Johnsson, G., and Regardh, C-G. Clinical pharmacokinetics of β-adrenoceptor blocking drugs. *Clin. Pharmacokinet.,* 1976, 1, 233.
42. Costain, D. W., and Green, A. R. β-Adrenoceptor antagonist inhibit the behavioural responses of rats to increased brain 5-hydroxytryptamine. *Br. J. Pharmacol.,* 1978, 64, 193.
43. Cruickshank, J. M., Neil-Dwyer, G., Cameron, M. M., and McAinsh, J. Beta-blockers and the central nervous system. Sixth Scientific Meeting International Society Hypertension, Goteborg, June 11–13, 1979.
44. Garvey, H. L., and Ram, N. Comparative antihypertensive effects and tissue distribution of beta-adrenergic blocking drugs. *J. Pharmacol. Exp. Ther.,* 1975, 194, 220–33.
45. Speizer, Z., and Weinstock, M. The influence of propranolol on abnormal behaviour induced in rats by prolonged isolation—an animal model for mania? *Br. J. Pharmacol.,* 1973, 48, 348.
46. Koella, W. P. Anatomical, physical and pharmacological findings relevant to the central nervous effects of the beta-blockers. In: *Beta-Blockers and the Central Nervous System,* edited by P. Kielholz. Hans Huber, Switzerland, 1977.
47. Axelrod, J., and Weinshilbaum, R. Catecholamines. *N. Engl. J. Med.,* 1972, 287, 237.
48. Hellenbrecht, D., Lemmer, B., Wiethold, G., and Grobecker, H. Measurement of hydrophobicity, surface activity, local anaesthesia and myocardial conduction velocity as quantitative parameters of the non-specific membrane affinity of nine β-adrenergic blocking agents. *Naunyn Schmiedebergs Arch. Pharmacol.,* 1973, 277, 211.
49. Wheatley, D. Timolol and bendrofluazide in the management of hypertension in general practice. *Eur. J. Clin. Pharmacol.,* 1978, 14, 319.
50. Snaith, R. P., Bridge, G. W. K., and Hamilton, M. The Leeds Scale for the Self-Assessment of Anxiety and Depression. *Br. J. Psychiatry,* 1976, 128, 156–65.

51. Gibbons, D. O., and Phillips, M. The effect of acebutolol on tachycardia and performance during competition rifle shooting. *Br. J. Clin. Pharmacol.* 1976, 3, 516.
52. Wheatley, D. A new beta-adrenergic blocking drug in hypertension. *Practitioner,* 1976, 216, 218.
53. Heidbreder, E., Pagel, G., Rockel, A., and Heidland, A. Beta-adrenergic blockade in stress protection. Limited effect of metoprolol in psychological stress reaction. *Eur. J. Clin. Pharmacol.,* 1978, 14, 391–398.
54. Conway, J. Beta-adrenergic blockade and hypertension. In: *Modern Trends Cardiol.,* edited by M. F. Oliver, Butterworth, London. 1975, 3, 376.
55. Annotation. Beta-blockers and the central nervous system. *Aust. Prescriber,* 1977, 2, 2, 37–38.
56. Abrams, W. B. Lipid solubility and CNS effects of timolol vs. propranolol. Timolol Intercontinental Symposium, Stockholm, October, 1979.
57. Turner, P., and Hedges, A. An investigation of the central effects of oxprenolol. In: *New Perspectives in Beta-blockade,* edited by D. M. Burley et al., p. 269. CIBA, Horsham, England, 1973.
58. Lader, M. H., and Tyrer, P. J. Central and peripheral effects of propranolol and sotalol in normal human subjects. *Br. J. Pharmacol.,* 1972, 45, 557.
59. Ogle, C. W., and Turner, P. The effects of oral doses of oxprenolol and of propranolol on CNS function in man. *J. Pharmacol. Clin. (Paris),* 1974, 1, 256.
60. Turner, P. Clinical and experimental studies on the central effects of beta-blockade in man. In: *Beta-Blockers and the Central Nervous System,* edited by P. Kielholz. Hans Huber, Switzerland, 1977.
61. Felix, R. H., Ive, F. A., and Dahl, M. G. C. Cutaneous and ocular reactions to practolol. *Br. Med. J.,* 1974, 4, 321.
62. Brown, P., Baddeley, H., Read, A. E., et al. Sclerosing peritonitis, an unusual reaction to a beta-adrenergic blocking drug (practolol). *Lancet,* 1974, 2, 1477.

Stress and the Heart, edited by D. Wheatley,
Raven Press, New York © 1981.

Propranolol in the Treatment of Schizophrenia

Neil J. Yorkston, John H. Gruzelier, and Saniha A. Zaki

Present evidence about the rate of improvement in patients with schizophrenia who benefit from beta-blockers is that the effects usually occur gradually over weeks or months, but the discovery of an antipsychotic effect of propranolol was in an acute illness that responded dramatically to the drug. In 1969, a woman with an acute attack of porphyria variegata, whose pulse and blood pressure kept rising, was given increasing doses of propranolol up to 400 mg in 24 hr. At this stage, all her symptoms, including those of psychosis, suddenly subsided. Withholding propranolol was followed by a relapse of symptoms and giving it again by another remission (1,2).

UNCONTROLLED CLINICAL TRIALS

Atsmon and his group (3), who reported this case, then gave propranolol openly to 44 patients with psychotic illnesses. Most improvement was seen in patients with mania, postpartum psychosis, and acute schizophrenia, less improvement with chronic schizophrenia, and virtually no change in those with psychosis due to organic brain damage. The role of propranolol in schizophrenia was not clear, partly because these patients' illnesses may have been difficult to classify. For example, three of five of their representative cases had visual hallucinations, one had mania, and the fifth had catatonia. Symptoms did not remit in patients with chronic schizophrenia (4), possibly because treatment was stopped after 3 weeks if there was not marked improvement (3).

The possible use of propranolol in the treatment of patients with florid symptoms of schizophrenia was explored by our group in an uncontrolled study of 55 adults (5,6). Propranolol was often maintained for many months.

Florid schizophrenic symptoms remitted, at least temporarily while propranolol was continued, in 28 of the 55 patients (see Fig. 7.1). Seventeen patients who lost all their florid symptoms of schizophrenia were on propranolol alone, while the other 11 received propranolol combined with a phenothiazine drug. In 22 patients whose symptoms remitted, the pattern of improvement was gradual and progressive, but in six patients the symptoms stopped suddenly on a given day. Individuals whose symptoms remitted felt and looked well, and the response rate was roughly inversely related to the duration of the illness, but chronicity was no contraindication. Florid schizophrenic symptoms remitted in two patients whose symptoms had continued for more than 20 years. Certain practical aspects of using propranolol in schizophrenia emerged from this study, including the

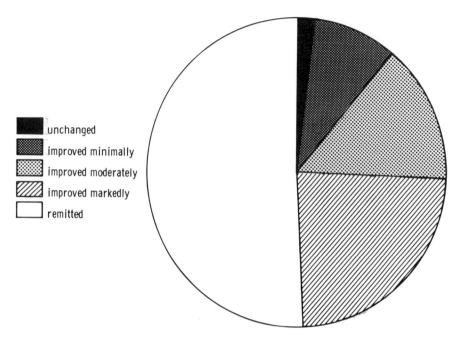

unchanged
improved minimally
improved moderately
improved markedly
remitted

FIG. 7.1. Response in 55 patients with florid symptoms of schizophrenia who were treated with propranolol alone or as an adjunct to a neuroleptic drug.

technique of increasing the dose gradually to avoid toxic effects and to find the optimal dose, which is then continued for many months in chronic cases (7,8). Toxic effects included ataxia, visual hallucinations, and confusional states. These seemed to be related to the rate of increase of the dosage of propranolol rather than to the absolute amounts given.

Atsmon and Blum (9) reviewed the uncontrolled studies of propranolol, oxprenolol, and pindolol in the treatment of patients with psychosis. Acebutolol has also been used (10). The great variations in diagnosis, drugs, dosage, and results emphasized the need for controlled studies. The remainder of this chapter is restricted to summarizing controlled studies of propranolol in patients with schizophrenia, because it is the only one of the beta-adrenoceptor blocking drugs whose effects in schizophrenia have been studied in a controlled manner. As the mechanism of action in schizophrenia is not known, the effects seen in schizophrenia may not necessarily be due to blocking beta-adrenoceptors.

CONTROLLED CLINICAL TRIALS

Four kinds of controlled study have been undertaken to show that propranolol benefits a useful proportion of patients with schizophrenia. Two of these studies have not yet been published, but we mention them to add the results of two more different approaches and to bring this review as up to date as possible.

The first study described the effects of adding propranolol to conventional neuroleptic treatment. The second reports the effects of withdrawing propranolol from a combination of propranolol and a neuroleptic. The third compares the effects of propranolol and chlorpromazine. The fourth measures some psychophysiologic effects.

Propranolol Added to Conventional Treatment

This controlled study was designed to compare the effects of adding either propranolol or a matching placebo to the treatment regimen of 14 patients with chronic schizophrenia whose florid symptoms had not remitted with conventional treatment (11,12). The mean age of these patients was 40 years. The average age of onset of the illness was 30 years, and the episode treated, which was usually the first, had continued for a mean of 9 years. The patients had been treated with major tranquillizers for almost a decade, with an average maximum dose expressed as the chlorpromazine equivalent (13) of 1,634 mg/24 hr. The mean dose on entering the study was 954 mg/24 hr, and the neuroleptic was maintained throughout the trial. The patients were randomly assigned to two groups of seven each and were given, in addition, either propranolol or placebo in a flexible dosage schedule for 12 weeks. After a test dose, propranolol or placebo was begun in a dose of 40 mg twice a day, the aim being to find the dose at which symptoms steadily improved. The dose was reviewed two or three times each week and was raised by no more than 80 mg/24 hr, provided that there were no early toxic effects and that the symptoms of schizophrenia were not improving.

The criterion for inclusion in the study was a score of at least "moderate" on two or more of the 10 "schizophrenia" scales of a modified (14) Brief Psychiatric Rating Scale (BPRS) (15). At least one of these was from the three "thought-disorder" scales, namely: conceptual disorganization, hallucinatory behavior, or unusual thought content. The seven "nonthought-disorder" schizophrenia scales were: blunted affect, emotional withdrawal, suspiciousness, grandiosity, mannerisms or posturing, hostility, and motor retardation. The sum of these 10 schizophrenia scales gave the "total schizophrenia" score. There were also nine "nonschizophrenia" scales: somatic concern, anxiety, feelings of guilt, tension, depressed mood, uncooperativeness, excitement, disorientation, and pressure of speech. At 4-week intervals, ratings were made of symptoms on this modified BPRS; in addition, global assessments of the severity of illness and clinical change were recorded. Nurses rated the patients' behavior before and at the end of the study, and the diagnosis of schizophrenia was confirmed with the Present State Examination (16).

Before treatment, the groups were closely comparable in demographic data and ratings of schizophrenia. As the trial progressed, the BPRS total schizophrenia scores for both groups improved significantly ($f = 11.35$, df $= 3.36$, $p <$

0.001), but the propranolol group improved significantly more than the placebo group (f = 3.06, df = 3.36, p < 0.04), see Fig. 7.2.

The sum of the three thought-disorder scales showed that both groups improved, but by week 12 the propranolol group had improved significantly more than the control group. A similar result was also recorded on the schizophrenia scales, but the nonschizophrenia scales showed no difference between the groups. The only one of the 19 individual items that improved significantly more in the propranolol group than in the placebo group was unusual thought content (delusions and bizarre ideas). Improvement in two other items, grandiosity and conceptual disorganization, approached significance. Global ratings of severity and of change both favored the propranolol group, while the nurses' ratings did not change in the placebo group but improved significantly in the propranolol

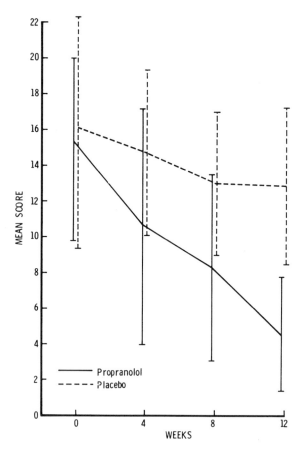

FIG. 7.2. Total schizophrenia scores (mean and SD) on a modified BPRS for two groups of patients with chronic, florid schizophrenia who had propranolol or placebo added to their neuroleptic treatment for 12 weeks.

group ($p < 0.01$). The individuals whose symptoms remitted often felt and looked well and relaxed and spoke more fluently and naturally. In most cases, schizophrenic symptoms improved slowly, both during and after the 12 week trial.

No significant toxic effects were seen, while the average dose of propranolol at the end of the present trial (500 mg/24 hr) was lower than the modal dose for remission in earlier studies (5,6). The investigation was limited to 14 patients for 12 weeks. Although the patients were few, the 12 weeks design is probably better for such a chronic illness than, for example, plans to treat 28 patients for 6 weeks or 56 patients for 3 weeks. It is noteworthy that the 12 weeks of the controlled trial itself were less than the median time for symptoms to remit in earlier studies (5,6).

Propranolol was continued openly for some months in the experimental group and was also given to five patients in the control group. Seven of the 12 patients in whom propranolol was maintained as an adjunct to their conventional treatment lost their florid schizophrenic symptoms. When followed-up by their usual psychiatrists who originally referred the patients, six of the 12 treated with propranolol were rated "as good as," and six as "better than," the best the psychiatrists had known them to be before the trial. Although the groups did not differ significantly in chronicity, the mean length of episode in the propranolol plus chlorpromazine group was 5 years 11 months, compared with 11 years 6 months in the placebo plus chlorpromazine group. (This probably occurred because the randomization procedure did not stratify for chronicity.) Whether or not this difference conferred any advantage on the propranolol group is uncertain; but it is unlikely because both groups of patients had long-standing illness, and some patients in the control group later responded to propranolol after the study.

It was concluded that propranolol contributed perceptibly to the treatment of chronic schizophrenia in patients whose illness had not responded to major tranquilizers.

Propranolol Withdrawal

Double-blind withdrawal of propranolol from patients with chronic schizophrenia who were taking both a neuroleptic and propranolol resulted in 15 of 20 cases deteriorating within 2 weeks. The relevant details of this study, which are yet to be published, are presented in abstract form as follows. Twenty patients with chronic schizophrenia, nine men and 11 women, were treated in the hospital for more than 1 year with propranolol as an adjunct to neuroleptic treatment. When a decision was made to stop propranolol, it was withdrawn at an unpredictable date over 7 days in a double-blind manner, while the neuroleptic was continued. Propranolol and placebo were dispensed so that the same number of apparently identical capsules were taken throughout three phases: full dosage, withdrawal, and placebo. The patients were in five different wards so that their influence on each other was dispersed. Obvious changes in behavior were observed and dated; if a progressive change was observed, the data from which improvement or deterioration occurred were decided before the code was broken.

The details of the 15 patients who deteriorated within 2 weeks of stopping propranolol follow. Three patients had weekend leave stopped by their relatives and also stopped going to work in the workshops. Four more also stopped the latter activity, for a cumulative total of seven. Three became physically aggressive, nine verbally aggressive, and five increasingly deluded, giving cumulative totals of nine, 13, and 15 persons, respectively, in each category. Changes in psychomotor activity were common: 10 of the 15 patients whose condition worsened became more restless, and four became more inert.

Ratings on the modified BPRS increased after withdrawal of propranolol. Four scales that showed significant worsening were: unusual thought content, suspiciousness, tension, and excitement.

Propranolol Versus Chlorpromazine

Propranolol and chlorpromazine were about equally effective in a study of 46 patients newly admitted with schizophrenia. As would be expected, no extrapyramidal reactions occurred in the propranolol group. This is a large interhospital study which has been completed but not yet published. Its essential result is recorded here for completeness.

PSYCHOPHYSIOLOGIC STUDIES

In conjunction with psychiatrists' and nurses' ratings of clinical change, objective psychophysiologic measures were obtained in patients treated with propranolol. Key psychologic deficits, long associated with schizophrenia, are disorders of selective and sustained attention (17–21). As a biologic index of attention, psychophysiologists have recorded the arousal reaction of the autonomic nervous system to a novel stimulus and the rate at which it habituates with repetition (22). This was termed the "orienting reflex" by Pavlov (23) (see also Chapter 12); it can be seen, for example, as a dog pricks up his ears at the sound of another dog barking. A reliable, noninvasive measure of this reaction in man can be obtained from changes in the electrical conductance of the skin due to increased sweating as the sympathetic nervous system is activated.

Electrodermal Orientating Responses

In previous studies of Gruzelier and Venables (24,25), schizophrenic patients on phenothiazines were found to exhibit one of at least two abnormalities in their electrodermal orienting responses. They either failed to respond (or responded only occasionally) or they tended to overreact, and their responses were slow in habituating. These abnormal forms of responding, together with the normal response, are shown schematically in Fig. 7.3. The abnormalities could not be attributed to medication, for they occurred after drug withdrawal; nor were they permanent features of the illness, for occasionally an individual patient switched from one extreme to the other (26,27).

Subsequently, we have undertaken three studies in which the effects of propranolol were evaluated on the skin conductance responses to moderate intensity tones in schizophrenic patients (28–30).

The first cross-sectional study involved four groups of subjects, 36 in each group. They comprised: (a) normal volunteers, (b) schizophrenic patients who were not on neuroleptics (either newly admitted to hospital and untreated, or chronic patients withdrawn from drug therapy), (c) schizophrenic inpatients treated with phenothiazines, and (d) schizophrenic inpatients treated with propranolol either as the sole drug or combined with phenothiazines.

The number of trials to habituation of the four groups are shown in Fig. 7.4, habituation being determined by the conventional criterion of no response to three successive stimuli. All but two of the 36 normal volunteers exhibited responses, and the majority habituated by trial six, although a small subgroup was slow in habituating and needed more than 10 trials to habituation. The patients with schizophrenia on no drug showed similar patterns of responding to those on phenothiazines: many did not react to the tones, and most of the others were slow in habituating. Group comparisons indicated that those on propranolol habituated faster than normal volunteers ($p < 0.002$) and faster than patients on other treatment ($p < 0.0001$) or no drugs ($p < 0.001$). At the same time, there were 50% fewer nonresponsive patients on propranolol than on phenothiazines or no drug. Propranolol appeared to influence both extreme forms of abnormal response: nonresponding and impaired habituation. This twofold effect occured whether propranolol was administered alone or combined with phenothiazines (Fig. 7.4).

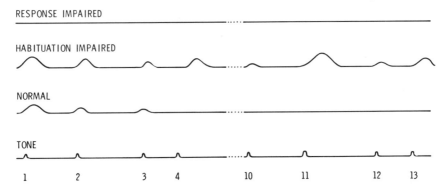

FIG. 7.3. Diagram to illustrate the normal pattern of electrodermal responses to repeated tones of moderate intensity, and two abnormal patterns: impaired response and impaired habituation.

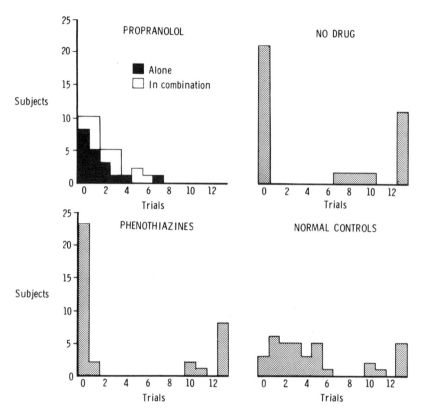

FIG. 7.4. Trials to habituation for patients on propranolol (alone or in combination with pheno-thiazines), on phenothiazines, on no drug, and for normal volunteers.

The results of the first study were confirmed in a second experiment in which patients were openly treated with either propranolol or chlorpromazine. Fourteen patients on no drugs or phenothiazines were tested before and after the addition of propranolol. They were compared with 14 patients tested either before and after phenothiazines or twice on phenothiazines. All these patients had been openly treated and had improved on BPRS ratings.

The distribution of trials to habituation was bimodal, indicating over- or underresponsiveness, except when the patients were treated with propranolol. Here responding and habituation returned to normal when propranolol was administered alone ($p < 0.0001$) but not when it was added to phenothiazines, in which case the results did not reach significance.

In the clinical trial comparing propranolol with chlorpromazine, the twofold influence of propranolol on electrodermal orienting response in schizophrenia was confirmed, this time under double-blind conditions. Twenty-seven patients newly hospitalized, who were part of the controlled comparison of propranolol and chlorpromazine as the sole drug, were examined before drug treatment and at the end of the trial 12 weeks later. Fifteen patients on propranolol and 12 on chlorpromazine had psychophysiologic examination, and all patients had their diagnosis confirmed by the Present State Examination (16). Before taking the drugs, most patients either showed no orienting responses or their responses were slow in habituation.

At the end of the trial 12 weeks later, orienting activity was categorized as (a) *improved,* if responses now occurred and habituated, or (b) *not improved,* if responding either remained the same or changed from one extreme to the other. Thus categorized, six patients improved on propranolol compared with one on chlorpromazine, while nine patients showed no improvement on propranolol compared with 11 on chlorpromazine. The influence of drug treatment favored propranolol ($p < 0.01$). Two of those who improved were nonresponders before treatment; the others were nonhabituators. A return to normal orienting activity was less frequent in this study, possibly because psychophysiologic measures may mirror therapeutic effectiveness. In the first two studies, it was necessary for patients to show a favorable clinical response to the drug before psychophysiologic testing took place. In the third study, however, retesting was determined by a time interval: the end of the trial. Here fewer patients showed a reduction in schizophrenic symptoms to the extent found in previous open (5) or controlled (11) studies. The precise relationships between the clinical and psychophysiologic changes on drug have yet to be determined.

In summary, in patients with schizophrenia on propranolol, unlike those on phenothiazines, the electrodermal orienting responses returned to normal in most who responded clinically to treatment.

Nature of the Propranolol Response

Propranolol had a powerful effect on habituation in all three studies. This might be thought to relate to its anxiolytic effects, since failure of habituation has been associated with preexamination stress in students (31), as well as with morbid anxiety (32). Should the anxiolytic explanation be sufficient, the influences of propranolol on the centrally mediated orienting reaction suggest that it may involve psychic components of anxiety in addition to somatic components with which its action has been associated in the past (33), as discussed in the preceding chapter.

A purely anxiolytic explanation does not explain the reinstatement of orienting responses in nonresponsive patients. This finding, coupled with the action of propranolol on habituation, indicates that propranolol influences two extreme modes of responding. An alternative explanation is that propranolol influences a sensory gating mechanism, which normally has a twofold function. It determines whether or not the orienting reaction occurs at all, and whether the orienting reaction recurs when the stimulus is repeated. Such a mechanism has been proposed to underlie the process of selective attention and has been attributed to subcortical limbic functions (22,34). In this regard, it is noteworthy that in animals, *dl*-propranolol is concentrated in the limbic brain areas, particularly in the hippocampus (35) (see Chapter 6).

A central action of propranolol is also implied by further evidence from our investigations. Neither the background levels of sweating nor the nonspecific fluctuations in the electrodermal tracing were influenced by propranolol (36). If the influences of propranolol on orienting activity were due to peripheral autonomic effects, one would expect corresponding changes in background levels of sweating and nonspecific responses. Furthermore, *d*-propranolol, which has minimal if any effects on peripheral adrenoceptors, has effects similar to those

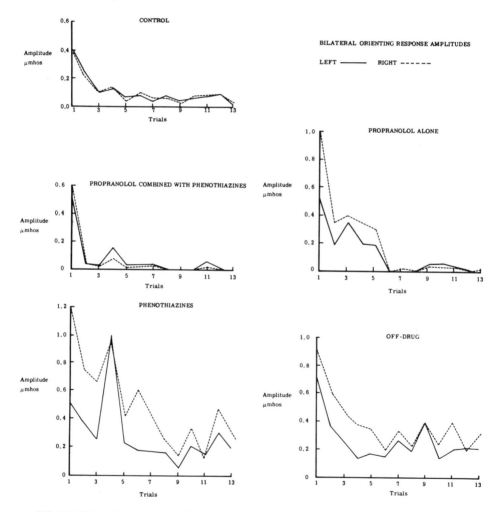

FIG. 7.5. Bilateral response amplitudes of patients on no drug, phenothiazines, or propranolol, showing higher right-hand responses, whereas normal volunteers and patients on propranolol combined with phenothiazines showed no lateral differences.

of racemic propranolol on the habituation of electrodermal orienting responses
(37).

In all three studies, electrodermal activity was recorded bilaterally to examine
hemisphere influences on orienting responses. A growing body of evidence impli-
cates lateralized dysfunction in schizophrenia, involving the hemisphere dominant for speech (38). Lesion studies suggest ipsilateral mediation of electrodermal
orienting responses to simple stimuli (39–41), so that a left-sided lesion results
in reduced electrodermal responding from the left hand and increased responding
on the right hand. Asymmetries in skin conductance responses to moderate
intensity tones, consistent with a left-sided dysfunction model, were found in
hospitalized schizophrenic patients, expecially those with a chronic illness

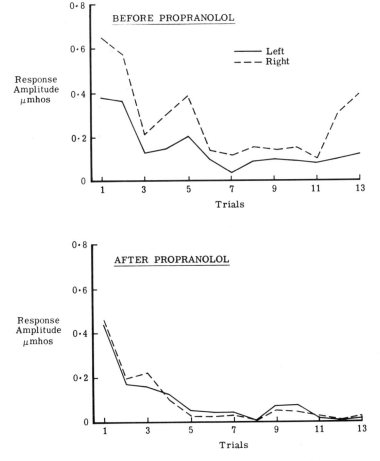

FIG. 7.6. Lateral differences in response amplitudes before propranolol, and no asymmetries
after the addition of propranolol.

(25,42,43). In the untreated and phenothiazine-treated patients, responses on the left hand were smaller than those on the right (Fig. 7.5). Normal volunteers had no asymmetries consistently in one direction. Propranolol administered alone usually did not influence asymmetries, but when combined with phenothiazines, the asymmetrical pattern, right higher than left, was no longer in evidence. Patients on the combined medication (propranolol and a phenothiazine drug) more closely resembled the control group (Fig. 7.5). This result was replicated in the second experiment (28). The asymmetries evident before administering propranolol were absent after propranolol treatment ($p < 0.03$) (Fig. 7.6).

The psychophysiologic results show differential effects of propranolol and phenothiazines on central attentional processes. The action of a drug on basic attentional mechanisms, including habituation, implies that propranolol may have a wide range of applications in psychiatry. That abnormal patterns of psychophysiologic responses were corrected by a combination of propranolol and a phenothiazine drug in a way in which neither drug alone could do, accords with clinical experience the value of the combination (5,6,11,12) and raises the question of the place for combined medication in the treatment of schizophrenia.

CONCLUSIONS

Adding propranolol to the treatment of patients with chronic schizophrenia, whose florid symptoms had not remitted with conventional neuroleptics, gave significantly more improvement than adding a placebo.

Double-blind withdrawal of propranolol from patients with chronic schizophrenia, who were taking both a neuroleptic and propranolol, resulted in 15 of 20 cases deteriorating within 2 weeks.

Propranolol and chlorpromazine were about equally effective in a study of 46 newly admitted inpatients with schizophrenia.

In psychophysiologic studies, propranolol often corrected the abnormal patterns of the orienting reflex found in schizophrenia. Combining propranolol with a phenothiazine drug corrected the imbalance between the left and right sides, unlike the effects of either treatment alone.

These four kinds of controlled study showed that propranolol benefits some patients with schizophrenia.

ACKNOWLEDGMENTS

We thank Ms. M. Johnstone for her organizing skills; Ms. E. Ames for her help with references; I.C.I. Pharmaceuticals Division, The Sir Jules Thorn Medical Research Endowment Trust, and The Scottish Rite Schizophrenia Research Programme, Massachusetts, for grants toward this research.

REFERENCES

1. Atsmon, A., and Blum, I. Treatment of acute porphyria variegata with propranolol. *Lancet,* 1970, i, 196–197.
2. Atsmon, A., Blum, I., and Fischl, J. Treatment of an acute attack of porphyria variegata with propranolol. *S. Afr. Med. J.,* 1972, 46, 311–314.
3. Atsmon, A., and Blum, I. The discovery. In: *Propranolol and Schizophrenia,* edited by E. Roberts and P. Amacher, pp. 5–38. Alan R. Liss, New York, 1978.
4. Atsmon, A. *Personal communication,* 1973.
5. Yorkston, N. J., Zaki, S. A., Themen, J. F. A., and Havard, C. W. H. Propranolol to control schizophrenic symptoms: 55 patients. *Adv. Clin. Pharmacol.,* 1976, 12, 91–104.
6. Yorkston, N. J., Zaki, S. A., and Harvard, C. W. H. Propranolol in the treatment of schizophrenia: An uncontrolled study with 55 adults. In: *Propranolol and Schizophrenia,* edited by E. Roberts and P. Amacher, pp. 39–67. Alan R. Liss, New York, 1978.
7. Yorkston, N. J., Zaki, S. A., Themen, J. F. A., and Havard, C. W. H. Safeguards in the treatment of schizophrenia with propranolol. *Postgrad. Med. J. [Suppl. 4],* 1976, 52, 175–180.
8. Yorkston, N. J., Zaki, S. A., and Havard, C. W. H. Some practical aspects of using propranolol in the treatment of schizophrenia. In: *Propranolol and Schizophrenia,* edited by E. Roberts and P. Amacher, pp. 83–97. Alan R. Liss, New York, 1978.
9. Atsmon, A., and Blum, I. Beta-adrenergic blocking drugs in psychiatry: Present status, future approaches and research. *L'Encephale,* 1978, iv, 1973–186.
10. Daskalopoulos, N. Th., Cottereau, M. J., and Deniker, P. A double-blind crossover trial: Acebutolol versus placebo in schizophrenic patients. Abstracts 11th Collegium Inter Neuro-Psychopharmacol. Congress, Vienna, p. 225, July 9–14, 1978.
11. Yorkston, N. J., Gruzelier, J. H., Zaki, S. A., Hollander, D., Pitcher, D. R., and Sergeant, H. G. S. Propranolol as an adjunct to the treatment of schizophrenia. *Lancet,* 1977, ii, 575–78.
12. Yorkston, N. J., Gruzelier, J. H., Zaki, S. A., Hollander, D., Pitcher, D. R., and Sergeant, H. G. S. Propranolol as an adjunct to the treatment of schizophrenia. In: *Propranolol and Schizophrenia,* edited by E. Roberts and P. Amacher, pp. 69–82. Alan R. Liss, New York, 1978.
13. Davis, J. M. Dose equivalent of the antipsychotic drugs. *J. Psychiatr. Res.* 1976, 11, 65–69.
14. Yorkston, N. J., Zaki, S. A., Malik, M. K. U., Morrison, R. C., and Havard, C. W. H. Propranolol in the control of schizophrenic symptoms. *Br. Med. J.,* 1974, 4, 633–635.
15. Overall, J. E., and Gorham, D. R. The brief psychiatric rating scale. *Psychol. Rep.,* 1962, 10, 799–812.
16. Wing, J. K., Cooper, J. E., and Sartorius, N. *The Measurement and Classification of Psychiatric Symptoms.* Cambridge University Press, London, 1974.
17. Bleuler, E. *Dementia Praecox or the Group of Schizophrenias. (1911).* International Universities Press, New York, 1950.
18. Kraepelin, E. *Dementia Praecox and Paraphrenia. (1919).* Livingstone, New York, 1977.
19. Shakow, D. Some psychological features of schizophrenia. (1950). In: *Schizophrenia: Selected Papers, Psychological Issues,* International Universities Press, New York, 1977.
20. McGhie, A. *Pathology of Attention.* Penguin Books, Harmondsworth, 1969.
21. Matthysse, S. Spring, B. J., and Sugerman, J., Attention and information processing in schizophrenia. *J. Psychiatr, Res.,* 1978, 14, 1–331.
22. Pribram, K. H., and McGuiness, D. Arousal, activation and effort in the control of attention. *Psychol. Rev.,* 1975, 82, 116–149.
23. Pavlov, I. P. *Conditioned Reflexes and Psychiatry.* International Publishers, New York, 1941.
24. Gruzelier, J. H., and Venables, P. H. Skin conductance orienting activity in a heterogeneous sample of schizophrenics: Possible evidence of limbic dysfunction. *J. Nerv. Ment. Dis.,* 1972, 155, 277–287.
25. Gruzelier, J. H., and Venables, P. H. Biomodality and lateral asymmetry of skin conductance orienting activity in schizophrenics: Replication and evidence of lateral asymmetry in patients with depression and disorders of personality. *Biol. Psychiatry,* 1974, 8, 55–73.
26. Gruzelier, J. H., and Hammond, N. V. Schizophernia: A dominant hemisphere temporal-limbic disorder? *Res. Commun. Psychol. Psychiatr. Behav.,* 1976, 1, 33–72.

27. Rubens, R. L., and Lapidus, L. B. Schizophrenic patterns of arousal and stimulus barrier functioning. *J. Abnorm. Psychol.,* 1978, 87, 199–211.
28. Gruzelier, J. H., and Yorkston, N. J. Propranolol and schizophrenia: Objective evidence of efficacy. In: *Biological Basis of Schizophrenia,* edited by W. Hemmings and G. Hemmings. MTP Press, Lancaster, 1978.
29. Gruzelier, J. H. Propranolol acts to modulate autonomic orienting and habituation processes in schizophrenia. In: *Propranolol and Schizophrenia,* edited by E. Roberts and P. Amacher, pp. 99–118. Alan R. Liss, New York, 1978.
30. Gruzelier, J. H. Bimodal states of arousal and lateralised dysfunction in schizophrenia: The effect of chlorpromazine. In: *Nature of Schizophrenia. New Approaches to Research and Treatment,* edited by L. Wynne, R. Cromwell, and S. Mattysse, pp. 167–187. Wiley, 1978.
31. Maltzman, I., Smith, M. J., Kantor, W., and Mandell, M. P. Effects of stress on habituation of the orienting reflex. *J. Exp. Psychol.,* 1971, 87, 207–214.
32. Lader, M. H., and Wing, L., Physiological measures, sedative drugs and morbid anxiety. In: *Institute of Psychiatry, Maudsley Monographs 14.* Oxford University Press, London, 1966.
33. Tyrer, P. J. Role of bodily feelings in anxiety. In: *Institute of Psychiatry, Maudsley Monographs 23.* Oxford University Press, London, 1976.
34. Pribram, K. H. The limbic system, efferent control of neural inhibition and behaviour. *Prog. Brain Res.,* 1967, 27, 318.
35. Masuoka, D., and Hansson, E. Autoradiographic distribution studies of adrenergic blocking agents. II. ^{14}C-propranolol, a beta-receptor-type blocker. *Acta Pharmacol. Toxicol.,* 1967, 25, 447–455.
36. Gruzelier, J. H., and Connelly, J. F. Differential actions of a pharmacological agent on electrodermal orienting responses as distinct from non-specific responses and electrodermal levels. In: *The Orienting Reflex in Humans,* edited by H. D. Kimmel, C. H. van Olst, and J. F. Orlebke. *(In press.)*
37. Gruzelier, J. H., Hirsch, S. R. Weller, M., and Murphy, C. The influence of d- or dl-propranolol and chlorpromazine on habituation of phasic electrodermal responses in schizophrenia. *Acta Psychiatr. Scand. (In press.)*
38. Gruzelier, J. H., and Flor-Henry, P. (eds.) *Hemisphere Asymmetries of Function in Psychopathology.* Elsevier, Amsterdam, 1980.
39. Schwartz, H. G. Effect of experimental lesions of the cortex on the "psychogalvanic reflex" in the cat. *Arch. Neurol. Psychiatry,* 1937, 38, 308–320.
40. Luria, A., and Homskaya, E. D. Frontal lobe and the regulation of arousal processes. In: *Attention: Contemporary Theory and Research,* edited by D. Mostofsky, pp. 303–330. Appleton-Century-Crofts, New York, 1970.
41. Sourek, K. *The Nervous Control of Skin Potential in Man.* Nakladetelstvi Ceskoslovenska Akademie Ved, Praha, 1965.
42. Gruzelier, J. H., and Venables, P. H. Bilateral asymmetry of skin conductance orienting activity and levels of schizophrenia. *J. Biol. Psychol.,* 1973, 1, 21–41.
43. Gruzelier, J. H., and Hammond, N. V. The effect of chlorpromazine upon bilateral asymmetries of bioelectrical skin reactivity in schizophrenia. *Stud. Psychol.,* 1977, 19, 40–50.

Prologue: Psychotropic Drugs and the Heart

In every Eden there lurks a snake, and nowhere is this truer than in the drug treatment of illness. The "perfect" drug, the outstanding therapeutic effect accompanied by no ill effects on the organism as a whole, does not exist. Nor is there any correlation between the degree of therapeutic effect and the severity of unwanted or side effects. Therefore, the most successful drugs are those that combine maximal clinical effectiveness with minimal side effects. Probably the outstanding example of such compounds are to be found in the range of antibiotics that are available to the practicing physician. At the other end of the scale are drugs whose effectiveness may be poorly defined or those that may carry with them the risk of serious toxic reactions. The latter type of drug may be found in systemic corticosteroids used in conditions other than those due to adrenal insufficiency, and antirheumatic compounds, such as phenylbutazone, which may carry the risk of serious blood dyscrasias. It is a matter of fine clinical judgment to determine when to use such compounds and to select the most appropriate type of case.

Many of the drugs in normal clinical use fall between these two extreme categories. With the accumulation of knowledge concerning their pharmacology within the body, the clinician is able, in most cases, to arrive at the correct decision concerning their use. It is a sobering fact, however, that no matter how careful the experimental and clinical pharmacology may be before a new drug is introduced for general use, serious toxic effects may not be recognized until that drug has been in use for some time. The recognition of serious toxic effects with practolol, after it had been in use for many years, is a particularly pertinent example.

Although the phenothiazine antipsychotic drugs can produce changes in the electrocardiogram (EKG), these would not appear to be of any practical importance and constitute no bar to their continued usage for the appropriate indications (1). The benzodiazepine antianxiety drugs have also become firmly established over a similar period of time and would not appear to exercise any harmful effects on the cardiovascular system but rather, as we have seen in previous chapters, may be of benefit in coronary heart disease (see Chapter 4) and hypertension (see Chapter 15). However, in the case of the tricyclic antidepressant drugs, cardiotoxicity is now recognized as constituting a potentially dangerous side effect, particularly when used in the elderly or in patients with underlying cardiovascular disorders. Although the tricyclics in normal dosage do not have any adverse effects in patients with normal cardiovascular systems, there is always the problem of overdosage, either deliberate or accidental, which may result in death due to cardiac depression.

In a recent review of the problem, Crome and Newman (2) examined all death certificates issued in 1976 in the United Kingdom where antidepressants were mentioned as the sole or a contributory factor in the patient's death. There were 345 deaths due to tricyclic antidepressants as the sole or contributory cause (11.6% of the total 2,984 deaths due to solid and liquid poisoning); 42.6% of these patients were aged between 40 and 59 years, women outnumbering men in the ratio of 1.6:1. This section of this edition is mainly concerned with the problem of cardiotoxicity in relation to antidepressants and the advantages of the newer antidepressant drugs in this respect.

Seldom can an animal model be produced that convincingly mimics the clinical situation in man. In the first chapter of this section, Davidson describes fascinating and highly credible animal experiments which he has devised to investigate the association between tricyclic antidepressants and stress in relation to their effects on the cardiovascular system. This work is particularly important because it provides a satisfactory parallel to the clinical situation, particularly as it may affect elderly patients under treatment with tricyclic antidepressants. Such patients may suffer additionally from various degrees and types of cardiovascular insufficiency and so present a particular therapeutic hazard. In the first section of this book, the role of the beta-adrenergic blocking drugs in the prevention of cardiovascular responses to emotional and physical stresses was outlined. It is of particular interest that Davidson found that these drugs also block the cardiotoxic effects of the combination of tricyclics and stress. Clearly, this group of drugs is of considerable interest to all those who are concerned with the treatment of psychiatric conditions that may have associations with circulatory disease.

From this specific example of the interactions between stress, cardiac disease, and tricyclic antidepressants, this section surveys the considerable experimental background, both in animals and humans, which provides precise information on the etiology of tricyclic cardiotoxicity. This chapter is a joint contribution from Leeds (Hughes) and Australia (Burrows and Norman). A major part of the original work in these fields has been undertaken by the authors of this chapter. The text provides an invaluable guide to understanding the mechanisms underlying the effects which tricyclic antidepressants exert on the cardiovascular system.

From the experimental background, the discourse proceeds to the clinical implications in the next chapter written by Burgess and Turner. This chapter comprehensively surveys the clinical situation in relation to the cardiotoxic effects of antidepressant drugs and the management of tricyclic overdosage in this context. From the point of view of the normal therapeutic use of antidepressant drugs, the observations of these authors concerning the safety of the newer nontricyclic compounds are of particular relevance to all clinicians employing drugs to relieve depression.

In the final chapter of this section, Kopera describes his studies with one of these newer antidepressants, namely, mianserin, not only in human volunteers but also in patients suffering from a variety of cardiac disorders and in depressed patients without such underlying abnormalities. It is apparent from these studies that this new antidepressant produces either no effect at all or minimal changes only on the cardiovascular system.

In view of their proven potential cardiotoxicity, there may well be a strong case in the future to discontinue using the tricyclic group of drugs in favor of the newer compounds now available. Of these, there is no doubt that mianserin has been the most extensively researched. As Crome and Newman, reporting from the National Poisons Information Service (U.K.), comment (3): "it [antidepressant medication] is also a significant clinical problem with a substantial proportion of both adults and children developing serious symptoms such as coma, convulsions, and myocardial depression." On the other hand, Crome and Chand (4) have also studied 42 patients suffering from nomifensine overdosage, reported from the introduction of the drug in 1977 to the end of September 1979. There were no reports of convulsions, cardiac arrhythmias, or other EKG abnormalities. These authors commented that this suggests that nomifensine is less toxic than conventional tricyclic antidepressants. These authors undertook a similar survey of cases of mianserin poisoning reported to the center from the introduction of the drug in the United Kingdom in May 1976 (5). Data were available on 100 such cases, and the authors commented: "Even at levels ten times the accepted therapeutic level, there are no convulsions, cardiac arrhythmias and respiratory depression, complications which are associated with the severe poisoning of tricyclic antidepressants."

REFERENCES

1. Holden, M., and Itil, T. Electrocardiographic changes with psychotropic drugs. In: *Stress and the Heart,* first edition, edited by D. Wheatley, p. 87. Raven Press, New York, 1977.
2. Crome, P., and Newman, B. Fatal tricyclic antidepressant poisoning. *J. R. Soc. Med.,* 1979, 72, 649.
3. Crome, P., and Newman, B. The problem of tricyclic antidepressant poisoning. *Postgrad. Med. J.,* 1979, 55, 528.
4. Crome, P., and Chand, S. *The Clinical Toxicology of Nomifensine: Comparison with Tricyclic Antidepressants,* 1980, Royal Society of Medicine. International Congress and Symposium Series, No. 25, p. 55.
5. Chand, S., Crome, P., and Dawling, S. *Mianserin Poisoning in 100 Patients. Neuropsy. Psychopharm.,* 1981, *(in press)*.

Stress and the Heart, edited by D. Wheatley,
Raven Press, New York © 1981.

Psychotropic Drugs, Stress, and Cardiomyopathies

William J. Davidson

Amitriptyline, imipramine, and other tricyclic compounds are currently the drugs used most commonly and most effectively in the treatment of depression (1,2). Nevertheless, attempted suicide and accidental overdose with these drugs are reported frequently in both adults and children (3,4). Such overdosage can produce multiple complications, and fatalities are usually due to cardiovascular effects, such as cardiac arrhythmias and conduction defects. A number of scientists have observed that hypertension followed by hypotension commonly occurs (5–9). These effects are fully reviewed in the next chapter.

Kristiansen (10) found that electrocardiographic (EKG) changes occurred in 16 of 85 patients suffering from endogenous depression who were being treated with imipramine. These EKGs were taken weekly during treatment, and the abnormal changes occurred during treatment, as compared to both the initial and final tracings taken after treatment had been withdrawn. This author also reported two cases of coronary thrombosis occurring during imipramine therapy, in 66- and 67-year-old patients, respectively. Kristiansen concluded:

> From a clinical viewpoint it is important that imipramine affects the heart both directly and indirectly. The effects are slight in healthy persons who are not submitted to circulatory stress, but in cases where there is hypertension or cardiac insufficiency and perhaps also in cases where the patient has to carry out strenuous work even if he is healthy, there appears to be an increased risk of myocardiac disease.

Accordingly, I tested the cardiotoxicity of amitriptyline and imipramine in normal rats, in rats with naturally occurring cardiac myopathies, and in rats with experimentally induced cardiomyopathies. We also investigated the effects of stress of a psychogenic nature, by means of a sudden unexpected noise test (q.v.).

MATERIALS AND METHODS

Mature male rats of the Long-Evans hooded strain were used in this study. Initial ages of animals were matched as closely as possible, and all rats were weighed every third day until the study was completed. As described by Siegel and Stuckley (11), Richter (12), and ter Haar (13), animals were weighed at the same time every day, between 9 and 10 a.m. to minimize fluctuations in body weight due to circadian rhythms of food and fluid intake.

Spontaneous cardiomyopathies occurred in a number of species. Weber et al. (14) described them in the baboon. Saunders (15), Webb (16), and Caufield and Shelton (17) in the guinea pig, and Selye (18) and Boorman et al. (19) in the rat. These cardiomyopathies were detected at autopsy. The incidence varied from species to species, between strains within a species, and in relation to the predominantly affected sex. The cause or pathogenesis of these cardiomyopathies was unknown, but the incidence had a tendency to increase with age. There is an obvious danger of confusing spontaneous cardiomyopathies with experimentally induced changes. However, a search of the cardiovascular literature clearly showed that most investigators rarely selected experimental animals with regard for age or the possibility of preexisting cardiac disease.

Approximately 7% of mature male rats in our colony show EKG abnormalities, such as elevated S-T segment, conduction defects, and arrhythmias (Davidson, *unpublished data*). To minimize chances of including animals with preexisting cardiac damage, only animals with normal EKGs (determined twice, 7 days apart) were classified as normal in our studies. EKGs were recorded via sterile hypodermic needle electrodes while animals were anesthetized by ether. No atropine or other preanesthetic medication was given, while tracheal and bronchial secretions were kept minimal by a slow induction of anesthesia. Heering (20) studied and discussed fully the problems of interpreting EKGs in the rat. We now have records from 6,000 rats of different ages and sex, obtained over a number of years from animals of the same strain. Basically, we have made a quality control chart of the standard EKG parameters in our strain of rat, as exemplified by the P-R interval; besides gross abnormalities, we can quickly assess if any rat falls outside the normal EKG standards. We are aware that in animals or man, normal EKGs can be obtained when cardiac damage is present, as described by Short and Stowers (21) and Maroko (22).

Rats were housed, one per standard cage, in a well-ventilated room kept at 23°C, on a controlled light-dark cycle, with illumination from 7 a.m. to 7 p.m. daily. All rats were supplied with normal rat food and water *ad libitum*. At the time of the first EKG screening, all animals in our colony are numbered by means of an earpunch system, so that each one is easily and permanently identified.

PRODUCTION OF EXPERIMENTAL CARDIAC MYOPATHIES

Isoprenaline- (Isoproterenol) Induced Cardiac Myopathies

Animals were given a single intraperitoneal injection of *dl*-isoprenaline hydrochloride (250 mg/kg of base). In the colony of rats used, this dose regimen reliably produces necrotic lesions of the myocardium in all (100%) male animals. Since endogenous catecholamines may play a role in the development of ischemic heart disease in man, catecholamine-induced cardiac myopathies produced in various species have been studied as a model of factors that may be important in the genesis of human myocardial disease (23–28).

Cobalt-Induced Cardiac Myopathies

Animals were given equal doses of cobalt chloride (20 mg/kg of the salt) by intraperitoneal injections on each of two successive days (total, 40 mg/kg/ animal). This dose regimen in the colony of rats used reliably produces cardiac myopathies in all (100%) male animals. The cardiac toxicity of cobalt was first reported by medical authorities who found that an unusual incidence of a previously unreported type of cardiac myopathy, characterized by sudden onset and a peculiar degeneration of the myocardium, had been produced by cobalt found in a local beer in Quebec (29,30). Since this report, several researchers have been investigating the pathogenesis of cobalt cardiomyopathies (31,32), while we have been investigating the use of cobalt-induced cardiac myopathies as a model for the study of antiarrhythmic agents.

Left Ventricular Hypertrophy

The animal was anesthetized with ether and, using standard aseptic operative techniques, a midline abdominal incision was made and the abdominal aorta exposed. A coarctation of the aorta was produced by placing a silk ligature around the abdominal aorta below the origin of the renal arteries. To ensure a uniform degree of constriction in all animals, the aorta was tightly ligated to a solid stainless steel rod (external diameter, 0.5 mm). On withdrawal of the rod from the ligature, an aortic constriction remained that was equal to the external diameter of the rod. After closure of the abdomen, animals were allowed to recover, sutures being removed on the fifth postoperative day.

This method of producing left ventricular hypertrophy is essentially that reported by Wachtlova et al. (33), Rogo-Ortega and Genest (34), Anversa et al. (35), Sybulski et al. (36), and Gamble et al. (37).

OTHER EXPERIMENTAL PROCEDURES

Noise Stress Test

Our stress test is produced by firing specially loaded blank cartridges giving a sound level of 200 dynes/cm^2 at a distance of 1 m (reproducible within 1%) (Fig. 8.1).

Injection Schedules

Animals were injected at 9 a.m. and 4 p.m. We chose to divide the daily dosage of drugs so that we might achieve smoother and maintained blood levels.

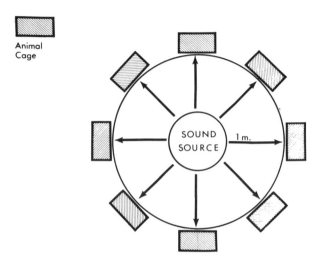

FIG. 8–1. Noise stress test.

The dosage regimen of amitryptyline and imipramine was the highest doses that we could use chronically without causing the animals to lose weight consistently. Fortuitously, the doses on a per kilogram basis approximate the clinical doses of these drugs. We adjusted the dosage of other drugs accordingly to approximate the clinically used dosage.

The total daily dosage of drugs given was: amitriptyline hydrochloride, 2 mg/kg; chlorpromazine, 6 mg/kg; diazepam, 0.6 mg/kg; imipramine hydrochloride, 2.4 mg/kg; sodium pentobarbital, 10 mg/kg; piperacetazine, 2 mg/kg; and propranolol, 2 mg/kg. All drugs were dissolved in physiologic saline, with the exception of diazepam, which was dissolved in 40% propylene glycol. Appropriate controls were injected with equivolumes of vehicle on the same time regimen. All injections were given intraperitoneally.

Histologic Techniques

After the animals were killed, the thorax was quickly opened, and the heart, severed at the conus from its attachments, was removed from the thorax and washed with physiologic saline. The heart was then weighed, and 10% formol saline was infused into the ventricles by way of the aorta and pulmonary vessels. After 48 hr fixation, the heart was cut into a series of parallel sections from the posterior auriculoventricular (A-V) sulcus to the apex. The resulting five cross sections were then placed in a coded Tissue-Tek capsule, processed in a Tissuematon, and embedded in paraffin blocks. Four slides were made from each tissue block (three sections per slide, cut at 6 μm). One slide was stained in hematoxylin-eosin and one with Milligan's trichrome stain.

With our two standard techniques, we can clearly determine the extent of fibrosis, myocytolysis, granulation of sarcoplasm, pyknosis, karolysis, and karyorrhexis in all myocardial areas. In addition, we can assess interstitial edema, focal hemorrhages, and collections of inflammatory cells.

EKG CHANGES

We had previously noted that in rats where we had produced experimental cardiomyopathies, some animals would die during the first 48 hr after insult. After this time period, there were no further deaths in surviving animals receiving no other treatment.

EKGs of animals insulted by aortic coarctation, cobalt, and isoprenaline were recorded 2 weeks postinsult. EKG changes were determined by comparison of recordings before and after insult. These changes varied from animal to animal but were usually: insult + aortic coarctation, inverted T-waves, and increased QRS voltages; insult + cobalt, marked elevation of S-T segments or conduction defects, usually 2:1 block; and insult + isoprenaline, inverted P-waves, elevated S-T segments, and in some animals very low QRS voltages with a wide QRS complex.

EKGs from a normal male rat and animals with spontaneous cardiac myopathies are shown in Fig. 8.2.

Male rats weighing approximately 250 g were divided into four main experi-

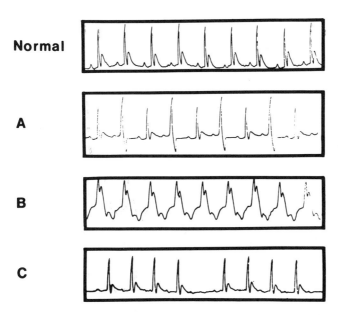

FIG. 8-2. Spontaneous cardiac myopathies: different types of EKG changes **(A, B, C)** as compared to normal tracing in rats.

mental groups. Each of these four groups was then further subdivided into five subgroups (10 animals per subgroup), according to the cardiac damage which might be present. The following were the designations of these subgroups in relation to cardiac damage: (a) none, (b) spontaneous cardiomyopathies, (c) isoprenaline cardiomyopathies, (d) cobalt cardiomyopathies, and (e) aortic coarctation cardiomyopathies. All animals in groups with experimentally induced cardiomyopathies had received their cardiac insult 21 days before the start of any other treatment. The four main groups were differentiated in relation to the nature of treatment as: (a) none, (b) vehicle alone, (c) amitriptyline, and (d) imipramine. Treatment was carried on for a period of 8 weeks.

HISTOPATHOLOGY

All animals were killed by an overdose of ether. The hearts were removed, visually examined for gross cardiac damage, and prepared for histologic evaluation. Hearts from noninsulted animals showed small traces of myocytolysis and fibrotic tissue which, as far as we could determine, were endogenous. Treatment with tricyclic antidepressants did not significantly increase these areas, and the hearts were used to establish baseline values for endogenous fibrotic tissue and myocytolysis.

Spontaneous Cardiomyopathies

Although the hearts from a few of these animals showed small focal hemorrhagic areas, we did not find any evidence of gross cardiac damage. Treatment with tricyclic antidepressants did not significantly change the histopathologic findings.

Isoprenaline Cardiomyopathies

The presence of invasive fibrotic hyperplasia in the myocardial wall was the most distinctive pathology found after isoprenaline insult. Fibrotic areas consisted of wavy bundles of collagen fibers which interdigitated with myocardial fibers undergoing varying stages of degeneration. Fibrosis was observed most often in the apex of the left ventricular subendocardial and endocardial regions, but the peripheral muscle fibers of the epicardium in the left apical region were seldom replaced by fibrotic tissue. Leukocytic invasions of polymorphonuclears occurred in areas showing muscle degeneration. Muscle fibers which lost their striations exhibited a granular mass that blended into a hyaline-clear zone before joining a tightly woven collagen fiber bundle. Fibrotic lesions occurred frequently in epicardial, subendocardial, and endocardial regions of the ventral wall of the left ventricle but infrequently on either the posterior wall of the left ventricle or the walls of both atria. In about half the animals examined, the interventricular septum and right ventricular wall had fibrotic lesions of varying size. The presence of healthy cardiac muscle fibers interdigitating with fibrotic lesions was noted as occurring in all isoprenaline-insulted animals.

Degeneration of contractile muscle protein, as evidenced by myocytolysis, was widespread in the myocardium. Lysis of cross-striations was focal within a single cardiac cell and was characterized by granulation sarcoplasm. Some cardiac cells showed an intracellular linear spread of myocytolysis in which the central core area was enlarged by an intrusion of clear fluid. Hemorrhagic lesions were intracellular and of small diameter and did not appear to contribute to any appreciable edema, but some evidence of cardiac cell fragmentation was present in the myocardium of the left ventricle.

Treatment with the tricyclic antidepressants did not significantly change the histopathologic findings.

Cobalt Cardiomyopathies

Cardiomyopathies induced by cobalt insult did not show fibrotic lesions. The main histologic finding was myocytolysis, in which cross-striations of cardiac cells were lost and replaced by granular cytoplasm. The lysis was focal within a cell and did not extend beyond 30 μm in the initial stage but extended up to several hundred microns in length during secondary stages. Nuclei of cardiac cells showing myocytolysis were generally unaffected histologically. Parallel histologic changes included interstitial edema of the myocardium in left and right ventricles, the interstitial spaces becoming enlarged and edematous and exhibiting fibrin network in laceform. Edematous areas were generally widespread within the epicardial and subendocardial regions.

Of equal importance as a diagnostic histologic feature of cobalt insult is the widespread occurrence of fragmentation of cardiac cells. Several microscopic tests were conducted to differentiate histologic artifact from this type of histopathology. Fragmented cells appeared irregularly sheared across the transverse plane, but signs of necrotic lesions accompanying fragmented areas were absent. This may be due to the multinucleated character of cardiac cells, in which the fragmented cell isolate also contains a nucleus. Hemorrhagic lesions were generally widespread throughout the myocardial wall and could be seen on gross examination as a distinct dark coloration on the epicardial surface.

Treatment with tricyclic antidepressants did not significantly change the histopathologic findings.

Aortic Coarctation—Left Ventricular Hypertrophy

Animals insulted by aortic coarctation did not develop myocardial fibrotic lesions. Aortic coarctation, however, as a model for the hypertensive damaged heart, resulted in several histologic changes; myocytolysis, cardiac cell fragmentation, hemorrhagic lesions, and small anomalous projections of the cell membrane of cardiac cells.

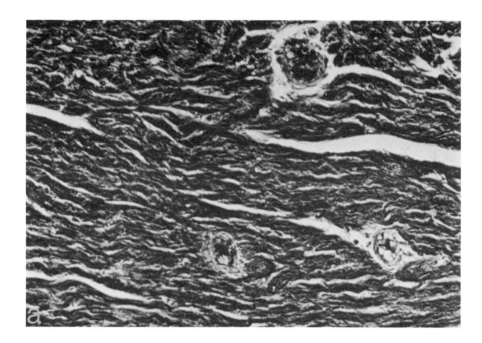

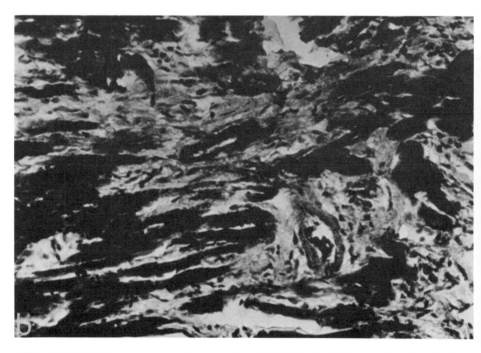

FIG. 8–3. Histologic appearance of myocardium. **(a)** No insult; **(b)** isoprenaline; **(c)** cobalt; **(d)** aortic coarctation. (×490. Stained with Milligan's trichrome.)

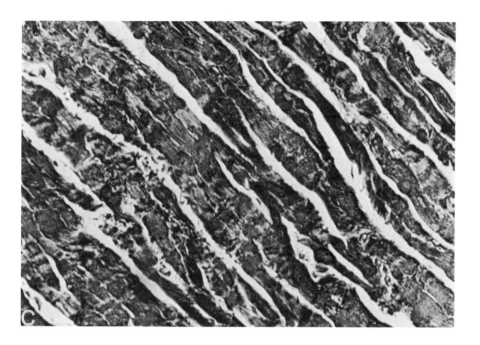

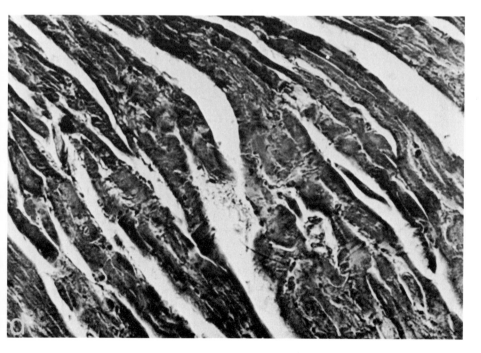

FIG. 8–3. (cont.)

Fragmentation of myocardial cells was most severe and widespread in animals insulted by aortic stenosis, when compared to the other insults in this study, muscle fibers being transversely sheared and separated. Hemorrhagic areas were scattered and irregular in size throughout the subendocardial regions of the heart.

Treatment with tricyclic antidepressants did not significantly change the histopathologic findings.

Typical appearance of the cardiac damage is shown in Fig. 8.3.

THE STRESS FACTOR

We were surprised that no deaths occurred in animals with cardiomyopathies and treated with tricyclic antidepressants. One major difference between our experimental animals and patients receiving antidepressant agents was stress. Depressed patients suffer emotional stress; indeed, stress (e.g., grief, financial worry) may be the precipitating factor in a depression.

Since similar emotional stress could not be produced in our experimental animals, we decided that we would expose them instead to a quantitative reproducible stress. Noise has recently been recognized as an environmental hazard producing alterations of the endocrine and cardiovascular systems (38). We had previously found that approximately 2% of rats with cardiomyopathies died immediately of ventricular fibrillation when exposed to a sudden noise stress of 200 dynes/cm².

We repeated the first experiment with the same number of animals in each group. The difference between the first and second experiment was that we treated the rats with tricyclic antidepressants for only 3 weeks before we exposed them to the noise stress. The animals with spontaneous cardiomyopathies were detected during our EKG screen, and the type and numbers of abnormalities occurring were outside our control.

The results of this experiment are shown in Table 8.1. The noise stress caused no deaths in normal rats given tricyclic antidepressants, and the incidence of deaths in rats with cardiomyopathies of various kinds was 2 to 6% among

TABLE 8-1. *Percent deaths on noise stress (200 dynes/cm²)*

Type of cardiac damage	None	Treatment for 3 weeks	
		Amitriptyline (1 mg/kg b.i.d.)	Imipramine (1.2 mg/kg b.i.d.)
None	0	0	0
Spontaneous	2	80	90
Isoprenaline	4	90	80
Cobalt	2	90	80
Aortic coarctation	6	70	90

untreated animals. In the groups of animals with cardiomyopathies and treated with tricyclic antidepressants, however, the death rate rose dramatically to 70 to 90%.

The animals that died did not convulse when exposed to the noise stress (this happens to rats during withdrawal from alcohol), and immediate poststress EKGs clearly showed ventricular fibrillation. We did not attempt any resuscitation, and the remaining animals that did not die were killed by an overdose of ether. The hearts from all the animals in this experiment were then processed and examined histologically, as in the previous experiment. No significant differences were noted in the type or extent of cardiac damage from that found in the first experiment.

Tricyclic antidepressants are known to potentiate the effects of the sympathetic nervous system (39–41), and this system plays an important role in mediating the cardiovascular responses to stress. We reasoned, therefore, that if the sudden deaths among our animals who had been exposed to noise stress were due to a potentiation of sympathetic cardiac effects, then we could effectively antagonize these effects by treatment with a beta-adrenoceptor antagonist. We chose propranolol for this purpose because it is an effective agent widely used to treat patients with heart disease, as described in the first section of this book. The results of concomitant treatment with this drug, i.e., effect on the incidence of noise-induced sudden cardiac deaths, are shown in Table 8.2.

Treatment with propranolol alone had no deleterious effects and completely abolished the noise stress deaths in animals with cardiomyopathies. In animals with cardiomyopathies treated with amitriptyline and receiving concomitant treatment with propranolol, the deaths after noise stress showed a striking reduction from 70 to 90% to 2 to 10%. (Results with imipramine were virtually identical.)

The results of these experiments strongly supported our ideas on the mechanism by which tricyclic antidepressants produced sudden deaths.

These agents are in common use; stress in one form or another is part of everyday life, and even the animals with relatively mild cardiomyopathies showed a high percentage of sudden deaths. It would not be unreasonable, therefore, to expect that in the clinical situation there would be a high incidence of sudden

TABLE 8-2. *Percent deaths on noise stress (200 dynes/cm²)*

Type of cardiac damage	None	Amitriptyline (1 mg/kg b.i.d.)	Propranolol (1 mg/kg b.i.d.)	Amitriptyline and propranolol
None	0	0	0	0
Spontaneous	2	80	0	8
Isoprenaline	4	90	0	10
Cobalt	2	90	0	6
Aortic coarctation	6	70	0	2

deaths associated with tricyclic antidepressant agents. However, although there have been a number of reports of isolated sudden cardiac deaths occurring possibly in association with tricyclic drugs, there is no evidence to suggest a high incidence of such deaths in patients being treated with tricyclics.

One possible explanation is that patients suffering from depression often receive concomitant treatment with other drugs which could reduce or exacerbate the potential cardiotoxicity of the tricyclic antidepressants. The drugs most commonly prescribed to patients treated with tricyclic antidepressants are benzodiazepines, phenothiazines, and barbiturates. Therefore, it occurred to us that these drugs might provide a protective effect against the development of tricyclic cardiotoxicity.

Accordingly, we undertook further experiments to investigate this possibility by repeating our experiments in animals who received concomitant treatment with diazepam together with imipramine. These results are shown in Table. 8.3.

As in the case of propranolol, diazepam alone produced no cases of sudden death; when given together with imipramine, however, it considerably reduced the incidence of sudden deaths due to the combination of imipramine and noise stress in all four groups of cardiac damage. Thus the incidence of these sudden deaths was reduced from 80 to 90% to 18 to 30%.

We also investigated the effect of sodium pentobarbital and found this to have a small but definite effect, the percentage range of deaths dropping from 80 to 90% to 45 to 60%. Concomitant treatment with a phenothiazine, chlorpromazine, and piperacetazine again had cardioprotective effects; the death rate ranges were reduced from 80 to 90% to 35 to 40%. The results of experiments where amitriptyline was used were not significantly different.

EKGs were recorded in this last experiment 1 week before the animals were exposed to the noise stress, i.e., after 2 weeks of drug treatment. The only changes noted were in animals with no cardiac damage treated with chlorpromazine and piperacetazine. These drugs each produced reduced T-wave voltages in approximately 40% of treated animals. Analysis of the data showed that the animals surviving after noise stress were equally distributed between those with and without T-wave changes. Histologic examination of the hearts of all

TABLE 8-3. *Percent deaths on noise stress (200 dynes/cm²)*

Type of cardiac damage	None	Imipramine (1.2 mg/kg b.i.d.)	Diazepam (0.3 mg/kg b.i.d.)	Imipramine and diazepam
None	0	0	0	0
Spontaneous	2	90	0	18
Isoprenaline	4	80	0	20
Cobalt	2	80	0	30
Aortic coarctation	6	90	0	20

animals was undertaken, but no significant differences were noted in the type or extent of cardiac damage compared to that found in the previous experiments.

CLINICAL IMPLICATIONS

The tricyclic antidepressants introduced by Kuhn (42) are now generally accepted as drugs of first choice in the treatment of unipolar depression, as described by Wheatley (2). Therapeutic doses of the tricyclic agents have marked effects on the cardiovascular system (41), and there have been reports of unexpected deaths. (These clinical effects in man are considered in more detail in the following chapters.)

The results of the present study indicate that in the rat, chronic administration of the tricyclic antidepressants amitriptyline and imipramine did not result in sudden deaths in normal animals or in those with cardiomyopathies. When these animals were treated with tricyclic antidepressants and exposed to noise stress, however, the incidence of sudden deaths in animals with cardiomyopathies increased 45 times, from 2 to 90%. These findings are in agreement with clinical data of Asmussen and co-workers (43), who reported that preexisting heart disease may influence cardiac complications.

Patients who are suffering from depression are already in a stress situation, and the symptoms exhibited may be psychic or somatic. Selye (18,45–47) first introduced the concept that stress was important in the production and prevention of pathologic conditions, as he describes in the introductory chapter to this volume. Studies in man and other species have shown that marked changes occur in the cardiovascular system during periods of various types of stress, as Taggart and Carruthers (Chapter 3) describe in their various experiments. Another study conducted by the same authors is of interest in that it showed some qualitative differences from those described in their chapter in this book. It concerned an investigation by Taggart et al. (48) into the effects of short exposures to the intense heat of a sauna bath. The authors studied 17 normal patients and 18 suffering from coronary heart disease. As in their previous experiments, they recorded EKGs before and after exposure, together with estimations of plasma catecholamines, free fatty acids (FFA), and triglycerides. As a control, they used patients from both groups and made similar recordings and estimations before and after exercise. They found that following exposure to heat, there was the expected increase in plasma epinephrine but not in plasma norepinephrine, FFA, or triglycerides. Exercise, on the other hand, produced the anticipated increase in both plasma epinephrine and norepinephrine.

The investigators found that both heat and exercise produced tachycardias with rates up to 180 beats/min, and that on the EKG, ST-T changes occurred frequently in both groups in response to heat, but there were few such changes following exercise. Furthermore, exercise was sufficient to produce an increase in heart rate comparable to that produced by exposure to heat. Bergamaschi et al. (49) investigated the effects of emotional stress on conscious dogs, measuring heart rate, cardiac output, and left ventricular work. As in our experiments, the stress was induced by firing a gun, and increases were found in all three parameters. These responses were all reduced by propranolol, practolol, and sotalol, and were completely abolished by alprenolol. Bergamasechi et al. also found that stress increased the mean blood flow through the left circumflex coronary artery, and that this effect could also be blocked, in a similar manner, by the same adrenergic beta-blocking drugs. These observations led to the suggestion that "stimulation of beta-adrenoceptors in the coronary arteries plays an important role in the coronary vasodilation produced by emotional stress."

Retrospective analysis of the sudden unexpected deaths in patients treated with tricyclic antidepressants indicated a possible causal relationship with preexisting cardiac disease. Unfortunately, we do not know if these patients were exposed to other forms of stress besides existing emotional problems. If so, the influence of various types of stress, including psychogenic factors, associated with sudden death is well documented. Perhaps one of the most intriguing of investigations was that reported by Engel (50), who probed deaths reported in the press as due to disrupting life events. Over a 6-year period, he was able to collect details of 170 such deaths and found that the causes, in order of frequency, were as follows:

1. Personal danger or threat of injury: 27%.
2. Collapse or death of a close person: 21%.
3. During a period of acute grief (within 16 days): 20%.
4. Threat of loss of a close person: 9%.
5. After danger is over (e.g., a car accident): 7%.
6. Reunion, triumph, "happy ending" (e.g., sudden meeting after long separation): 6%.
7. Loss of status or self-esteem (e.g., failure to get expected promotion): 6%.
8. During mourning or anniversary of a death: 3%.

Engel made the following comment on his investigation:

Common to all is that they involve events impossible for the victims to ignore and to which their response is overwhelming excitation or giving up, or both. It is proposed that this combination provokes neurovegetative responses, involving both the flight-fight and conservation-withdrawal systems, conducive to lethal cardiac events, particularly in individuals with pre-existing cardiovascular disease. Other modes of death, however, were also noted.

In a further communication, Engel goes on to speculate (57): "Whether ventricular fibrillation and death can be induced by neurogenic influences alone in the absence of cardiac abnormality, remains a moot point."

Geha et al. (52) investigated the effects of catecholamine-induced stress in dogs, in which they had previously produced a stable, compensated left ventricular hypertrophy. Sudden death in such animals often follows bursts of physical activity, but the catecholamine-induced stress did not result in any functional impairment compared to normal controls. Geha et al. found that oxygen consumption in the heart was increased to the same level in both groups, whereas oxygen extraction increased 63% in normal animals but not at all in the dogs with left ventricular hypertrophy. They concluded that "the intact stable hypertrophed myocardium shows no functional impairment during catecholamine-induced stress, but the increased oxygen requirements of stress can be met only by an increase in coronary flow, since oxygen extraction in left ventricular hypertrophy is already maximal." In other words, they demonstrated in the laboratory that it is the combination of stress and prior cardiac damage that may result in sudden death.

This theme is affirmed by Doyle et al. (53) who reported a case of sudden death in a young patient with congenital aortic stenosis who was running after being frightened by lightning. Rahe et al. (54) adopted a different approach and in a retrospective survey recorded recent life-change data (mainly adverse events) collected from 279 survivors of documented myocardial infarction, as well as from relatives of 226 patients who had suffered an abrupt coronary death. Using a rating system, the authors found marked elevation in the mean magnitude of life changes during the 6 months immediately prior to infarction, as compared to the same time interval 1 year earlier. Finally, Lown et al. (55) described the interesting case of a 39-year-old man suffering from serious psychiatric problems, who twice experienced spontaneous ventricular fibrillation and also exhibited numerous ventricular premature beats. His coronary arteries were normal, and no impairment of cardiac functioning could be found even on cardiac catheterization. It was discovered that the ventricular premature beats could be provoked by psychophysiological stress, and that they also increased during REM sleep. On the other hand, they could be reduced by meditation and completely controlled by beta-adrenergic blocking drugs. Lown et al. concluded that "psychologic and neurophysiologic factors may predispose to life-threatening cardiac arrhythmias in the absence of organic heart disease." Therefore, although the bulk of the evidence suggests that sudden cardiac death due to stress is more likely to occur in patients with preexisting cardiac disease, it may also occur in patients with normal cardiovascular function. Although stress in one form or another has been cited as a causal factor, mechanisms involved vary from changes in monoamine oxidase levels, as described by Maura et al. (56), to the development of hypertension, as described by Smookler et al. (57) (see ensuing chapters), to the occurrence of intravascular platelet aggregation in the heart, as described by Haft and Fani (58).

The importance of the sympthetic nervous system in the production of fatal cardiac arrhythmias is unanimously accepted by workers in this field. It was not too surprising that concomitant treatment with the beta-adrenergic blocking drug propranolol strikingly reduced the incidence of stress-related deaths in our experiments. Propranolol has been used frequently in the treatment of cardiac arrhythmias associated with amitriptyline and imipramine poisoning (4,59) and has been shown by Ruel et al. (60) to protect against ventricular fibrillation in cardiopulmonary bypass surgery. Our histologic findings that propranolol had no effect on the histologic appearance of animals without cardiomyopathies are in agreement with the findings of Allin et al. (61). Indeed, we did not expect, nor did we find, any histologic evidence of a beneficial effect from treating animals with propranolol alone. In this context, of course, it will be recalled that experimentally induced cardiomyopathies were already fully established before treatment with any other drugs began. On the other hand, we have noticed that rats whose spontaneous cardiomyopathy, as determined by EKGs, consisted of ectopic ventricular foci could be normalized by treatment with propranolol. A clinical counterpart has been reported by Fox et al. (62) to the effect that beta-adrenoceptor blockade may protect patients from the development of a myocardial infarction.

Although propranolol has been successfully used in anxiety states (2,63,64), as described in Chapter 6, we suggest that the reports of exacerbation of cardiac symptoms on sudden withdrawal of propranolol therapy should not be forgotten (65,66).

The remarkable effects of diazepam were at first quite puzzling. A literature search then clearly showed that the benzodiazepines have considerable antiarrhythmic properties. Kernohan (67) used intravenous diazepam to induce narcosis for shock therapy in 312 cases of atrial arrhythmias. He noted that this procedure did not produce any adverse effects on conversion to normal rhythm but did not adduce any evidence for a direct effect of diazepam in achieving this. In the laboratory, Gillis et al. (68) induced cardiac arrhythmias in cats with digitalis and found that chlordiazepoxide reestablished normal rhythm in nine of 12 animals. However, the authors were not able to demonstrate any similar effects from this drug in a parallel experiment in spinal-sectioned dogs. In another experiment, they produced coronary occlusion in dogs and found that chlordiazepoxide significantly reduced the number of abnormal ectopic beats while simultaneously increasing the number of sinus beats and significantly slowing the pulse rate. In further animal experiments, de Jong and Heaver (69) investigated pretreatment with diazepam in cats whose central nervous and cardiovascular systems were subject to the effects of lidocaine. Lidocaine induces seizures, and these were reduced by half when diazepam was given. In the cardiovascular system, lidocaine produces hypotension and ventricular tachycardia; although pretreatment with diazepam did not prevent them from developing, the EKG signs of ventricular irritation were fewer when diazepam had been used.

Benzodiazepines can have a beneficial effect on coronary blood flow in patients, as demonstrated by Côté et al. (70), who used intravenous diazepam prior to coronary angiography in 12 patients with coronary insufficiency and in eight controls. These investigators recorded various measurements of cardiac function and found that diazepam produced "a nitroglyrcerin-like action on the coronary and systemic circulation." Furthermore, this group of drugs will successfully reduce the effects of stress in experimental animals (71,72). It has been suggested that the mechanism involved in these antiarrhythmic effects consists of membrane stabilization (73,74). Thus Langslot (73), investigating the effects of D,L- and D-propranolol and chlorpromazine on the isolated hearts of rats, found that all three compounds decreased cardiac excitability and contractility as well as potassium efflux. In other words, they produced all the effects of membrane stabilization, as evidenced by other drugs known to act in this way. Langslot also found that all three drugs increased the coronary flow after certain blood concentrations had been reached. Similar effects of phenothiazines and barbiturates have been produced in isolated animal tissues, and membrane stabilization and reduced calcium permeability have been suggested as possible mechanisms of action (75–80).

Phenothiazines are now used in combination with tricyclic antidepressant drugs in the treatment of depression. However, there have been reports of EKG abnormalities produced by the phenothiazines themselves, as described in the next chapter. Indeed, in our experiments, chlorpromazine and piperacetazine alone did produce some minor T-wave changes in a few animals. Nevertheless, we found no histologic evidence of any cardiac damage produced by treatment with these agents. There was no increase in the number of deaths in animals with cardiomyopathies treated with the phenothiazines, even when these animals were exposed to our noise stress. From this result and the protection offered to some animals receiving concomitant treatment with the tricyclic antidepressants, we conclude that such combination therapy may be beneficial in clinical situations.

We cannot ignore the possibility that the cardioprotective effects of agents we used might be due to effects on metabolism of the tricyclic antidepressants. At present, reports vary from those recording no effect at all, to others recording inhibition of the metabolism of tricyclic drugs when given concomitantly, to yet others recording stimulation of that metabolism. Fuller et al. (81) administered combined nortriptyline and thioridazine to rats, and found that the combination resulted in higher plasma concentrations of nortriptyline than when the tricyclic was given alone. Furthermore, the concentration of nortriptyline in the brain was elevated and the half-life in the brain prolonged. On the other hand, in a human study involving five patients, Gram et al. (82) used nortriptyline in combination with benzodiazepines (diazepam or chlordiazepoxide) and also in combination with neuroleptics (haloperidol, perphenazine). They found that the benzodiazepines had no influence on the metabolism of nortriptyline, but that the neuroleptics actually inhibited it. These experiments were carried out using [^{14}C]-labeled nortriptyline. Silverman and Braithwaite (83) confirmed that there was no significant alteration in plasma levels of nortriptyline that could be attributed to the addition of various benzodiazepines (nitrazepam, chlordiazepoxide, diazepam, and oxazepam). In their study of 12 patients under treatment with nortriptyline, they did find that amobarbital caused a reduction of the plasma level of nortriptyline. Stevenson et al. (84) investigated various hypnotics in human volunteers and found that "Mandrax" (methaqualone + diphenhydramine) increased the rate of drug metabolism, presumably by enzyme induction.

Nitrazepam, however, had no such effect, and this led to the conclusion that it was unlikely that benzodiazepines were the cause of drug interactions generally. Finally, Ballinger et al. (85) gave either amobarbital or nitrazepam to depressed patients who were being treated with imipramine. They concluded that there was no evidence of adverse effects from either of these two drugs given in combination with imipramine. Therefore, the picture is somewhat confused, although it appears that the benzodiazepines, at least, are devoid of any adverse effect when combined with the tricyclic antidepressants.

The beneficial effects of the tricyclic agents in the treatment of depression clearly justify their widespread clinical use. Further investigation of the potential cardiotoxicities of these agents could reveal patients for whom there is a relative contraindication to their use, particularly patients with uncertain cardiac states. Our results indicate a need for further studies on the effects of various types of stress on the cardiotoxic effect of tricyclic antidepressants. Studies on the mechanisms of cardioprotective effects of agents commonly given as concomitant treatment in depressed patients, and on metabolic transactions, could provide important clinically relevant data.

Effects of Cold and Exercise

We have recently undertaken some preliminary studies in rats with preexisting cardiac infarction who were treated with amitriptyline. We assessed the application of cold and exercise as separate stress factors and found some increase in the death rate with each of these stressors individually. The combination of cold and exercise together, however, produced a much higher death rate in these animals being treated with tricyclics, compared to control animals who were not receiving any drugs. Nevertheless, the most spectacular results were obtained with the noise-stress experiments described in this chapter. The difference is probably attributable to the fact that noise stress is sudden, while cold and exercise have a more gradual impact.

These more recent experiments with cold and exercise have a direct clinical implication in man and in particular to the climatic conditions existing in Winnipeg in the winter. It is not unusual for middle-aged men to go outside into the cold to shovel snow; clearly, our experiments suggest that such individuals, who may well have underlying coronary heart disease, may be particularly at risk of a sudden cardiac incident, such as myocardial infarction. Since a number of such individuals may also be taking tricyclic antidepressants, it will be of interest to collect comparative data to determine whether the incidence of such acute cardiac events under these conditions of cold and exercise may be higher in the patients taking tricyclics as compared to those who are not. Furthermore, it would be an interesting therapeutic exercise to administer a benzodiazepine or beta-blocking drug to such patients on tricyclics, to determine whether this might reduce the incidence of these adverse cardiac effects. It may be that the introduction of the newer antidepressant agents (see succeeding chapters) renders such an investigation unnecessary.

CONCLUSIONS

We have conducted experiments in rats with various types of cardiomyopathies, including those spontaneously occurring and those induced by isoprenaline, cobalt, and experimental left ventricular hypertrophy, respectively. Characteristic histologic and EKG changes were produced in the hearts of these animals, who were then treated with amitriptyline and imipramine. Treatment with these tricyclic antidepressants, however, did not significantly change any of the histologic findings. In addition to treatment with tricyclic antidepressants, these various experimental groups of animals were also subjected to a standard noise stress test. Sudden unexpected cardiac deaths occurred in 2 to 6% of the untreated animals, but there were no deaths among normal rats given tricyclic antidepressants and subjected to the noise stress. However, in the groups of animals with cardiomyopathies to which tricyclic antidepressants were given, the death rate rose dramatically to 70 to 90% on exposure to noise stress. The cause of death was ventricular fibrillation.

The experiments were then repeated following concurrent treatment with the beta-adrenergic blocking drug propranolol and various tranquilizing drugs. The deaths after the combination of tricyclic antidepressant with noise stress were strikingly reduced, from 70 to 90% to 2 to 10%, by concurrent treatment with propranolol. Furthermore, similar effects were achieved with the various tranquilizing drugs used, although the reductions in death rate were not as great. Sodium pentobarbital reduced the death rate from 80 to 90% to 45 to 60%, chlorpromazine and piperacetazine from 80 to 90% to 35 to 40%, and diazepam from 80 to 90% to 18 to 30%.

There would seem to be a direct parallel between these animal experiments and tricyclic cardiotoxicity in man. Preexisting cardiac disease, such as commonly occurs in the elderly, may present a particular hazard when tricyclic antidepressants are used in clinical practice. Concomitant treatment with beta-adrenergic blocking drugs or tranquilizing drugs would seem to be based on sound experimental evidence and may result in reduction or abolition of possible cardiotoxic effects of tricyclic drugs in man.

ACKNOWLEDGMENTS

This investigation was supported by a grant from the Medical Research Council of Canada. The following companies generously donated drugs used in this investigation: Amitriptyline, Merck, Sharp and Dohme; chlorpromazine, Poulenc; diazepam, Roche; imipramine, Geigy; piperacetazine, Dow; propranolol, Ayerst.

REFERENCES

1. Hordern, A., Burt, C. G., Holt, N. S., and Cade, J. F. J. *Depressive States: A Pharmacotherapeutic Study.* Charles C Thomas, Springfield, Ill., 1965.
2. Wheatley, D. *Psychopharmacology in Family Practice.* William Heinemann, London, 1973.
3. Freeman, J. W., Ryan, C. A., and Beattie, R. R. Epidemiology of drug overdosage in Southern Tasmania. *Med. J. Aust.,* 1970, 2, 1168.
4. Sesso, A. M., Snyder, R. C., and Schott, C. E. Propranolol in imipramine poisoning. *Am. J. Dis. Child.,* 1973, 126, 847.
5. Goel, K. M., and Shanks, R. A. Amitriptyline and imipramine poisoning in children. *Br. Med. J.,* 1974, i, 261.
6. Greenblatt, D. J., Koch-Weser, J., and Shader, R. I. Multiple complications and death following protriptyline overdose. *JAMA,* 1974, 229, 556.
7. Vohra, J., Burrows, G. D., and Sloman, G. Assessment of cardiovascular side effects of therapeutic doses of tricyclic antidepressant drugs. *Aust. N.Z. J. Med.,* 1974, 5, 7.
8. Thorsand, C. Cardiovascular effects of poisoning with tricyclic antidepressants. *Acta Med. Scand.,* 1974, 195, 505.
9. Kantor, S. J., Bigger, T., Glassman, A. H., Macken, D. L., and Perel, J. M. Imipramine induced heart block. *JAMA,* 1975, 231, 1364.
10. Kristiansen, E. S. Cardiac complications during treatment with imipramine. *Acta Psychol. Neurol. Scand.,* 1961, 36, 427.
11. Siegel, P. S., and Stuckley, H. L. The diurnal course of water and food intake in the normal rat. *J. Comp. Physiol. Psychol.,* 1947, 40, 365.
12. Richter, C. P. In: *Biological Clocks in Medicine and Psychiatry.* Charles C Thomas, Springfield, Ill., 1965.
13. ter Haar, M. B. Circadian and estrous rhythms in food intake in the rat. *Horm. Behav.,* 1972, 3, 213.
14. Weber, H. W., Van Der Walt, J. J., and Greef, M. J. *Cardiomyopathies.* University Park Press, Baltimore, 1971.
15. Saunders, I. Z. Myositis in guinea pigs. *J. Natl. Cancer Inst.,* 1958, 20, 899.
16. Webb, J. N. Naturally occurring myopathy in guinea pigs. *J. Pathol.,* 1970, 100, 155.
17. Caufield, C. S., and Shelton, R. W. Spontaneous cardiomyopathy in guinea pigs. In: *Cardiomyopathies.,* University Park Press, Baltimore, 1971.
18. Selye, H. *Experimental Cardiovascular Diseases,* Springer-Verlag, Berlin, 1970.
19. Boorman, G. A., Zurcher, C., Hollander, C. F., Rijswijk, Z. H., and Feron, V. J. Naturally occurring endocardial disease in the rat. *Arch. Pathol.,* 1973, 96, 39.
20. Heering, H. Das elektrokardiogram der wachen und narkotisierten Ratte. *Arch. Int. Phamacodyn.,* 1970, 185, 308.
21. Short, D., and Stowers, M. Earliest symptoms of coronary heart disease and their recognition. *Br. Med. J.,* 1972, 2, 387.
22. Maroko, P. R. Assessing myocardial damage in acute infarcts. *N. Engl. J. Med.,* 1974, 290, 158.
23. Rona, G., Chappel, C. I., Balasz, T., and Gaudry, R. An infarct like myocardial lesion and other toxic manifestations produced by isoproterenol in the rat. *Arch. Pathol.,* 1959, 67, 443.
24. Rona, G. Zosoter, T., Chappel, C., and Gaudry, R. Myocardial lesions, circulatory and electrocardiographic changes produced by isoproterenol in the dog. *Rev. Can. Biol.,* 1959, 18, 83.
25. Handforth, C. P. Isoproterenol-induced myocardial infarction in animals. *Arch. Pathol.,* 1962, 73, 761.
26. Maruffo, C. A. Fine structural study of myocardial changes induced by isoproterenol in rhesus monkeys (Macaca mulatta). *Am. J. Pathol.,* 1967, 50, 27.
27. Ostadel, B., and Rychterova, U. V. Effect of nectrogenic doses of isoproterenol on the heart of the trench (Tinca tinca-Osteoichthyes), the frog (Rana temporaria-Anura) and the pigeon (columbia lives-aves). *Physiol. Bohemoslov.,* 1971, 20, 541.
28. Balags, T., Ohtake, S., and Noble, J. F. The development of resistance to the ischaemic cardiopathic effect of isoproterenol. *Toxicol. Appl. Pharmacol.,* 1972, 21, 200.
29. Morin, Y. L., and Daniel, P. Quebec beer drinkers cardiomyopathy: Etiological considerations. *Can. Med. Assoc. J.,* 1967, 97, 926.

30. Morin, Y. L., Foley, A. R., Martineau, G., and Roussel, J. Quebec beer drinkers cardiomyopathy: Forty-eight cases. *Can. Med. Assoc. J.,* 1967, 97, 881.
31. Huy, N. D., Morin, P. J., Mohiuddin, S. M., and Morin, Y. Acute effects of cobalt on cardiac metabolism and mechanical performance. *Can. J. Physiol. Pharmacol.,* 1973, 51, 46.
32. Rona, G., and Chappel, C. I. Pathogenesis and pathology of cobalt cardiomyopathies. *Recent Adv. Stud. Cardiac Struct. Metab.,* 2, 1973.
33. Wachtlova, M., Rakusan, K., and Roth, Z., The terminal vascular bed of the myocardium in the wild rat (Rattus norvegicus) and the laboratory rat (Rattus norvegicus lab). *Physiol. Bohemoslov.,* 1967, 16, 548.
34. Rogo-Ortega, J. M., and Genest, J. A method for production of experimental hypertension in rats. *Can. J. Physiol. Pharmacol.,* 1968, 46, 883.
35. Anversa, P., Vitali-Mazza, L., Vidioli, O., and Marchetti, G. Experimental cardiac hypertrophy: A quantitative ultrastructural study in the compensatory stage. *J. Mol. Cell. Cardiol.,* 1971, 3, 213.
36. Sybulski, S., Omay, Y., and Maughan, G. B. Pregnancy outcome in rats with aortic ligation. *Obstet Gynecol.,* 1972, 40, 391.
37. Gamble, W. J., Phornphutkul, A., Kumar, E., Sanders, G. L., Manasek, F. G., and Monroe, R. G. Ventricular performance, coronary flow, and MVO$_2$ in aortic coarctation hypertrophy. *J. Physiol.,* 1973, 224, 877.
38. Welch, B. L., and Welch, A. S. *Physiological Effects of Noise.* Plenum Press, New York, 1970.
39. Dannert, F., and Rosen, A. Massive imipramin-intoxikation med langdraget, periodvis kirstiskt forlopp. *Svenska Lak. Tidn.,* 1967, 64, 80.
40. Alexander, C. S., and Nino, A. Cardiovascular complications in young patients taking psychotropic drugs. *Am. Heart J.,* 1969, 78, 757.
41. Raisfield, I. K. Cardiovascular complications of antidepressant therapy. *Am. Heart J.,* 1972, 83, 129.
42. Kuhn, R. Uber die Behandlung depressiver Zustande mit eineim Imidobenzyderwat. *Schweiz. Med. Wochenschr.,* 1957, 87, 1135.
43. Asmussen, I., Uhrenholdt, A., and Dich, B. Cardiomyopathi udviklet under behandling med tricycliske antidepressiva. *Ugeskr. Laeger,* 1974, 57, 55.
44. Kiev, A. Somatic manifestation of depressive disorders. *Excerpta Medica,* 3, 1974.
45. Selye, H. Interactions between various steroid hormones. *Can. Med. Assoc. J.,* 1940, 42, 113.
46. Selye, H. *Stress.* Acta Inc. Med., Montreal, 1950.
47. Selye, H. *The Pluiricausal Cardiomyopathies.* Charles C Thomas, Springfield, Ill., 1961.
48. Taggart, P., Parkinson, P., and Carruthers, M. Cardiac responses to thermal, physical and emotional stress. *Br. Med. J.,* 1972, 3, 71.
49. Bergamaschi, M., Carravagi, A., Mandelli, V., and Shanks, R. The role of beta adrenoceptors in the coronary and systemic haemodynamic responses to emotional stress in conscious dogs. *Am. Heart J.,* 1973, 86, 216.
50. Engel, G. L. Sudden and rapid death during psychological stress: Folklore or folk wisdom? *Ann. Intern. Med.,* 1971, 74, 771.
51. Engel, G. L. Psychologic factors in instantaneous cardiac death. *N. Engl. J. Med.,* 1976, 294, 664.
52. Geha, A. S., Malik, A. G., Abe, T., and O'Kane, H. O. Response of the hypertrophied heart to stress. *Surgery,* 1973, 74, 276.
53. Doyle, E. F., Arumugham, P., Lara, E., Rutkowski, M. R., and Kiely, B. Sudden death in young patients with congenital aortic stenosis. *Pediatrics,* 1974, 53, 481.
54. Rahe, R. H., Romo, M., Bennett, L., and Stilanen, P. Recent life changes, myocardial infarction and abrupt coronary death. *Arch. Intern. Med.,* 1974, 133, 221.
55. Lown, B., Temte, J. V., Reich, P., Gaughan, C., Regestein, Q., and Hai, H. Basis for recurring ventricular fibrillation in the absence of coronary heart disease and its management. *N. Engl. J. Med.,* 1976, 294, 623.
56. Maura, G., Vaccari, A., Gemignani, A., and Cugurra, F. Development of monoamine oxidase activity after chronic environmental stress in the rat. *Environ. Physiol. Biochem.,* 1974, 4, 64.
57. Smookler, H. H., Goebel, K. H., Sieger, M. I., and Clarke, D. E. Hypertensive effects of prolonged auditory, visual, and motion stimulation. *Fed. Proc.,* 1973, 32, 2105.
58. Haft, J. I., and Fani, K. Stress and the induction of intravascular platelet aggregation in the heart. *Circulation,* 1973, XLVIII, 164.

59. Roberts, R. J., Mueller, S., and Lauer, R. Propranolol treatment of cardiac arrhythmias associated with amitriptyline intoxication. *J. Pediatr.*, 1973, 82, 65.
60. Ruel, J. G., Romagnoli, A., Sandiford, F. M., Wukasch, D. C., and Norman, J. C. Protective effect of propranolol on the hypertrophied heart during cardiopulmonary bypass. *J. Thorac. Cardiovasc. Surg.*, 1974, 68, 283.
61. Allin, E. P., Miller, J. M., Rowe, G. G., and Will, J. A. Effects of intraperitoneal administration of propranolol on the mouse heart. *Am. J. Cardiol.*, 1974, 33, 639.
62. Fox, K. M., Chopra, M. P., Portal, R. W., and Aber, C. P. Long-term beta-blockade: Possible protection from myocardial infarction. *Br. Med. J.*, 1975, 1, 117.
63. Wheatley, D. Comparative effects of propranolol and chlordiazepoxide in anxiety states. *Br. J. Psychiatry*, 1969, 115, 1411.
64. Tyrer, P. J., and Lader, M. H. Responses to propranolol and diazepam in somatic and psychic anxiety. *Br. Med. J.*, 1974, 2, 14.
65. Alderman, E. D., Coltart, J., Wettach, G. E., and Harrison, D. C. Coronary artery syndromes after sudden propranolol withdrawal. *Ann. Intern. Med.*, 1974, 81, 625.
66. Miller, R. R., Olson, H. G., Amsterdam, E. A., and Mason, D. T. Propranolol-withdrawal rebound phenomenon. *N. Engl. J. Med.*, 1975, 293, 416.
67. Kernohan, R. J. Diazepam in cardioversion of supraventricular arrhythmias. *J. Ir. Coll. Phys. Surg.*, 1972, 1, 88.
68. Gillis, R. A., Thibodeaux, H., and Barr, L. Antiarrhythmic properties of chlordiazepoxide. *Circulation*, 1974, XLIX, 272.
69. de Jong, R. H., and Heaver, J. E. Diazepam and lidocaine-induced cardiovascular changes. *Anethesiology*, 1973, 39, 633.
70. Côte, P., Guéret, P., and Bourassa, M. G. Systemic and coronary hemodynamic effects of diazepam in patients with normal and diseased coronary arteries. *Circulation*, 1974, 50, 1210.
71. Dantzer, R., and Baldwin, B. A. Effects of chlordiazepoxide on heart rate and behavioural suppression in pigs subjected to operant conditioning procedures. *Psychopharmacology*, 1974, 37, 169.
72. Lahti, R. A., and Barsuhn, C. The effect of minor tranquillizers on stress-induced increases in rat plasma corticosteroids. *Psychopharmacology*, 1974, 35, 215.
73. Langslot, A. Membrane stabilization and cardiac effects of D,L-propranolol, D-propranolol and chlorpromazine. *Eur. J. Pharmacol.*, 1970, 13, 6.
74. Liebeswar, G. The depressant action of flurazepam on the maximum rate of rise of action potentials recorded from guinea-pig papillary muscles. *Naunyn Schmiedebergs Arch. Pharmacol.*, 1972, 275, 445.
75. Beaulnes, A., and Lavallee, M. Differential effects of some phenothiazine derivatives against calcium-induced ventricular arrhythmias in the isolated rabbit heart. *Can. J. Physiol. Pharmacol.*, 1964, 42, 845.
76. Haacke, H., and Van Zwieten, P. A. The influence of hexobarbitone on calcium ion movements in isolated heart muscle. *J. Pharm. Pharmacol.*, 1970, 23, 425.
77. Landmark, K. The action of promazine and thioridazine in isolated rat atria. 1. Effects on automaticity, mechanical preformance refractoriness and excitability. *Eur. J. Pharmacol.*, 1971, 16, 1.
78. Haffner, J. F., and Landmark, K. Opposing anticholinergic and cardiodepressive effects of promazine and thioridazine in isolated rat atria. *Acta Pharmacol. Toxicol.*, 1972, 31, 529.
79. Haffner, J. F. The effects of promazine and thioridazine on the response to noradrenaline in isolated rat atria. *Acta Pharmacol. Toxicol.*, 1972, 32, 148.
80. Naylor, W. G., and Szeto, J. Effect of sodium pentobarbital on calcium in mammalian heart muscle. *Am. J. Physiol.*, 1972, 222, 339.
81. Fuller, R. W., Snoddy, H. D., and Slater, I. S. Metabolic interactions between nortriptyline and thioridazine in rats. *Toxicol. Appl. Pharmacol.*, 1974, 29, 259.
82. Gram, L., Over, K. F., and Kirk, L. Influence of neuroleptics and benzodiazepines on metabolism of tricyclic antidepressants in man. *Am. J. Psychiatry*, 1974, 131, 863.
83. Silverman, G., and Braithwaite, R. Interaction of benzodiazepines with tricyclic antidepressants. *Br. Med. J.*, 1972, 4, 111.
84. Stevenson, I. H., Browning, M., Crooks, J., and O'Malley, K. Changes in human drug metabolism after long-term exposure to hypnotics. *Br. Med. J.*, 1972, 4, 322.
85. Ballinger, B. R., Presly, A., Reid, A. H., and Stevenson, I. H. The effects of hypnotics on imipramine treatment. *Psychopharmacology*, 1974, 39, 267.

Stress and the Heart, edited by D. Wheatley,
Raven Press, New York © 1981.

Cardiotoxicity of Antidepressants: Experimental Background

Graham Burrows, Ian Hughes, and Trevor Norman

The introduction of the tricyclic antidepressants has been of great benefit to the patient suffering from depressive illness, although this benefit has not been without an attendant cost. Misuse of these drugs has led to an epidemic of tricyclic antidepressant poisoning, which shows little sign of abating. Examination of the Registrar General's figures (1) for fatal poisonings in England and Wales from 1961 to 1977 (Fig. 9.1) shows that deaths involving a tricyclic antidepressant have contributed a steadily increasing percentage (over 14% in 1977) to the total poisoning deaths, which have themselves been relatively constant in more recent years.

This should not be taken to imply that the tricyclic antidepressant was the cause of death in every case, since suicide attempts often involve self administration of several types of drug at the same time. Nevertheless, 14% is a large proportion of fatal poisonings to be associated with one group of drugs, even if the group is used in the treatment of the suicide-prone condition of depressive illness. Furthermore, it is relevant to note that all types of antidepressants accounted for less than 3% of the total number of prescriptions issued in England for the corresponding year (2).

ANIMAL STUDIES

The implicit purpose of most animal investigations into the relative cardiotoxicity of antidepressants is to predict or define their relative cardiotoxicity in man; the critical question in all these investigations: "How well does the model mimic man?" The previous chapter provides a relevant example of this proposition.

Animal models may measure effects dissimilar from those seen in man and may be totally divorced from the clinical situation. Nevertheless, they may still be effective in predicting relative activities in man. For example, screening tests for antidepressant activity, such as the rat swimming test (3) or the bulbectomized rat (4), do not bear an immediate and obvious relevance to the depressive syndrome in man, but these tests are reasonably effective in predicting antidepressant activity. With respect to the tests for cardiotoxicity, it is difficult to make a critical assessment of the various animal models which have been used, mainly because it is hard to obtain a single quantitative expression of the true cardiotoxic-

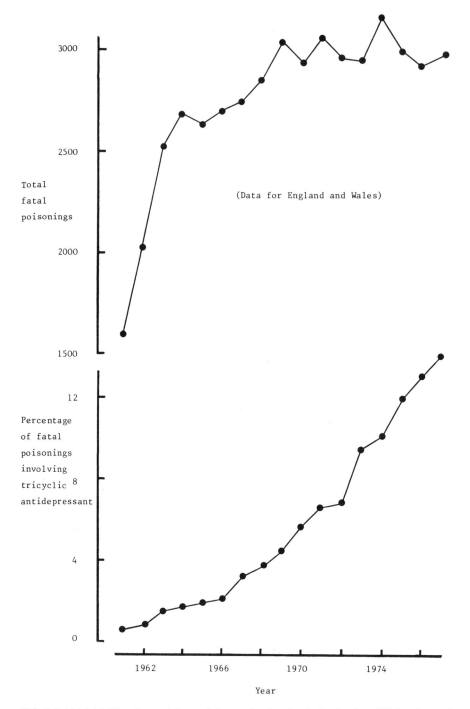

FIG. 9.1. Total fatalities **(upper)** from all forms of poisoning in England and Wales for each year from 1961 to 1977 and **(lower)** poisoning deaths involving a tricyclic antidepressant expressed as a percentage of the total fatal poisonings for each year in the same period. Note the increasing contribution of tricyclic antidepressants to the total poisonings (1).

ity of these compounds in man. In the absence of data to demonstrate that results in a particular animal model reflect clinical experience in man, no single method of testing for cardiotoxicity has become accepted, and a great variety of experimental approaches have been adopted by different workers.

IN VITRO MODELS

The isolated tissue is cut off completely from the normal neuronal and hormonal influences present in the body and may therefore give a misleading result, if cardiotoxicity is a consequence of modification of these controlling mechanisms. In this context, it should be noted that tricyclic antidepressants are known to affect the sympathetic nervous system at a variety of levels. In addition to their well-known ability to block norepinephrine reuptake, tricyclic antidepressants can cause α-adrenoceptor blockade at both postsynaptic (5) and presynaptic (6) sites and also have an atropinic action on muscarinic receptors. Sympathetic dominance may be produced not only because of potentiation of the effects of norepinephrine due to uptake blockade but also because of reduced opposing parasympathetic activity. Increased norepinephrine release may also occur as a result of blockade of presynaptic α-adrenoceptors and presynaptic muscarinic receptors, both of which may be involved in the control of norepinephrine output (7). The interplay between these effects is both complex and unclear, and the relevance of these actions to the cardiotoxicity seen in man is uncertain. The isolation of the tissue from the body is a disadvantage in this respect, but at least it ensures that biotransformation of the antidepressant is unlikely to complicate the picture. Thus the cardiotoxicity of the individual parent compound, but not that of its metabolites, will be assessed, although the relevance of this to the clinical situation, where biotransformation is likely to be extensive, is debatable.

Another factor which must be considered is that the physiologic saline solutions most frequently used in isolated tissue work are lacking in serum albumin, which is one of the plasma constituents (8) highly effective in binding tricyclic antidepressants. A measured plasma concentration of 300 μg 1^{-1} ($\approx 1 \times 10^{-6}$ M) in man would be equivalent to about 30 μg 1^{-1} (1×10^{-7} M) in physiologic saline. Although not all authors agree (9), protein binding is usually about 90% (10,11). This being absent, only the free drug molecules are pharmacologically active. Tricyclic antidepressants have also been shown to equilibrate slowly (12) with tissues and at different rates. In atria, for example, amitriptyline reaches a distribution equilibrium within 1 hr, while chlorimipramine is still accumulating in the tissue after 2 hr exposure to a fixed concentration (13). Any extrapolation of *in vitro* animal results to the human situation should be made with these factors in mind; also, consideration must be given to the problem of species difference. Species differences in biotransformation may be largely irrelevant to isolated tissue work, but different species may show other disparities in their biochemistry, which may influence the effects of the tricyclic antidepressants.

Imipramine, for example, reverses the adrenergic neuron-blocking action of gua-nethidine in the dog but not in the rat (14), whereas desmethylimipramine potentiates the effects of norepinephrine on mouse isolated vas deferens but antagonizes its effect on guinea pig vas deferens (5). The cause of these differences is unclear, partly because species difference is not an area of pharmacology which has received extensive study. Indeed, a complete understanding of this area would remove a convenient "last straw" at which pharmacologists clutch when faced with anomolous data.

Tricyclic Compounds

The effects of several tricyclic antidepressants have been compared in a number of relatively uncomplicated isolated preparations, such as the guinea pig (15,16), rat (13), and rabbit (17) atria, cat papillary muscle (18,19), and rat ventricle (20). There is general agreement among workers that at high concentrations ($> 300 \mu g \ l^{-1}; > 1 \times 10^{-6}$ M), the tricyclic antidepressants produce a negative inotropic response and, in preparations showing spontaneous activity, a negative chronotropic effect. This forms the basis for the quinidine-like actions these compounds are said to possess (21) (see Chapter 10). Although some differences have been observed in the effects of tricyclic antidepressants when applied to isolated tissues in low concentrations (13), there is general agreement that at high concentrations, any differences between the compounds are small (22–24).

In isolated guinea pig atria, for example, Dumovic and co-workers (22) found that at equal concentrations (1×10^{-5} M; ≈ 3 mg l^{-1}), there were some statisti-cally significant differences in the abilities of nortriptyline, protriptyline, des-methylimipramine, amitriptyline, imipramine, and doxepin to reduce rate and force of contraction. The maximum mean effect on rate (doxepin and imipramine) was a reduction of about 5%; the maximum mean effect on force (doxepin) was a reduction of about 13%. Differences of this size are unlikely to be clinically significant, especially in view of the fact that in an *in vivo* guinea pig model, doxepin was found to be equivalent to amitriptyline, imipramine, and nortripty-line with respect to effect on the electrocardiogram (EKG) (22).

New Antidepressants

Maprotiline appears to be similar (23) or slightly less cardiodepressant than imipramine, whereas nomifensine has been found to be significantly less cardiode-pressant than either drug (18). Figure 9.2 presents some previously unpublished data produced by one of us (I.H.) at Leeds on the effects of various antidepres-sants on isolated guinea pig atria.

Two preparations were used: the spontaneously beating right atrium (to deter-mine the effects of the antidepressants on heart rate) and the electrically driven or paced left atrium to examine the effects on contractile force. In these prepara-tions, nomifensine was significantly less cardiodepressant than any of the other

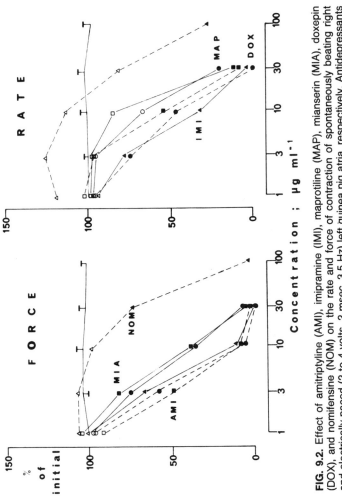

FIG. 9.2. Effect of amitriptyline (AMI), imipramine (IMI), maprotiline (MAP), mianserin (MIA), doxepin (DOX), and nomifensine (NOM) on the rate and force of contraction of spontaneously beating right and electrically paced (2 to 4 volts, 2 msec, 3.5 Hz) left guinea pig atria, respectively. Antidepressants were added cumulatively to the tissue bath; force and rate were measured after 20 min exposure and expressed as a percentage of the initial value in each tissue. The initial rate and force of contraction were 153 ± 4 beats min^{-1} and 0.49 ± 0.03 g, respectively (mean $\pm$ SE, $N = 27$). Four tissues usually contributed to each mean value. Solid points represent values which are statistically significantly different ($p < 0.05$; Student's t-test) from the controls (C; plotted with standard errors), which were not exposed to any drug (Hughes and Lapping, *unpublished*).

drugs. This confirms and extends the results obtained by Biamino (18). With respect to the other drugs, our data support the results of Dumovic et al. (22), who found little difference between several antidepressants in isolated guinea pig atria. Our data suggests, however, that maprotiline and mianserin may be less cardiodepressant than the remaining drugs, since at particular concentrations these newer compounds produced significantly less effect on rate or force than did imipramine or doxepin. The differences are small, and it must be remembered that while these uncomplicated preparations give useful information about the effect of antidepressants on the individual components of the heart, cardiac performance is an expression of the integrated activity of several components, some of which are interdependent to a greater or lesser degree. For this reason, whole hearts isolated form the animal may be more useful in the study of antidepressant cardiotoxicity.

Experiments with Whole Hearts

Whole hearts are usually perfused through the coronary arteries by the technique of Langendorff. Under these conditions, the work output and fluid dynamics of the heart are by no means normal. The small volume of perfusion fluid which reaches the chamber of the right ventricle is vented through the severed pulmonary artery; the left atrium and left ventricle do not receive sufficient fluid to fill; and the aortic valves are maintained closed by the pressure from the perfusion canula inserted in the aorta. These factors may or may not be significant in studies of the cardiotoxicity of antidepressants, but the pressure in the left ventricle is certainly highly significant in the study of the cardiac effects of halothane and epinephrine in isolated hearts (25). In these experiments, dysrhythmias could be induced by epinephrine in the presence of halothane only when the pressure in the left ventricle was raised and ceased when the pressure was returned to the original level, illustrating the importance of this factor under these conditions. It would be interesting to obtain an assessment of the relative cardiotoxicity of tricyclic antidepressants in the isolated heart which is performing work and pumping fluid (26); under these conditions, the fluid dynamics are much closer to the *in vivo* situation.

Antidepressants can be applied to isolated perfused hearts as a bolus dose injected into the perfusion fluid at the entrance to the heart or can be premixed at low concentration in the bulk of the perfusion fluid. Application of the drugs as a bolus dose presents certain problems, since the concentration to which the heart is exposed is not known to any degree of accuracy. This is highly dependent on the speed with which the bolus is injected, its mixing characteristics, and the perfusion flow rate. While these factors are likely to be relatively constant within a given set of experiments, they do complicate comparisons between results obtained by different workers.

A considerable variety of parameters can be recorded from the isolated perfused heart preparation. Workers have recorded various combinations of atrial or ventricular contractile force, dF/dT_{max}, heart rate, coronary flow or perfusion pressure, the interval between peak atrial and peak ventricular tension, EKG, and His bundle electrograms. Using such measurements, there is little difference between the tricyclic antidepressants in the perfused guinea pig (27,28) or rat (29) heart. At concentrations of about 1 mg l^{-1} (3 × 10^{-6} M), desipramine, imipramine, trimipramine, and amitriptyline all produced a negative inotropic effect, a decrease in coronary flow, and a negative chronotropic effect, which was not markedly different for the different drugs (28). Nomifensine, however, has less effect on contractile force than either amitriptyline or imipramine (30). In a similar series of experiments, Dumovic et al. (27) confirmed that imipramine, desipramine, and amitriptyline had similar cardiodepressive actions and showed that nortriptyline and protriptyline were quantitatively similar, while doxepin was slightly more cardiodepressive. EKG records were also taken from these isolated guinea pig hearts and showed that the P-R and QRS intervals were prolonged by all the drugs tested and that the size of the effect was not significantly different for the different drugs. At higher concentrations, a negative chronotropic effect, A-V block, and bizarre QRS complexes were apparent.

Similar types of effect are seen in rabbit heart, which can discriminate between the cardiodepressive actions of some antidepressants. Thus amitriptyline, doxepin, imipramine, noxiptiline, and opipramol (1 to 3 mg l^{-1}; 5 to 10 × 10^{-6} M) all produced reductions in atrial and ventricular systolic tensions, although only doxepin and opipramol produced a negative chronotropic effect, and none of the drugs reduced coronary flow (31). Desipramine and iprindole did not significantly affect atrial or ventricular systolic tensions in these experiments, although earlier work from the same laboratory (under slightly different conditions) had shown that desipramine reduced atrial and ventricular systolic tensions, while iprindole reduced ventricular systolic tension only (32). In the rabbit heart model, some of the newer antidepressants were less cardiotoxic than the traditional tricyclic antidepressants. Figure 9.3 shows results obtained in perfused rabbit heart, by methods described elsewhere (33), with maprotiline and mianserin in comparison with amitriptyline and imipramine.

Clearly, at equal concentrations (1.5 mg l^{-1}; 4.8 × 10^{-6} M), amitriptyline and imipramine reduced ventricular and atrial systolic tensions, while maprotiline affected only ventricular systolic tension, and mianserin affected neither. The lengthening of the interval between peak atrial and peak ventricular tension, which could be interpreted as a slowing of a A-V conduction, was quite marked with imipramine and amitriptyline but was not seen to the same extent with maprotiline; in contrast, mianserin produced a slight shortening of this interval.

Production of Dysrhythmias

Barth and co-workers (31,32) have investigated the interaction between norepinephrine and tricyclic antidepressants on the heart. It has been suggested that the ability of the tricyclic antidepressants to block norepinephrine uptake may

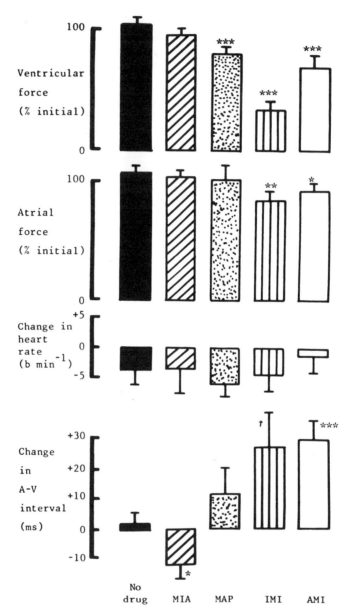

FIG. 9.3. Effects in isolated rabbit heart of a 15-min perfusion with amitriptyline, imipramine, maprotiline, or mianserin, each at a concentration of 4.8×10^{-6}M, on ventricular systolic force, atrial systolic force, heart rate, and the interval between peak atrial and ventricular tensions (A-V interval). Solid columns show the changes produced by perfusion with physiologic saline alone. Statistically significant differences are represented as follows (Student's *t*-test): ***p < 0.001; **p < 0.01 > 0.001; *p < 0.05 > 0.01; †p < 0.1 > 0.05. For detailed methods, see ref. 51.

sensitize the heart to the dysrhythmogenic actions of norepinephrine (34), and that this may account for the dysrhythmias produced by these drugs. The authors found that when sympathetic nerve stimulation or concentrations of norepinephrine which were not in themselves dysrhythmogenic were applied in the presence of various tricyclic antidepressants at concentrations which were also not dysrhythmogenic, the combination did precipitate dysrhythmias. Thus, in the presence of tricyclic antidepressants, the heart was sensitized to the production of dysrhythmias by norepinephrine. Dysrhythmias were not precipitated by combinations of norepinephrine with either atropine (indicating that cholinoceptor blocking properties are not involved) or with cocaine applied in concentrations that were effective in blocking norepinephrine uptake. The relationship between the relative ability of the tricyclic antidepressants to block norepinephrine uptake and to precipitate norepinephrine-induced dysrhythmias was not a close one, leading Barth and his co-workers to conclude that the abilities to inhibit norepinephrine uptake and to precipitate norepinephrine-induced dysrhythmias were not causally related.

This conclusion is supported by other evidence. If the dysrhythmias are due to a blockade of norepinephrine uptake, producing increased concentrations of norepinephrine within the tissue, then the application of very high concentrations or norepinephrine alone should have the same effect, but this is not so (31,33). Occasionally, when dysrhythmias did occur with high concentrations of norepinephrine, they were not of the same type as those seen with the norepinephrine-tricyclic antidepressant combination. In addition, mianserin, in a concentration that greatly inhibits the uptake of $[^3H]$-(-)-norepinephrine (33), did not predispose the heart to the dysrhythmogenic action of norepinephrine. This can be seen from Fig. 9.4, where the effect is shown of perfusion of the rabbit heart with increasing concentrations of norepinephrine in the presence of amitriptyline, imipramine, maprotiline, or mianserin. In control tissues receiving no drug and in those perfused with mianserin, norepinephrine produced a shortening of the interval between the peak atrial and peak ventricular tensions; no dysrhythmias were seen. In contrast, with amitriptyline, imipramine, and maprotiline, norepinephrine lengthened the interval between peak tensions and induced dysrhythmias in most hearts.

Comparative Effects of Different Antidepressants

Experiments on isolated tissues indicate that many of the older tricyclic antidepressants have a similar degree of cardiotoxicity, while some of the newer agents, e.g., nomifensine and mianserin, have less harmful effects on the heart at similar concentrations. One disturbing feature of all the work done in isolated tissues with respect to cardiotoxicity at therapeutic plasma levels is the concentration used in the experiments. In poisoning, plasma levels of amitriptyline may be very high (35) but in therapeutic use only rarely exceed 300 μg 1^{-1} (1×10^{-6} M) and are usually much lower (36,37). Allowing for 90% plasma binding

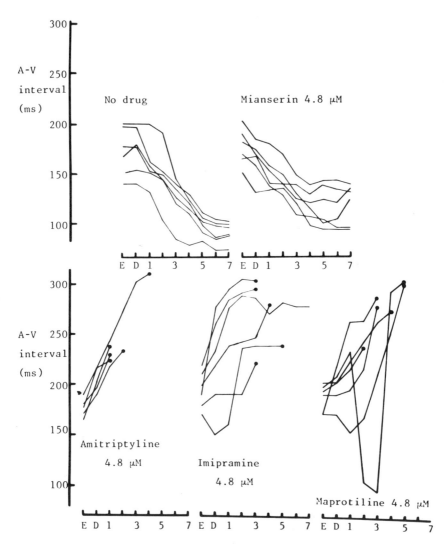

FIG. 9.4. Interval between peak atrial and peak ventricular tensions (A-V interval) in individual isolated perfused rabbit hearts after equilibration with physiologic saline (E), after 15 min perfusion with a drug when appropriate (D), and after further perfusion for 5 min each with seven concentrations of (-)-norepinephrine (1 to 7; 0.0059, 0.019, 0.059, 0.19, 0.59, 1.9, and 5.9 × 10⁻⁶M). Note the effect of norepinephrine to shorten the A-V interval in the absence of drugs or in the presence of mianserin, while in the presence of amitriptyline, imipramine, or maprotiline, this interval is lengthened. Solid points show when dysrhythmias developed in each heart (after which the A-V interval could not be determined). Note that dysrhythmias were not seen during norepinephrine treatment of hearts perfused with physiologic saline alone or with mianserin but were frequently seen in hearts perfused with amitriptyline, imipramine, or maprotiline. For methodology, see ref. 51.

(10,11), this represents a concentration in physiologic saline of about 1×10^{-7} M (30 μg l^{-1}), at least 10-fold less than that used in most experiments. One other feature of these experiments, particularly in relation to cardiotoxicity at therapeutic dose levels, is that all these isolated tissue experiments involve acute administration of the antidepressants, whereas chronic exposure is the rule in the human therapeutic situation. Despite these reservations, some of the newer antidepressants are significantly less toxic in these models than the more traditional tricyclic antidepressants.

IN VIVO MODELS

As with isolated tissue experiments, a number of considerations are particularly pertinent to cardiotoxicity studies in vivo in the whole animal.

Routes of Administration

The oral route is the usual route of administration of tricyclic antidepressants in man. After therapeutic doses, plasma levels peak at between 2 and 8 hr, depending on the particular antidepressant (37–40). Presumably, plasma levels follow a similar time course after a massive oral overdose, and oral dosing of animals with tricyclic antidepressants has been used (41) to try to mimic this situation. The inherent variability of absorption from the gastrointestinal tract, however, is likely to introduce considerable variation into the experimental results and necessitate the use of large groups to obtain useful comparative data. The intraperitoneal and intramuscular routes are likely to give peak plasma levels more quickly than the oral route; intravenous bolus dosing will give high plasma levels very quickly. None of these parenteral routes will mimic the plasma concentration/time picture seen in man.

A slow intravenous infusion, extending over several hours, is likely to produce steadily rising plasma levels, which will mimic the situation in man after tricyclic antidepressant overdose. This method of administration will also give comparatively constant results from animal to animal by eliminating the variability associated with gastrointestinal absorption; for these reasons, it has been used by several workers. The route of administration will not only affect the plasma concentration/time picture but may also affect the biotransformation of the antidepressant. Extensive hepatic biotransformation can be expected after oral administration of tricyclic antidepressants; a first pass effect has been demonstrated for a number of such drugs (see ref. 42 for references). Biotransformation in the liver may be less extensive after parenteral administration, since the portal circulation is effectively bypassed. This may have a bearing on the cardiotoxicity, as metabolites may play an important role in the overall cardiotoxicity of a drug (43).

Biotransformation may not only be affected by the route of administration but is also markedly different in different species (44). The dog, for example, excretes about three times more 10-hydroxyamitriptyline than 10-hydroxynor-triptyline, whereas in man, the 10-hydroxynortriptyline metabolite predominates after amitriptyline administration (45). In the rat, rabbit, and mouse, the plasma half-life of imipramine is approximately 2½, 2, and 1 hr, respectively, and all three species produce the active metabolite desmethylimipramine to some extent. The plasma half-life of desmethylimipramine in the three species is approximately 9, 1, and 0.9 hr, respectively, which means that desmethylimipramine will accu-mulate in the rat but not in the rabbit or mouse.

The metabolism of imipramine in man is closer to that in the rat, since man also accumulates desmethylimipramine after treatment with imipramine (46). The difficulties this type of problem creates are further complicated by the fact that what is really important is the tissue burden of the parent compound and/or metabolites, which will be determined not only by absorption and by various biotransformations but also by excretion rates, which may again be species dependent. Age may also play a role in that cardiac effects in old rats are more severe than those seen in younger rats (47); in the case of nortriptyline, however, that is probably related to the higher plasma levels found in older animals (48).

The initial hemodynamic state of the animal may also be important in that dogs with moderate hypertension showed EKG changes at lower doses of imipra-mine than did control animals (49). Part of this effect could be due to a stress factor. The interaction between tricyclic antidepressants and stress is described in the previous chapter, wherein Davidson showed that when rats with cardiomy-opathies were treated with tricyclic antidepressants, the application of a noise stress increased the incidence of death from 2 to 6% to 70 to 90%, a very dramatic effect.

Experimental Methods

One fundamental decision that must be made at the start of any *in vivo* animal work is whether to use an anesthetic and, if so, which anesthetic. Con-scious animals are usually more difficult to handle technically; other toxic effects of the antidepressants, such as convulsions, may interfere with the recording of cardiac parameters (50). The use of drugs, such as neuromuscular blocking agents, to produce paralysis and eliminate this problem is closely restricted in some countries and may produce unsuspected additional complications (51–53). The procedure may so stress the animal that results become grossly distorted. The presence of an anesthetic may materially alter the cardiotoxicity of tricyclic antidepressants. Urethane, for example, has been shown to greatly reduce the signs of cardiotoxicity seen in dogs after large doses of imipramine (54). Some halogenated hydrocarbons, such as halothane, are known to sensitize the heart to the dysrhythmogenic action of the catecholamines (55) and are probably best avoided even for preexperimental insertion of canulae; halothane, in particu-lar, is known to remain in the body for extended periods of time (56). Barbiturates may produce enhanced respiratory depression with tricyclic antidepressants (57), and particular care must be taken to maintain adequate respiration.

Animal experiments designed to assess cardiotoxicity in overdose present fewer problems than those designed to assess cardiotoxicity at therapeutic dose levels. Although the acute overdose situation can reasonably be mimicked in naive animals, therapeutic doses are given chronically, and animal experiments should mimic this situation. Chronic treatment may alter metabolite and parent drug levels in tissues (58). Glisson and co-workers (59) have shown that chronic treatment of cats with 1.5 mg kg^{-1} i.m. amitriptyline twice daily produced ST and T wave abnormalities which developed only in the second and third weeks of treatment. It is not clear if the basic cause underlying this observation is pharmacokinetic or if some tissue change was produced by chronic administration.

Finally, species variations in the control of cardiac function may play an important role. Primary neuronal tone to the heart in man is vagal, and atropinics increase heart rate by vagal release. In the rat, primary neuronal tone is sympathetic, and atropinics will have little effect on heart rate. All these factors must be considered when interpreting the applicability to man of cardiotoxicity data derived from animal work *in vivo*.

ASSESSMENT OF CARDIOTOXICITY

As with isolated tissues, no single *in vivo* method has become accepted as the best method to assess cardiotoxicity; many methods have been used, and experiments have been carried out in mice (60), rats (47,48), guinea pigs (61), rabbits (50), cats (62), and dogs (63,64). At very low doses, the tricyclic antidepressants produce an increase in heart rate, contractility, blood pressure, coronary and aortic flow, and automaticity (60,64). Both the atropinic and the norepinephrine uptake blocking properties of these drugs may be involved in these effects (65). At higher doses, there is general agreement that heart rate is reduced, blood pressure falls, automaticity is decreased, the PQ and PR intervals lengthen, the width of the QRS complex is increased, and changes in the T wave occur (47,64,66–68). Ventricular extrasystoles, bigeminy, trigeminy, A-V block, and ventricular fibrillation may all be seen (47,67).

The EKG changes and dysrhythmias found in animals are similar to those seen in man and occur at plasma levels within the range found in overdose patients (69,48). Quantitatively, imipramine, amitriptyline, nortriptyline, and doxepin appear to be only marginally different in their cardiotoxicity (61,47,64), although not all workers concur (70). Chlorimipramine (71) and protriptyline (72) have both been claimed to be less cardiotoxic in the models in which they were tested. Of the newer tricyclics, iprindole has less effect on ventricular and atrial conduction velocity or ventricular excitability than does imipramine, but iprindole is not without cardiotoxicity, since a significant prolongation of the A-V conduction time has been seen (73). Nomifensine is required in higher dose and produces smaller changes in the PQ interval in the guinea pig EKG than does either amitriptyline or imipramine (30). Table 9.1 shows the relative activity of imipramine and amitriptyline and two of the newer antidepressants, maprotiline and mianserin, on the cardiovascular system during continuous slow intravenous infusion into barbiturate-anesthetized rabbits.

Clearly, much higher doses of mianserin were needed to produce similar changes in the PR interval and in the width of the QRS complex than were needed with any of the other three drugs. It might be expected that with mianserin a similar low level of cardiotoxicity would be seen in man. Clinical experience to date indicates that this is indeed so. A comparison of the doses required to produce standard changes in heart rate and blood pressure indicates that the cardiovascular toxicity is also of a low order.

With respect to the production of dysrhythmias by the antidepressants, in these anesthetized rabbits, different types of dysrhythmia were seen, as is the case in man after gross overdose with tricyclic antidepressants. The number of experimental animals was too small and the variety of dysrhythmias too large to allow a proper analysis of the incidence of the different dysrhythmias with the different antidepressants; ventricular ectopic beats were seen least frequently with mianserin, which was required in much larger doses before any dysrhythmias were seen. In conscious rabbits (74), missing QRS complexes were seen in the EKG records from six of six animals infused with amitriptyline, in six of six with maprotiline, in two of six with imipramine, but in none in mianserin-treated rabbits; the potential to induce cardiac dysrhythmias is comparatively low with mianserin.

TABLE 9.1. *Effect of various antidepressants on PR interval, width of the QRS complex, heart rate, and blood pressure in barbiturate-anesthetized rabbits*

Dose required to produce	Amitriptyline ($N = 7$)	Imipramine ($N = 7$)	Maprotiline ($N = 6$)	Mianserin ($N = 6$)
20% Increase in the PR interval	12.2 ± 2.5 (6)	18.7 ± 7.6 (6)	21.4 ± 3.0 (6)	161.4 ± 2.0 (2)
20% Increase in the width of the QRS complex	2.6 ± 0.8 (7)	11.2 ± 6.0 (7)	7.1 ± 1.0 (6)	80.0 ± 1.0 (6)
50% Increase in the width of the QRS complex	7.4 ± 2.0 (7)	19.9 ± 5.8 (7)	18.0 ± 3.0 (6)	165.1 ± 1.0 (4)
30 Beat min⁻¹ reduction in heart rate	12.2 ± 3.1 (7)	12.8 ± 3.7 (7)	33.9 ± 7.5 (6)	41.9 ± 6.0 (6)
15 mm Hg fall in mean arterial blood pressure	15.0 ± 4.0 (7)	29.0 ± 10.5 (7)	33.9 ± 6.5 (6)	144.0 ± 3.0 (4)

The values shown represent the mean ± SE of the dose (mg kg⁻¹) which produced the given effect in the number of animals shown by the figures in parentheses. Note that very high doses of mianserin were required compared with the other drugs, and that not all experimental animals (particularly in the mianserin group) showed an effect of the required magnitude before the experiment was terminated. For detailed methods, see ref. 69.

Role of Catecholamines

A number of workers have investigated the involvement of catecholamines in the cardiac changes produced by tricyclic antidepressants in the whole animal. Élonen et al. (75) have shown that the relative ability to potentiate the pressor effect of norepinephrine in rabbits (i.e., to sensitize to the actions of catecholamines) is: protriptyline > nortriptyline > amitriptyline > doxepin, while the relative ability to induce changes in the EKG is: amitriptyline > doxepin > nortriptyline > protriptyline. Thus the author failed to show any direct correlation between these two effects.

Furthermore, the EKG changes produced by these drugs were not markedly altered by administration of the drugs during an infusion of norepinephrine, in contrast to the result which might be expected if sensitization to the effects of norepinephrine was involved (72). Forika and her co-workers (62) have shown that imipramine antagonizes norepinephrine-induced extrasystoles in rabbits and that electrographic repolarization perturbances caused by norepinephrine and ·isoprenaline are not affected by imipramine in cats. Finally, Thorstrand and co-workers (66) have shown that lengthening of the PQ interval and widening of the QRS complex produced by amitriptyline are unaffected by prior administration of propranolol, indicating that β-adrenoceptors are not involved in these effects. However, other workers have found that pretreatment with propanolol is effective in preventing some of the cardiotoxic effects of amitriptyline (76), which is in keeping with Davidson's experimental findings described in the previous chapter.

This evidence, together with the evidence derived from experiments on isolated tissues, casts doubt on the suggestion that the cardiotoxicity of the tricyclic antidepressants is entirely due to their ability to block norepinephrine uptake and thus sensitize the heart to the dysrhythmogenic action of the catecholamines. It seems more likely that the primary effect is through a direct depressant effect on the heart to slow atrial, atrioventricular, and intraventricular conduction (77). If these systems are not affected equally, then endogenous catecholamines may provoke increased rates of pacemaker firing at various levels. Combined with the quinidine-like effects outlined above, these will be sufficient to induce a variety of dysrhythmias, depending on the particular balance of influences exerted on the heart at the particular time.

Whatever the mechanism, the animal studies confirm the considerable cardiotoxic potential of the tricyclic antidepressants. The studies also indicate that not all anitdepressants are likley to show an equivalent cardiotoxicity in man. Although many of the older tricyclic antidepressants show approximately equal cardiotoxicity, this is not true of the newer antidepressants. The experiments with mianserin, for example, indicate a substantially reduced cardiotoxicity on a weight for weight basis, compared with other antidepressants. This reduced toxicity is likely to be reinforced by the fact that the daily dose of mianserin is somewhat lower than that of other antidepressants. If there is a risk of overdose, mianserin would provide a safer alternative than the more traditional tricyclic antidepressants.

HUMAN STUDIES

It has been said that the proper study of mankind is man; this statement has a certain relevance to studies on the cardiotoxicity of the tricyclic antidepressants. From the above sections, it is clear that unambiguously relevant experiments on cardiotoxicity can only be performed in man, but only in more recent years have suitable methods become available for this purpose.

Pharmacokinetic Background

Detailed pharmacokinetic investigations of the antidepressants have been carried out for relatively few of the drugs currently available, and only nortriptyline and imipramine have been well evaluated. This subject has been reviewed by Gram (78). Studies of absorption, distribution, elimination, and metabolism of bi-, tri-, and tetracyclic antidepressants show wide interindividual differences, as well as wide differences between drugs. These are some general unifying principles.

After oral administration, the tricyclics are almost completely absorbed from the gastrointestinal tract. Within 30 min blood levels of the drug are detectable, and peak plasma concentrations are observed within 2 to 6 hr after dosing (79). A significant first-pass effect has been demonstrated for the tricyclics. The systemic availability of these drugs is low, usually less than 80% but in some cases less than 50%. Most tricyclics have a large apparent volume of distribution, in the range of 10 to 60 liters/kg, indicating a significant degree of tissue binding, and also are usually highly bound to plasma proteins. Up to 90% of the drug present in plasma may be bound to protein, but protein binding of the tricyclics is significantly altered in the presence of other drugs. All tricyclics undergo extensive metabolic degradation in the liver (the first-pass effect). Tertiary amine tricyclics are demethylated to their corresponding secondary amine, hydroxylation and conjugation to glucuronic acid occurs, N-oxidation occurs to a minor extent, and secondary amines are demethylated to their primary amine counterpart. Complete side chain dealkylation may also occur (80). The pharmacologic activity of all of these metabolites has not been systematically investigated.

Most of an oral dose of a tricyclic is excreted in the urine, of which about 70 to 90% is recovered, largely as the glucuronide, while fecal elimination accounts for the rest of the dose. The tricyclics undergo a relatively slow elimination from the body, plasma elimination half-lives ($t\frac{1}{2}\beta$) varying widely, depending on the drug. Some representative ranges are: imipramine, 10 to 16 hr; desipramine, 12 to 77 hr; amitriptyline, 40 to 75 hr; and nortriptyline, 15 to 90 hr. Steady state levels of tricyclics are usually achieved within 7 to 10 days after commencing an oral dosage regimen (81,82), and therapeutic response is normally achieved at about this time (83). There is a wide range of steady state plasma levels of the tricyclics in different individuals receiving the same dose. Much of this variability can be accounted for by genetic factors (84).

TOXICITY IN MAN

A great variety of symptoms have been reported after the ingestion of an overdose of a tricyclic antidepressant. Typically, these include disorientation, ataxia, vomiting, coma, convulsions, EKG changes, and dysrhythmias (85). Since some of the tricyclic antidepressants show an affinity for myocardial tissue (69,86,87), it is not surprising that a large proportion of individuals experiencing overdose of these drugs show signs of cardiotoxicity. Thorstrand (88), for example, found that 49 and 42% of 153 unselected patients hospitalized because of tricyclic antidepressant overdose showed changes in the QT interval and in the width of the QRS complex, respectively. Freeman et al. (89) found in similar patients that 10 of 10 showed a prolonged QT time. In a further series of 30 admissions for tricyclic antidepressant poisoning (90), EKG records were taken in 21 patients; 19 were abnormal (mainly prolonged QT), and at least eight were not within normal limits 24 to 48 hr later. This is compelling evidence for a serious cardiotoxicity in overdose. Even at therapeutic dose levels, there is strong evidence to show that changes in cardiac parameters may occur with nortriptyline (91,61), imipramine (92,93), clomipramine (94), and amitriptyline (95,96), although these changes are not apparent in all patients (86,97). Using surface EKG recording and in other studies using His bundle electrocardiography, one of us (61) found that intracardiac conduction was prolonged in patients taking therapeutic doses of tricyclic antidepressants. Taylor and Braithwaite (91), using systolic time interval measurements, found changes indicating that a deterioration in cardiac function occurred with nortriptyline which was correlated with the plasma level.

Possible changes in cardiac parameters occurring at therapeutic dose levels are, of course, highly relevant to the problem of treating the depressed patient with a preexisting cardiac disorder. In tricyclic antidepressant overdose, the effects produced by the cardiotoxicity of these drugs can be most dangerous and may be difficult to correct (98) (see also Chapter 10). This necessitates continuous cardiac monitoring of the patient for many days, as sudden death, possibly associated with cardiac problems, has been reported as long as 4 to 6 days after the ingestion of an overdose of tricyclic antidepressant (99,100).

Effects of Therapeutic Doses

Epidemiologic studies have documented the cardiovascular side effects of the tricyclics, and these have been the subject of a number of reviews (65,86,88, 89,101–103). For example, the Boston Collaborative Drug Surveillance Program (101) reported on 260 patients who received tricyclic antidepressant therapy for depression (81% of patients), anxiety (13%), and other indications (6%). Of these, 237 patients received amitriptyline or imipramine, and the remainder received desipramine, protriptyline, or nortriptyline. The incidence of sudden death and the death rate did not differ between these patients and a similar group of hospitalized patients from the same wards, who did not receive antidepressants. Similarly, the survey found no difference in cardiotoxicity between 80 patients with cardiovascular disease receiving tricyclics and 3,994 patients with cardiovascular disease not receiving tricyclics. The incidence of arrhythmias, shock, syncope, heart block, hypotension, and congestive cardiac failure was the same. Mortality for the tricyclic-treated group was 5%; for the untreated group, it was 8%.

This apparent lack of cardiotoxic effects of the antidepressants is in contrast to the Aberdeen General Hospital Group studies (102,103). A group of 864 inpatients who were admitted during a 40-month period and who received amitriptyline were observed. Of these, 119 had a diagnosis of cardiac disease and were matched by age, sex, cardiac diagnosis, and length of hospitalization with a group of patients not taking antidepressants. In the amitriptyline group, there were 23 deaths (19% patients), compared with 15 deaths (12%) in the control group. This difference was not statistically significant. When compared for sudden unexpected cardiac death, 13 of 23 amitriptyline deaths met the criteria, compared with three of 15 controls, a significant difference. A further investigation of 87 cardiac patients receiving imipramine compared with 87 control patients revealed four unexpected deaths in the imipramine group, compared with two in the control group.

These retrospective studies have several methodologic flaws, such as the definition of sudden unexpected death, the use of appropriate controls, and the lower than usual average daily dose of 72 mg, compared to 150 mg in the Boston study. Both studies serve to point out the dangers associated with chronic tricyclic administration. Some earlier studies and some which followed these surveys have concentrated on changes seen in the EKG in patients receiving tricyclics.

EKG Changes

Numerous individual case reports of EKG abnormalities during tricyclic antidepressant therapy have been documented, but many of these cases are of patients who received multidrug administration during treatment. In such cases, it is difficult to decide which agent caused the observed change; such cases are not discussed here. There are fewer studies of EKG changes during pure tricyclic therapy. These are summarized in Table 9.2.

The general pattern of EKG changes which emerges from these studies is of ST-T wave changes, increases in PR and QRS width, bundle branch block, and sinus tachycardia. These changes are reversible in patients without preexisting heart disease when the drugs are withdrawn.

TABLE 9.2. *EKG effects of therapeutic doses of tricyclic antidepressant drugs*

Patient population	Drug[a] and dose	EKG findings	Ref.
23 Patients	IMI up to 200 mg/day	In 15 patients, there were alterations in the EKG which were often first manifest or were aggravated by physical exercise: "stress or cardiovascular disease may predispose to IMI-induced EKG changes."	92
82 Patients	IMI 75–200 mg/day	Serial EKGs over a treatment period of 30 days revealed no direct drug effect. The "changes that did occur could be explained by the presence of complicating factors."	163
36 Adults 15 Adults	AMI DMI "Ordinary therapeutic doses"	T wave changes (flattening, isoelectricity, inversion) in two patients on AMI. These changes were fully reversible and "did not produce any cardiac symptoms." There were no changes with DMI. Ten patients with an abnormal control EKG had no changes during treatment.	154
65 Patients (x̄ = 60 yr age)	AMI 75–225 mg/day	Treatment of 3 weeks or more during which one or more EKG was taken revealed EKG changes in 18% of patients. These included isoelectric T waves, ST segment depression, and frequent extrasystoles. "Possible changes in 32%, no changes in 50%."	164
40 Patients (20–72 yr)	NT 75–150 mg/day	After 3 weeks of drug therapy, the EKG at rest and during exercise revealed no direct effects except in one patient who developed a right bundle branch block during the work test (EKG response to exercise testing after drug withdrawal was normal).	105
40 Patients (x̄ = 50 yr age)	DOX range of daily doses (x̄ = 150 mg/day)	One or more EKG over 18 to 41 months revealed some transient tachycardia in five patients. Otherwise, "no adverse cardiac effects were detected clinically or electrographically."	165
14 Children with enuresis (5–10 yr)	IMI 25–75 mg/day	No significant changes in serial EKGs.	166
30 Patients	"Recommended" doses of tricyclics for >3 weeks	Nonspecific flattening of T waves. Two patients developed primary heart block (reversible in one case).	167
27 Children with enuresis (5–12 yr)	IMI 25–75 mg/day	"No substantial EKG changes."	168

TABLE 9.2. (cont.)

Patient population	Drug[a] and dose	EKG findings	Ref.
32 Patients (19–57 yr)	NT IMI AMI DOX 75–400 mg/day (x̄ = 175 mg/day)	Moderate increase in heart rate; mild increase in PR interval; and no significant effect on the QTc. Repolarization changes in four patients.	97
12 Patients	NT 150 and 200 mg/day	Distal atrioventricular conduction (H-V interval) increased in five patients after 2 weeks of therapy.	107
Seven children with hyperkinetic/aggressive behavior disorders (7–10 yr)	IMI 5 mg/kg/day	In all cases, the repolarization phase was affected (decreased T wave amplitude and increased T wave width). Three children evidenced primary A-V block.	169
Nine patients (>65 yr)	IMI 75–100 mg/day	An increased heart rate: "clinical meaningful changes were observed in four patients." Two developed sinus tachycardia, one developed nonspecific ST-T wave abnormalities, and one developed left axis deviation and complete bundle branch block.	170
47 Patients (x̄ = 43 yr age)	AMI IMI MAP MIA TRI 40–300 mg/day	No serious disturbances of cardiac rhythm after 3 weeks of therapy. Increases in PR and QRS proved reversible after drug withdrawal.	171
15 Patients (18–50 yr)	AMI 75–200 mg/day (x̄ = 132 mg/day)	Significant increase in heart rate (mean increase, 16/min). Those patients having rate change >16/min had significantly higher AMI and AMI + NT plasma levels.	109
17 Patients (20–65 yr)	NT 50–150 mg/day	Significant increases in heart rate and nonspecific ST-T wave changes during treatment. Weak positive correlation between the change in heart rate and the plasma NT level ($r = 0.46$; $p < 0.05$; one-tailed test).	108

Subjects	Drug/dose	Results	Ref.
27 Female patients ($\bar{x}$ = 32 yr age)	AMI (100–200 mg/day, $N = 14$) MIA (80–100 mg/day, $N = 13$)	EKGs recorded before and after 3 weeks of drug treatment revealed an increase in heart rate and PR interval in 12 and 11 of the 14 AMI patients, respectively.	137
Eight healthy male volunteers (20–40 yr)	IMI 0.5 mg/kg i.v. infused/30 min.	Slight increase in heart rate. H-V interval increased to pathologic values in two volunteers; there was prolongation of repolarization in the ventricle.	172
66 Patients (20 men, 46 women)	AMI IMI MAP MIA TRI (40–300 mg/day)	After 3 weeks of therapy, heart rate and PR interval were increased ($p < 0.02$; $p < 0.05$). Significant flattening of the T wave was also noted. When therapy was maintained for 13 months, only heart rate continued to be increased; all other values had returned to normal.	139
Seven patients (six had prior ECG abnormalities)	IMI 175–400 mg/day ($\bar{x}$ = 271 mg/day)	Slight increases in heart rate, PR, QRS, and QTc intervals (see text).	111

[a] AMI, amitriptyline; DMI, desipramine; DOX, doxepin; IMI, imipramine; MAP, maprotiline; MIA, mianserin; NT, nortriptyline; TRI, trimipramine.

Influence of Drug Plasma Levels

In addition to monitoring EKG changes, some studies have monitored drug plasma levels, since it has been suggested by some authors that plasma levels of the tricyclics are correlated with their clinical effect. Others have found no correlation, and the subject has recently been reviewed in detail (104). There is a general consensus that there must be a lower limit of plasma concentrations, below which no clinical response is manifest, and an upper limit, beyond which toxic symptoms become apparent. The debate revolves around the key issue of the upper limit to the therapeutic range. In this respect, the cardiologic studies may resolve the issue.

Freyschuss et al. (105) studied 40 depressed patients (19 males and 21 females) treated with nortriptyline (either 75 mg/day, eight cases, or 150 mg/day, 32 cases). Mean steady state nortriptyline levels were 47 ng/ml for the 75 mg group and 93 ng/ml for the 150 mg group. Heart rate and blood pressure increased during drug treatment. In one patient (a 51-year-old male), a right bundle branch block appeared, but when drug therapy was withdrawn, his EKG returned to normal. In the remaining patients, the EKG records showed no signs of adverse effects of nortriptyline. Plasma levels did not correlate with the increase in pulse rate observed.

EKG changes were studied by one of us (106) in a group of 32 patients receiving various doses of amitriptyline, nortriptyline, imipramine, and doxepin. Plasma levels were determined in the 20 patients who received nortriptyline, the mean plasma concentration being 182 ng/ml (range, 60 to 392 ng/ml). Heart rate increased in 26 of the 32 patients. This increase tended to be greater when the pretreatment heart rate was slow. The PR interval increased in all subjects after drug administration; there were no significant changes in the QT interval; and the ST-T wave changes were considered unremarkable. Three patients on nortriptyline showed prolongation of the QRS, which did not occur with the patients receiving other drugs. There was no correlation between plasma nortriptyline levels and increased heart rate or PR interval. It was tentatively suggested that doxepin had less effect on the cardiovascular system than nortriptyline.

Relative Cardiotoxicity of Different Tricyclics

We also undertook intracardiac conduction studies using His bundle electrography (HBE). These provide some support for the hypothesis that doxepin is less cardiotoxic than nortriptyline and suggest that plasma levels of nortriptyline in excess of 200 ng/ml are more often associated with cardiac abnormalities (107). The relationship between the HBE and the standard EKG is shown in Fig. 9.5.

HBE studies were carried out in 12 patients before and at least 2 weeks

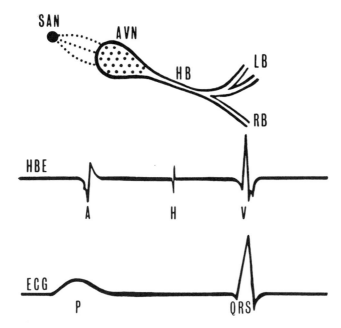

FIG. 9.5. HBE with the standard EKG. An anatomic model of the conduction system at the top of the figure is orientated to show the sites of origin of the electrical waves. The A-H and H-V intervals represent proximal and distal intracardiac conduction, respectively.

after they had been on therapeutic doses of nortriptyline (150 mg/day, 11 cases; 200 mg/day, one case). Plasma for nortriptyline determination was collected at the same time as the HBE recordings were made; the mean nortriptyline level was 209 ng/ml (range, 75 to 490 ng/ml). Five patients showed significant prolongation of the H-V interval, and of these four had plasma levels in excess of 200 ng/ml. The effect on the A-V conduction was variable. We suggest that prolongation of the H-V interval may account for the increased incidence of sudden deaths that have been reported in cardiac patients taking tricyclics (102, 103).

This study also provided some tentative evidence for the comparative safety of doxepin. In one patient initially treated with 200 mg nortriptyline daily and later changed to 200 mg doxepin daily, HBEs were performed before and after 2 weeks on each drug. Initial A-H and H-V intervals were normal but increased markedly on nortriptyline (plasma level, 260 ng/ml) and returned to normal on doxepin. QRS width also returned to normal on doxepin.

In a subsequent study (106), we compared the effects of therapeutic doses of doxepin and nortriptyline on intracardiac conduction. After a 1-week placebo period, 17 depressed patients with no history of cardiac disease were randomly allocated to treatment with 150 mg nortriptyline or 150 mg doxepin daily. After 3 weeks of treatment, patients were allowed a 10-day washout period and then crossed over to the other drug. Pretreatment EKGs showed no significant abnormalities.

In six cases, there was a significant prolongation of the QRS complex while receiving nortriptyline, but this was only observed in one case on doxepin; there was no correlation between plasma levels with either drug and QRS prolongation. Doxepin plasma levels were, on the whole, much lower than those of nortriptyline. This may explain the apparent lack of effect *in vivo. In vitro* doxepin has been shown to be at least as cardiotoxic as the other tricyclics, if not more so (22,27,32). Levels of the desmethyl metabolite of doxepin were also low (mean, 22 ng/ml), so that total levels of active compounds did not approach the nortriptyline levels. A lower bioavailability of doxepin might account for its apparent lack of cardiotoxicity.

Ziegler et al. (108) also noted cardiographic abnormalities in a study of 17 depressed patients treated with nortriptyline for 3 weeks. In two patients, clinically significant EKG abnormalities developed during treatment, while in a 65-year-old male, a first degree heart block developed (plasma nortriptyline, 129, ng/ml). Premature ventricular contractions were observed in a 33-year-old female (plasma nortriptyline, 176 ng/ml), but this abnormality disappeared when her dose was halved and her plasma level fell to 80 ng/ml. There was a significant correlation between plasma nortriptyline level and change in heart rate for the group as a whole. In another study by the same investigators (109), 15 patients were treated with amitriptyline (75 to 200 mg/day) for 3 weeks. Heart rate increased significantly, and patients with high plasma amitriptyline or high total plasma tricyclic levels (amitriptyline + nortriptyline) were those who most often experienced the greatest increase in heart rate.

Kantor et al. (110) reported the case of a 74-year-old man with a 3-year history of right bundle branch block treated with 200 mg imipramine daily. Heart block occurred when total plasma tricyclic level was 220 ng/ml. The drug was stopped, and intermittent 2:1 atrioventricular block occurred as the plasma level fell. Finally, the block disappeared as the plasma level fell to 150 ng/ml. On recommencing treatment, however, heart block occurred at almost an identical plasma drug concentration. In a further study of seven depressed patients (six with prior EKG abnormalities) treated with imipramine daily (111), mean heart rate, determined by computer analysis of the continuous 24-hr EKG recordings, increased significantly but slightly in each patient. There were also significant increases in PR, QRS, and QT intervals, although plasma tricyclic levels in these patients remained within the therapeutic bounds for this compound.

As a general conclusion from these studies, usual doses of the tricyclics can lead to EKG changes in some patients, and these changes are most likely to be associated with high plasma levels of the drug. Plasma level monitoring, on the other hand, is not necessarily a guide to EKG changes.

EFFECTS OF OVERDOSAGE

Overdosages with the tricyclics were reported as soon as the drugs were introduced into clinical practice, the first lethal one in 1959 (112), just 1 year after Kuhn introduced imipramine therapy (113). The subsequent increase in tricyclic overdosage (see Fig. 9.1 for the English experience) has prompted at least one author to say: "poisoning with this class of drugs is no longer a rare curiosity but rather a serious problem with which many emergency physicians, toxicologists or forensic scientists are confronted" (114).

The EKG features of tricyclic overdosage include prolongation of intra- and atrioventricular conduction, sinus tachycardia, prolongation of the corrected QT interval, ST-T wave abnormalities, including ST deviation, which may stimulate acute myocardial infarction, ventricular arrhythmias, profound bradycardia, supraventricular tachycardia, and asystole (115). Some or all of these complications are observed in tricyclic overdosage, but it is apparent from the studies reported that tricyclic poisoning is unpredictable. Severe complications are often seen in patients who ingest only small amounts of the drugs, while mild or no symptoms may occur in some patients who ingest 2 g or more. This uncertainty may be related to pharmacokinetic differences between patients, to which reference has already been made. Some individual cases of tricyclic antidepressant overdosage are presented in Table 9.3.

EKG Changes and Plasma Levels

We (116) have described intracardiac conduction defects and EKG changes in four patients hospitalized with an overdosage of nortriptyline (two cases) and imipramine (two cases). Both EKG and HBE were recorded within 2 hr of admission to hospital, the A-H interval being normal in all cases. In three patients, QRS width increased to between 100 and 120 msec, and their H-V intervals ranged from 70 to 90 msec. After 8 days, all values returned to within normal limits. Plasma imipramine levels were not measured, but the plasma nortriptyline levels were 820 and 500 ng/ml. Both these patients had prolonged QRS and H-V intervals. We suggest that there is a direct drug action on His-Purkinje and intraventricular conduction, which would be a potential hazard for patients with preexisting impairment of atrioventricular conduction. In a further report (107), we studied 14 patients admitted with an overdosage of doxepin (six cases), nortriptyline (three cases), imipramine (two cases), and amitriptyline (three cases). None of the doxepin patients had prolongation of the H-V interval, but seven of the eight patients with overdoses of the other drugs did. Average dosage in both cases was the same (1.3 versus 1.4 g). Plasma doxepin levels in one patient were > 2 μg/ml (see Fig. 9.6) soon after admission and rapidly fell over the next 24 hr (117). Plasma levels in other patients were not reported.

EKG parameters and plasma tricyclic levels were determined in a study by

TABLE 9.3. Selected cases of tricyclic antidepressant overdosage

Age (years)	Sex	Drug[a]	Amount ingested	EKG findings	Ref.
19	F	IMI	3.75 g	Intraventricular conduction block; complete right bundle branch block; death 13 hr after overdose(O/D).	112
1.5	M	IMI	1.5 g	Prolonged QRS width, depressed ST, ventricular beats, complete heart block.	173
70	F	IMI	2.5 g	Cardiac arrest after 17 hr.	174
2	M	IMI	600–650 mg	Irregular beat 60/168/min, AV dissociation, prolonged QRS, depressed ST segments.	175
59	F	DMI	2.5 g	Prolonged QRS (0.14 sec c.f. 0.08 sec before O/D).	176
2	F	DMI	2.5 g	Progressive slowing of the heart, death after O/D.	177
59	M	NT	1.25 g	Lengthening of PR interval, inverted T waves.	178
2	F	DBZ	160 mg	Supraventricular and ventricular tachycardia, ST-T wave changes.	179
27	F	IMI	1.6 g	Cardiac arrest after 30 hr.	180
22	F	AMI	1.5 g	Supraventricular tachycardia, nonspecific ST-T wave changes.	181
2.5	F	IMI	760 mg	First degree AV and intraventricular block.	182
1.8	M	IMI	500 mg	Supraventricular tachycardia.	182
1.5	M	DBZ	1.5 g	Prolonged QRS width; supraventricular tachycardia; first degree AV block.	182
30	F	AMI	2.5 g		183
29	M	AMI	2.5 g	Prolonged QRS width.	183
27	F	AMI	2.5 g		183
35	M	AMI	600 mg		183
1.5	?	AMI	400 mg	Ventricular premature beats.	184

2.3	?	IMI	500 mg	Right bundle branch block; complete heart block.	184
27	F	NT	2.0 g	Intraventricular conduction defects; prolonged QRS width and prolonged H-V conduction time.	116
20	F	IMI	2.0 g		
35	F	NT	1.5 g		
17	M	NT	625 mg	Right ventricular conduction defect; first degree A-V block.	118
22	F	DMI	2.0 g	Sinus tachycardia; ST-T wave abnormalities.	
16	F	AMI	1.5 g	Intraventricular conduction defect.	
36	F	AMI	2.5–3.0 g	No abnormal findings.	
26	F	AMI	750 mg	Prolonged QRS width.	185
22	F	AMI	750–1,000 mg	Sinus tachycardia.	186
22	M	AMI	1.0 g	Sinus tachycardia.	186
45	F	AMI	500 mg	ST-T wave changes.	186
49	F	AMI	500 mg	No abnormal findings.	186
59	F	AMI	750 mg	No abnormal findings.	186
39	F	AMI	500 mg	Sinus tachycardia.	132
28	F	NOM	1.5 g	Sinus rhythm; minor T wave flattening.	133
43	F	NOM	3.5 g	QRS widening; ST-T wave abnormalities.	187
54	M	AMI	?	First degree heart block.	144
39	F	MIAN	580 mg	Left axis deviation.	143
53	F	MIAN	600 mg		

[a] AMI, amitriptyline; IMI, imipramine; DBZ, dibenzepine; NT, nortriptyline; DMI, desipramine; NOM, nomifensine; MIAN, mianserin.

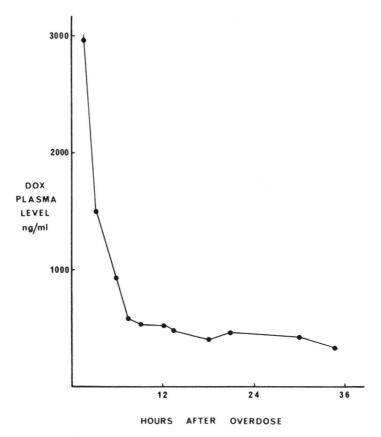

FIG. 9.6. Plasma doxepin levels in a 41-year-old female following an overdose of 1.5 g doxepin. The first plasma sample was taken 4 hr after the overdose. The patient was unconscious for 24 hr following the overdose.

Spiker et al. (118) of 15 patients with overdoses of various tricyclics. There was no correlation between total plasma tricyclic levels and maximum heart rate, lowest diastolic or systolic blood pressure, level of consciousness, pupil size, or P-R interval. Maximum QRS duration showed a strong positive correlation ($r = 0.75$ $p < 0.01$) with total tricyclic levels; excluding one patient with preexisting bundle branch block, intraventricular conduction delays were more often associated with plasma levels in excess of 1,000 ng/ml. As plasma levels decreased, the QRS width returned to normal. This study was confirmed in a group of 36 overdosed patients, all of whom had a QRS width ▷ 100 ms and a total plasma tricyclic level in excess of 1,000 ng/ml (119). The same investigators (120) found that tricyclic plasma levels could remain above 1,000 ng/ml for up to 96 hr after overdose; they suggest that sustained plasma levels may play a role in sudden death 3 to 6 days after overdose.

In contrast to Spiker's findings, no relationship between plasma tricyclic concentration and EKG changes was observed in another study of eight patients with overdoses of amitriptyline (six cases) and imipramine (two cases) (121). Maximum plasma concentration did not exceed 750 ng/ml in any patient, and apart from one patient in whom ventricular ectopic beats developed at a plasma concentration of 320 ng/ml, EKG findings were not reported in detail. In Spiker's studies, broadening of the QRS width to 100 msec or more was associated with plasma levels in excess of 1,000 ng/ml.

Forty patients ingesting tricyclic antidepressants overdoses were studied by Petit et al. (35), cases being grouped into those with total plasma tricyclic levels above (13 cases) and below (27 cases) 1,000 ng/ml. The mean plasma level of all those patients who died, had cardiac arrest, required respiratory support, in whom unconsciousness or grand mal seizures developed was $> 1,000$ ng/ml. Similarly, the mean plasma level of all patients in whom EKG abnormalities occurred (ventricular rate ≥ 120/min; QRS width ≥ 100 msec; cardiac arrhythmia; bundle branch block) was $> 1,000$ ng/ml. When each of these groups was analyzed individually, significantly more patients with the specific major adverse effect had plasma levels above than below 1,000 ng/ml. These authors again demonstrated the trend for cardiotoxic symptoms of the tricyclics to be associated with elevated plasma levels.

Bailey et al. (90) studied EKG changes following amitriptyline (19 cases) and imipramine (11 cases) overdosage. Within 2 to 4 hr after admission, the total tricyclic plasma levels ranged from 29 to 1,260 ng/ml for amitriptyline and from 123 to 1,732 ng/ml for imipramine. Prolonged QT intervals, widened QRS complexes, abnormal ST segments, and flattened T waves were observed 4 to 6 hr after admission, and there was a significant difference between total tricyclic levels for patients with widened QRS complex and those without widening (821 ng/ml and 396 ng/ml, respectively). There was no correlation between plasma level and the extent of QRS widening. Furthermore, the range of plasma levels observed in this study overlap with those observed in patients receiving chronic oral doses, making the use of plasma levels alone an unreliable index of tricyclic overdosage.

Indices of Overdosage

On the basis of the studies described, the most reliable and readily available clinical index of tricyclic antidepressant overdosage is prolongation of the QRS width by 100 msec or more. This will almost certainly be associated with elevated plasma levels of the drug. Plasma levels per se are not indicative of cardiotoxicity, but a parent drug-to-metabolite (P/M) ratio may be a better predictor of overdosage. A P/M ratio of less than 2 is more usual in steady state levels, while a P/M of greater than 2 strongly suggests an overdose, but its absence does not exclude it. Bailey et al. (90) conclude that QRS widening, arrhythmia, and increased total plasma tricyclic levels represent serious cardiotoxicity. Treatment of tricyclic overdose has been described (115) and is elaborated upon in Chapter 10.

STUDIES WITH NEW ANTIDEPRESSANTS

Nomifensine

Nomifensine is a new antidepressant of unique chemical structure unrelated to the monoamine oxidase inhibitors or the tricyclics. It is a tetrahydroisoquinoline derivative which blocks the reuptake of norepinephrine and dopamine and has a direct agonist effect on dopaminergic receptors (122–125). The drug is metabolized by hydroxylation at the 4-position to give the M_1 metabolite, which is a potent serotinin uptake inhibitor. Subsequent methoxylation of the phenyl ring leads to the inactive M_2 and M_3 metabolites (126). In controlled clinical studies, the drug has been shown to be an effective antidepressant with few side effects, particularly those of a cardiovascular nature (127–130).

We have investigated the effects of nomifensine on the cardiovascular system in 10 inpatients suffering from depressive illness (131). Each patient was studied before treatment and at the end of a 3-week period of nomifensine. The results of the study are shown in Table 9.4.

Nomifensine was associated with an increase in heart rate in seven of the 10 patients, which was not statistically significant. Nomifensine had no effect on H-V interval, QRS width, or other EKG parameters (A-H, PR, QT, and ST intervals and T waves); nor did the drug significantly affect blood pressure. There was no significant correlation between free or total plasma levels of nomifensine and any of the parameters measured in the study. The mean level

TABLE 9.4. *Effects of nomifensine on distal intracardiac conduction, heart rate, and QRS width in 10 patients receiving up to 200 mg/day of the drug*

Case no.	Age (years)	Sex	Dose (mg/day)	H-V interval (msec)		Heart rate (beats/min)		QRS width (sec)	
				Pre	Post	Pre	Post	Pre	Post
1	34	F	100	48	50	81	76	0.08	0.08
2	62	M	100	60	60	92	100	0.08	0.08
3	18	F	100	50	55	84	95	0.07	0.07
4	54	M	100	40	40	63	60	0.10	0.10
5	40	M	100	45	45	86	92	0.06	0.06
6	31	F	200	45	45	67	57	0.09	0.09
7	33	F	200	40	40	67	77	0.08	0.08
8	38	F	200	45	50	89	99	0.06	0.06
9	59	F	200	45	45	65	92	0.08	0.08
10	63	F	200	60	60	82	86	0.08	0.08

of free nomifensine was 45 ng/ml and of total drug (free plus conjugated) 185 ng/ml for the group of patients who received 100 mg daily, and 75 and 370 ng/ml, respectively, for those on 200 mg daily. Wide interindividual variations in plasma levels were demonstrated in this study. On the basis of this investigation, nomifensine appears to be without serious effect on the cardiovascular system of man at these doses.

Reports of nomifensine overdosage in man also suggest that the drug is without serious cardiotoxic properties. After an overdose of 1.5 g nomifensine, a 28-year-old woman had a normal EKG recording (132); the plasma nomifensine concentration 3 hr after the overdose was 2,780 ng/ml. Similarly, in a 43-year-old woman who ingested 3.5 g nomifensine together with 20 mg nitrazepam and 200 mg chlorpromazine, only minor EKG changes occurred, and the QRS width remained within normal limits (133); the plasma nomifensine level 17 hr after the overdose was 3,710 ng/ml. Of 26 cases of nomifensine overdose reported in another study, only six patients experienced any effect on the cardiovascular system (134), the average dose of nomifensine being 1.15 g. Nomifensine is apparently without serious effect on the cardiovascular system in both therapeutic doses and overdosage.

Mianserin

Mianserin is a tetracyclic piperazinoazepine compound, effective in the treatment of depressive illness (135,136). In addition to the animal studies already described, cardiovascular effects of mianserin have been examined in healthy volunteers and depressed patients. Studies in this latter group have most relevance clinically and are described here (see also Chapter 11).

No consistent effect on heart rate, PR interval, QRS width, or T wave amplitude was observed when mianserin was administered to 13 depressed patients in doses of 80 to 120 mg for 3 weeks (137). In two depressed patients, mianserin prolonged the QT interval after 1 week of treatment; by the second week, however, this had returned to normal, and no other effects on the EKG were noted (138). In a comparative study of the long-term effects of antidepressant treatment, four patients treated with 40 mg mianserin daily showed increased PR intervals, QT and QRS widening, and T wave flattening after 3 weeks of treatment (139). These EKG changes returned to normal after 13 months of treatment, and only heart rate remained raised. In another study of 60 patients with preexisting heart disease, 35 received mianserin (30 to 60 mg/day) for 3 weeks in a double-blind trial, while 15 patients received a placebo (140). Heart rate, blood pressure, and EKG were monitored at various intervals throughout the trial. There were no sudden unexpected deaths and no differences between groups on the cardiovascular parameters monitored (this study is described in more detail in Chapter 11).

We have measured intracardiac conduction in 10 depressed inpatients by

HBE before and after 3 weeks of treatment with 60 mg mianserin daily (141). Heart rate increased in 6 of the 10 patients, but this was not considered to be clinically significant, and no other significant changes in cardiovascular parameters were observed during the study. This investigation supports the other studies described and suggests that mianserin is without significant effects on the cardiovascular system.

On overdosage, mianserin does not cause the severe complications of most other antidepressants. A study of 44 cases (5 children and 39 adults) has been reported (142); in 21 adults who ingested mianserin alone, there were no serious cardiovascular problems. In another report, no EKG abnormalities, apart from left axis deviation, were observed in a 53-year-old female who overdosed on 600 mg mianserin and 10 g carbromal-like monoureides (143). Plasma mianserin level was 780 ng/ml 5 hr after ingestion (about seven to eight times in excess of that found in patients using therapeutic doses). In another case, however, first degree heart block was observed in a 39-year-old woman who overdosed on 580 mg mianserin, 35 mg diazepam, and 30 mg nitrazepam (144). The serum mianserin level 3½ hr after the overdose was 439 ng/ml, again well in excess of levels found in patients receiving therapeutic amounts. After 9 hr, the serum level fell to 157 ng/ml (an upper therapeutic level?[1]), and the EKG returned to normal. Finally, one death has been reported in a woman who ingested 600 mg mianserin and a large dose of lorazepam (147). Plasma mianserin was within normal limits (110 ng/ml), while the lorazepam level was 500 ng/ml, about two to three times the levels observed with chronic dosing. The time that had elapsed between blood sampling and overdosage was not known.

The cardiovascular safety of mianserin in both therapeutic and overdoses is established by these studies. Mianserin may be of particular value in the treatment of the depressed patient with heart disease and represents a significant advance in the treatment of depressive illness.

Zimelidine

Zimelidine (Astra H102/09) is a selective serotonin uptake inhibitor with a bicyclic structure. Limited clinical studies have shown that it possesses antidepressant effects (148,149). Burgess et al. (150) compared the cardiovascular effects of amitriptyline, mianserin, and zimelidine by using high speed surface EKG and systolic time intervals (see Chapter 10) and, on the basis of the eight mianserin and seven zimelidine patients studied, concluded that both drugs are safer than amitriptyline. In another report of two cases of overdosage with zimelidine, both patients experienced few adverse reactions (151). The safety of zimelidine awaits further studies.

---

[1] Some authors (145) suggest a curvilinear relationship between clinical response and plasma mianserin concentration with 70 ng/ml as an upper therapeutic limit. Others (146) find no relationship.

CARDIOVASCULAR EFFECTS OF LITHIUM

The use of lithium for the treatment of manic-depressive disorders is well established, although its mechanism of action is not known (152). Although the effects of lithium on the heart are generally regarded as being infrequent, innocuous, and reversible (153), several actions have been noted. In order of decreasing frequency of occurrence they are: T wave flattening (154,155), sinus node abnormalities (156), ventricular arrhythmias (157,159), myocarditis (157,159), and first degree AV block (158).

Most reports describing the cardiovascular effects of lithium have been anecdotal or retrospective, and controlled investigations are few. However, we have investigated the effects of therapeutic levels of lithium in six healthy male volunteers, aged 18 to 23 years (160). Subjects were studied before and after 2 weeks of lithium treatment, when steady state plasma levels were obtained. In addition to the standard 12-lead EKG, a high-speed, high-fidelity EKG was used to record electrical activity of the heart. Some minor T wave flattening occurred in three subjects, but there was no effect on any other EKG parameters. Furthermore, there was no correlation between plasma lithium levels and the magnitude of T wave depression. Serum potassium levels remained within normal limits for all volunteers throughout the study. It has been proposed that slow, partial intramyocardial depletion of potassium and its replacement by lithium may explain the T wave flattening seen on the EKG (153). The observations in this study do not exclude this possibility. Systolic time intervals were not affected by lithium treatment.

This study supports the contention that lithium is without serious cardiotoxicity, at least in short-term use. Clearly, more systematic studies of the effects of long-term administration of lithium on the heart are required. In view of the question of the nephrotoxicity of chronic lithium treatment, which has recently been raised (161,162), serious consideration should be given to the use of lithium in patients with preexistent heart disease.

CONCLUSIONS

The cardiotoxicity of antidepressant drugs can be studied in animals both *in vitro* (isolated tissues or whole hearts) and *in vivo* (intact animals). Although animal models may measure effects different from those seen in man and unrelated to the clinical situation, they may be effective in predicting relative activities in man.

Experiments *in vivo* show that the tricyclic antidepressants slow the heart rate, reduce blood pressure and automicity, lengthen PQ and PR intervals on the EKG, and widen the QRS complex and changes in the T wave. Ventricular extrasystoles, bigeminy, trigeminy, A-V block, and ventricular fibrillation may all be seen. In comparative experiments, the potential to induce cardiac dysrhythmias and other EKG changes is comparatively low with mianserin.

In human studies, the antidepressants exert significant effects on the cardiovascular system, as demonstrated by the characteristic changes observed in the EKG or by HBE.

Studies of the EKG effects in relation to plasma levels of the tricyclics, after either therapeutic doses or overdosage, have failed to demonstrate toxic levels of these drugs, EKG changes occurring with both therapeutic doses and overdoses. At present, the best indication of tricyclic overdose is a significant prolongation ($>$ 100 msec) of the QRS complex on the EKG. Significant cardiotoxicity is associated with elevated plasma levels of the tricyclics.

Studies with newer antidepressants, such as nomifensine, mianserin, and zimelidine, have shown that these compounds lack the cardiotoxicity of the older drugs. Further studies to confirm these preliminary findings are required. If they are less cardiotoxic, they represent a significant advance in the treatment of depression, especially in patients with preexistent heart disease. The risk of suicide, a significant component of the depressive syndrome, by overdose with these agents is markedly reduced.

Regular monitoring of cardiovascular status in patients receiving prophylactic treatment with antidepressants is to be advised.

REFERENCES

1. Office of Population Censuses and Surveys. (1961–1976). Deaths from poisoning by solid and liquid substances. OPCS, London.
2. Health and Personal Social Service Statistics for England. (1976). Department of Health and Social Security, HMSO, 1977.
3. Porsolt, R. D., Le Pichon, M., and Jalfre, M. Depression; a new animal model sensitive to antidepressant treatments. *Nature,* 1967, 266, 730–732.
4. Cairncross, K. D., Cox, B., Forster, C., and Wren, A. F. The olfactory bulbectomised rat; a simple model for detecting drugs with antidepressant potential. *Br. J. Pharmacol.,* 1977, 61, 497P.
5. Hughes, I. E., Kneen, B., and Main, V. The use of desipramine in studies of noradrenergic nerve function. *J. Pharm. Pharmacol.,* 1974, 26, 903–904.
6. Hughes, I. E. The effect of amitriptyline on presynaptic mechanisms in noradrenergic nerves. *Br. J. Pharmacol.,* 1978, 63, 315–321.
7. Langer, S. Z. Presynaptic receptors and their role in the regulation of transmitter release. *Br. J. Pharmacol.,* 1977, 60, 481–497.
8. Danon, A., and Chen, Z. Binding of imipramine to plasma proteins: Effect of hyperlipoproteinemia. *Clin. Pharmacol. Ther.,* 1979, 25, 316–321.
9. Borga, O., Azarnoff, D. J., Forshell, G. P., and Sjoqvist, F. Plasma protein binding of tricyclic antidepressants in man. *Biochem. Pharmacol.,* 1969, 18, 2135–2143.
10. Glassman, A. H., Hurwic, M. J., and Perel, J. M. Plasma binding of imipramine and clinical outcome. *Am. J. Psychiatry,* 1973, 130, 1367–1369.
11. Potter, W. Z., Muscettola, G., and Goodwin, F. K. Binding of imipramine to plasma proteins and to brain tissue. Relationship to CSF tricyclic levels in man. *Psychopharmacology,* 1979, 63, 187–192.
12. Babulova, A., Bareggi, S. R., Bonaccorsi, A., Garattini, S., Morselli, P. L., and Pantarotto, C. Correlation between desmethylimipramine levels, (-)-noradrenaline uptake and chronotropic effect in isolated atria of rats. *Br. J. Pharmacol.,* 1973, 48, 464–474.
13. Mundo, A. S., Bonaccorsi, A., Bareggi, S. R., Franco, R., Morselli, P. L., Riva, E., and Garattini, S. Relationships between tricyclic antidepressant concentration. L-^{3}H-noradrenaline uptake and chronotropic effects in isolated rat atria. *Eur. J. Pharmacol.,* 1974, 28, 368–375.

14. Gokhale, S. D., Gulati, O. D., and Udwadia, B. P. Antagonism of the adrenergic neurone blocking action of guanethidine by certain antidepressants and antihistamine drugs. *Arch. Int. Pharmacodyn.*, 1966, 160, 321–329.

15. Greeff, K., and Wagner, J. Cardiotoxic effects of thymoleptics in animals. *Dtsch. Med. Wochenschr.* 1971, 96, 1200–1201.

16. Kato, H., Noguchi, Y., and Takagi, K. Comparison of cardiovascular toxicities induced by dimetacrine, imipramine and amitriptyline in isolated guinea-pig atria and anesthetised dogs. *Jpn. J. Pharmacol.*, 1974, 24, 885–891.

17. Hughes, M. J., and Coret, I. A. Effects of tricyclic compounds on the response of isolated atria. *J. Pharmacol. Exp. Ther.*, 1974, 191, 252–261.

18. Biamino, G. Comparative studies on the cardiovascular effects of tricyclic antidepressants as well as nomifensine. An *in vivo* and *in vitro* study. *Alival Symp. Ergeb. Exp. Klin. Pruef.*, 1976, 129–140.

19. Biamino, G., Fenner, H., Schuren, K.-P., Neye, J., Ramdohr, B., and Lohmann, F.-W. Cardiovascular side effects of tricyclic antidepressants—a risk in the use of these drugs. *Int. J. Clin. Pharmacol. Biopharmacol.*, 1975, 11, 253–261.

20. Prudhommeaux, J. L., Streichenberger, G., and Lechat, P. An experimental study of the effects of imipramine on the rat ventricle strip. *C. R. Soc. Biol. (Paris)*, 1968, 162, 346–351.

21. Auclair, M. C., Gulda, O., and Lechat, P. Electrophysiological analysis of the effects of imipramine on ventricular muscle fibers. *Arch. Int. Pharmacodyn.*, 1969, 181, 218–231.

22. Dumovic, P., Burrows, G. D., Vohra, J., Davies, B., and Scoggins, B. A. The effect of tricyclic antidepressants on the heart. *Arch. Toxicol.*, 1976, 35, 255–262.

23. Brunner, H., Hedwall, P. R., Meier, M., and Bein, H. J. Cardiovascular effects of CIBA 34, 276-Ba and imipramine. *Agents Actions,* 1971, 2, 69–82.

24. Greeff, K., and Wagner, J. Cardiodepression and local anaesthetic effects of thymoleptics. *Arzneim. Forsch.*, 1969, 19, 1662–1664.

25. Reynolds, A. K., Chiz, J. F., and Tanikella, T. W. On the mechanism of coupling in adrenaline-induced bigeminy in sensitized hearts. *Can. J. Physiol. Pharmacol.*, 1975, 53, 1158–1171.

26. Flynn, S. B., Gristwood, R. W., and Owen, D. A. A. An isolated guinea-pig working heart; preliminary studies with histamine and noradrenaline. *Br. J. Pharmacol.*, 1977, 59, 530P.

27. Dumovic, P., Trethewie, E. R., and Burrows, G. D. The effect of tricyclic antidepressant drugs on the isolated perfused guinea-pig heart. *Clin. Exp. Pharmacol. Physiol.*, 1977, 4, 421–424.

28. Marmo, E., Coscia, L., and Cataldi, S. Cardiac effects of antidepressants. *Jpn. J. Pharmacol.*, 1972, 22, 283–292.

29. Langslet, A., Johansen, W. G., Ryg, M., Skomedal, T., and Oye, I. Effect of dibenzepine and imipramine on the isolated rat heart. *Eur. J. Pharmacol.*, 1971, 14, 333–339.

30. Hoffmann, I. A comparative review of the pharmacology of nomifensine. *Br. J. Clin. Pharmacol.*, 1977, 4, 69S–75S.

31. Barth, N., Manns, M., and Muscholl, E. Arrhythmias and inhibition of noradrenaline uptake caused by tricyclic antidepressants and chlorpromazine on the isolated perfused rabbit hearts. *Naunyn Schmiedebergs Arch. Pharmacol.*, 1975, 288, 215–231.

32. Barth, N., and Muscholl, E. The effects of the tricyclic antidepressants desipramine, doxepin and iprindole on the perfused rabbit heart. *Naunyn Schmiedebergs Arch. Pharmacol.*, 1974, 284, 215–232.

33. Harper, B., and Hughes, I. E. A comparison in isolated rabbit hearts of the dysrhythmogenic potential of amitriptyline, maprotiline and mianserin in relation to their ability to block noradrenaline uptake. *Br. J. Pharmacol.*, 1977, 59, 651–660.

34. Byck, R. Drugs and the treatment of psychiatric disorders. In: *The Pharmacological Basics of Therapeutics,* edited by L. S. Goodman and A. Gilman, p. 177. Macmillan, New York, 1975.

35. Petit, J. M., Spiker, D. G., Ruwitch, J. F., Ziegler, V. E., Weiss, A. N., and Biggs, J. T. Tricyclic antidepressant plasma levels and adverse effects after overdose. *Clin. Pharmacol. Ther.*, 1977, 21, 47–51.

36. Braithwaite, R. A., and Widdop, B. A specific gas chromatographic method for the measurement of steady state plasma levels of amitriptyline and nortriptyline in patients. *Clin. Chim. Acta,* 1971, 35, 461–472.

37. Jørgensen, A. A gas chromatographic method for the determination of amitriptyline and nortriptyline in human serum. *Acta Pharmacol. Toxicol.,* 1975, 36, 79–90.

38. Riess, W., Dubey, L., Funfgeld, E. W., Imhof, P., Hurzeler, H., Matussek, N., Rajagopalan, T. G., Raschdor, F., and Schmid, K. The pharmacokinetic properties of maprotiline (Ludiomil) in man. *J. Int. Med. Res. [Suppl. 2], 1975, 3, 16–41.*

39. Coppen, A., and Kopera, H. Workshop on the clinical pharmacology and efficacy of mianserin. *Br. J. Clin. Pharmacol.,* 1978, 5, 91S–99S.

40. Dencker, S. J., and Nagy, A. Single versus divided daily doses of clomipramine. Plasma concentration and clinical effect. *Acta Psychiatr. Scand.,* 1979, 59, 326–334.

41. Zaitseva, K. A. Comparative effects of pyrazidol and imazine (imipramine) on the ECG and some other aspects of cardiac activity. *Farmakol. Toksikol.,* 1977, 40, 400–403.

42. Gram, L. F., and Overo, K. F. First pass metabolism of nortriptyline in man. *Clin. Pharmacol. Ther.,* 1975, 18, 305–314.

43. Jandhyala, B. J., Steenberg, M. L., Perel, J. M., Manian, A. A., and Buckley, J. P. Effect of several tricyclic antidepressants on the haemodynamics and myocardial contractility of anaesthetised dogs. *Eur. J. Pharmacol.,* 1977, 42, 403–410.

44. Dreyfuss, J., Shkosky, J. M., Ross, J. J., and Schreiver, E. C. Species differences in metabolism of a tricyclic psychotropic agent. *Toxicol. Appl. Pharmacol.,* 1972, 22, 105–114.

45. Hucker, H. B., Balletto, A. J., Demetriades, J., Apison, B. H., and Zacchei, A. G. Urinary metabolites of amitriptyline in the dog. *Drug Metab. Dispos.,* 1977, 5, 132–142.

46. Dingell, J. V., Sulser, F., and Gillette, J. R. Species difference in the metabolism of imipramine and desmethylimipramine. *J. Pharmacol. Exp. Ther.,* 1964, 143, 14–22.

47. Nemec, J. Cardiotoxic effects of tricyclic antidepressants imipramine, amitriptyline and dosulepin (Prothiaden) in acute experiments in rats. *Acta Nerv. Super.,* 1974, 16, 182–183.

48. Bonaccorsi, A., Franco, R., Garattini, S., Morselli, P. L., and Pita, E. Plasma nortriptyline and cardiac responses in young and old rats. *Br. J. Pharmacol.,* 1977, 60, 21–27.

49. Cairncross, K. D., and Gershon, S. A pharmacological basis for the cardiovascular complications of imipramine medication. *Med. J. Aust.,* 1962, 2, 372–375.

50. Hughes, I. E., and Radwan, S. The relative toxicity of amitriptyline, imipramine, maprotiline and mianserin in rabbits *in vivo. Br. J. Pharmacol.,* 1979, 65, 331–338.

51. Quintana, A. Effect of pancuronium bromide on the adrenergic responsivity of the isolated rat vas deferens. *Eur. J. Pharmacol.,* 1977, 46, 275–277.

52. Vercruysse, P., Bossuyt, P., Hanegreefs, G., Verbeuren, T. J., and Vanhoutte, P. M. Gallamine and pancuronium inhibit pre- and postjunctional muscarinic receptors in canine saphenous veins. *J. Pharmacol. Exp. Ther.,* 1979, 209, 225–230.

53. Edwards, R. P., Miller, R. D., Roizen, M. F., Ham, J., Way, W. L., Lake, C. R., and Roderick, L. Cardiac responses to imipramine and pancuronium during anaesthesia with halothane of enflurane. *Anesthesiology,* 1979, 50, 421–425.

54. Forika, M., Feszt, Gh., and Forika, Gh. Effect of reserpine and urethane on the cardiovascular disturbances produced by large doses of imipramine. *Fiziol. Norm. Patol.,* 1972, 18, 363–375.

55. Joas, T. A., and Stevens, W. C. Comparison of the arrhythmic dose of epinephrine during forane, halothane and fluroxene anaesthesia in dogs. *Anesthesiology,* 1971, 35, 48–53.

56. Corbett, T. H., and Ball, G. L. Respiratory excretion of halothane after clinical and occupational exposure. *Anesthesiology,* 1973, 39, 342–345.

57. Stockley, I. Interactions with phenytoin, phenobarbitone and other antiepileptic agents. In: *Drug Interactions and Their Mechanisms.* The Pharmaceutical Press, London, 1974.

58. Corona, G. L., Facino, R. M., and Santagostino, G. Influence of chronic treatment on the distribution of amitriptyline and metabolites in the rabbit brain. *Biochem. Pharmacol.,* 1971, 20, 2768–2771.

59. Glisson, S. N., Fajardo, L., and El-Etra, A. A. Amitriptyline increases ECG changes during reversal of neuromuscular blockade. *Anesth. Analg. Curr. Res.,* 1978, 57, 77–83.

60. Elonen, E. Correlation of the cardiotoxicity of tricyclic antidepressants to their membrane effects. *Med. Biol.,* 1974, 52, 415–423.

61. Burrows, G. D., Vohra, J., Hunt, D., Sloman, J. G., Scoggins, B. A., and Davies, B. Cardiac effects of different tricyclic antidepressant drugs. *Br. J. Psychiatry,* 1976, 129, 335–341.

62. Forika, M., Feszt, Gh., and Repoiski, E. Effect of imipramine on ECG disorders provoked by isoprenaline and noradrenaline. *Rev. Med.,* 1971, 17, 281–286.

63. Dhumma-Upakorn, P., and Cobbin, L. B. Cardiovascular effects of amitriptyline in anaesthetised dogs. *Clin. Exp. Pharmacol. Physiol.*, 1977, 4, 121–129.
64. Baum, T., Peters, J. R., Butz, F., and Much, D. R. Tricyclic antidepressants and cardiac conduction; changes in ventricular automaticity. *Eur. J. Pharmacol.*, 1976, 39, 323–329.
65. Bonaccorsi, A., and Garattini, S. Cardiac effects of nortriptyline and other tricyclic antidepressant drugs. *Gen. Pharmacol.*, 1978, 9, 81–84.
66. Thorstrand, C., Bergsyrom, J., and Castenfors, J. Cardiac effects of amitriptyline in rats. *Scand. J. Clin. Lab. Invest.*, 1976, 36, 7–15.
67. Kurioka, Y., and Taniwa, M. Effects of imipramine on the ECG in the rabbit. *Igaku to Seibutsugaku,* 1974, 88, 201–204.
68. Desager, J. P., Leonard, J. P., Vanderbist, M., and Harvengt, G. Reduced cardiac output and renal blood flow during amitriptyline intoxication in conscious rabbits. *Toxicol. Appl. Pharmacol.*, 1979, 47, 445–449.
69. Bianchetti, G., Bonaccorsi, A., Chiodaroli, A., Franco, R., Garattini, S., Gomeni, R., and Morselli, P. L. Plasma concentrations and cardiotoxic effects of desipramine and protriptyline in the rat. *Br. J. Pharmacol.*, 1977, 60, 11–19.
70. Ribeiro, C., Silva Neves, L., Bordalo, A. D. B., Ajaujo, A., and Longo, A. Psychopharmaceuticals and intraventricular conduction disorders. *Boll. Soc. Ital. Cardiol.*, 1975, 20, 1385–1390.
71. Simon, P., Boissier, J. R., and Witchitz, S. Cardiotoxicity of some tricyclic antidepressants in the guinea-pig and the rat. *J. Eur. Toxicol.*, 1969, 2, 288–290.
72. Elonen, E., and Mattila, M. J. Cardiovascular effects of amitriptyline, nortriptyline, protriptyline and doxepin in conscious rabbits after subacute treatment with protriptyline. *Med. Biol.*, 1975, 53, 238–244.
73. Baum, T., Shropshire, A. T., Rowles, G., and Gluckman, M. I. Antidepressants and cardiac conduction: Iprindole and imipramine. *Eur. J. Pharmacol.*, 1971, 13, 287–291.
74. Hughes, I. E., and Radwan, S. Relative toxicity of amitriptyline, imipramine, maprotiline and mianserin after intravenous infusion in conscious rabbits. *Br. J. Clin. Pharmacol.*, 1978, 5, 19S–20S.
75. Elonen, E., Mattila, M. J., and Saarnivaara, L. Cardiovascular effects of amitriptyline, nortriptyline, protriptyline and doxepin in conscious rabbits. *Eur. J. Pharmacol.*, 1974, 28, 178–188.
76. Nymark, M., and Rasmussen, J. Effects of certain drugs upon amitriptyline induced electrocardiographic changes. *Acta Pharmacol. Toxicol.*, 1966, 24, 148–156.
77. Junien, J. L., Lakatos, C., and Padioleau, F. Studies of the effects of imipramine on cardiac conduction in anaesthetised dogs by His bundle electrogram recording. *J. Pharmacol.*, 1976, 7, 133–145.
78. Gram, L. F. Plasma level monitoring of tricyclic antidepressant therapy. *Clin. Pharmacokinet.*, 1977, 2, 237–251.
79. Garattini, S., and Morselli, P. L. Metabolism and pharmacokinetics of psychotropic drugs. In: *Principles of Psychopharmacology,* edited by W. G. Clark and J. deGiudice, pp. 169–182. Academic Press, New York, 1978.
80. Gram, L. F. Metabolism of tricyclic antidepressants. A review. *Dan. Med. Bull.*, 1974, 21, 218–231.
81. Alexanderson, B. Pharmacokinetics of desmethylimipramine and nortriptyline in man after single and multiple oral doses. *Eur. J. Clin. Pharmacol.*, 1972, 5, 1–10.
82. Alexanderson, B. Pharmacokinetics of nortriptyline in man after single and multiple oral doses: The predictability of steady-state concentrations from single dose plasma level data. *Eur. J. Clin. Pharmacol.*, 1972, 4, 82–91.
83. Scoggins, B. A., Coghlan, J. P., Maguire, K. P., Burrows, G. D., and Davies, B. The measurement of plasma levels of tricyclic antidepressant drugs. *Aust. N.Z. J. Psychiatry,* 1976, 10, 7–12.
84. Alexanderson, B., and Sjoqvist, F. Individual differences in the pharmacokinetics of monomethylated tricyclic antidepressants: Role of genetic and environmental factors and clinical importance. *Ann. N.Y. Acad. Sci.*, 1971, 179, 739–751.
85. Hamilton, M., and Mahapatre, S. B. Antidepressant drugs. In: *Side Effects of Drugs,* edited by L. Meyler and A. Herxheimer, pp. 17–37. Excerpta Medica, Amsterdam, 1972.
86. Jefferson, J. W. A review of the cardiovascular effects and toxicity of tricyclic antidepressants. *Psychosom. Med.*, 1975, 37, 160–179.

87. Elonen, E., Linnoila, M., Lukkari, I., and Mattila, M. J. Concentrations of tricyclic antidepressants in plasma, heart and skeletal muscle after intravenous infusion to anaesthetised rabbits. *Acta Pharmacol. Toxicol.*, 1975, 37, 274–281.

88. Thorstrand, C. Clinical features in poisoning by tricyclic antidepressant drugs with special reference to the ECG. *Acta Med. Scand.*, 1976, 199, 337–344.

89. Freeman, J. W., Mundy, G. R., Beattie, R. R., and Ryan, C. Cardiac abnormalities in poisoning with tricyclic antidepressant drugs. *Br. Med. J.*, 1969, 2, 610–611.

90. Bailey, D. N., van Dyke, C., Langou, A., and Jatlow, P. I. Tricyclic antidepressant plasma levels and clinical findings in overdose. *Am. J. Psychiatry*, 1978, 135, 1325–1328.

91. Taylor, D. J. E., and Braithwaite, R. A. Cardiac effects of tricyclic antidepressant medication; a preliminary study of nortriptyline. *Br. Heart J.*, 1978, 40, 1005–1009.

92. Kristiansen, E. S. Cardiac complications during treatment with imipramine (Tofranil). *Acta Psychiatr. Neurol.*, 1961, 36, 427–442.

93. Bigger, J. T., Giardina, E. G. V., Perel, J. M., Kantor, S. J., and Glassman, A. H. Cardiac antiarrhythmic effect of imipramine hydrochloride. *N. Engl. J. Med.*, 1977, 296, 206–208.

94. Singh, G. Cardiac arrest with clomipramine. *Br. Med. J.*, 1972, 3, 698.

95. Smith, R. B., and Rusbatch, B. J. Amitriptyline and heart block. *Br. Med. J.*, 1967, 3, 311.

96. Scollins, M. J., Robinson, D. S., and Nies, A. Cardiotoxicity of amitriptyline. *Lancet*, 1972, 2, 1202.

97. Vohra, J., Burrows, G. D., and Sloman, G. Assessment of cardiovascular side effects of therapeutic doses of tricyclic antidepressant drugs. *Aust. N.Z. Med. J.*, 1975, 5, 7–11.

98. Manoguerra, A. S., and Weaver, L. C. Poisoning with tricyclic antidepressant drugs. *Clin. Toxicol.*, 1977, 10, 149–158.

99. Barnes, R. J., Kong, S. M., and Wu, R. W. Y. Electrocardiographic changes in amitriptyline poisoning. *Br. Med. J.*, 1968, 3, 222.

100. Masters, A. B. Delayed death in imipramine poisoning. *Br. Med. J.*, 1967, 3, 866–867.

101. Boston Collaborative Drug Surveillance Program. Adverse reactions to tricyclic antidepressant drugs. *Lancet*, 1972, I, 529–531.

102. Coull, D. C., Crooks, J., Dingwall-Fordyce, I., Scott, A. M., and Weir, R. D. Amitriptyline and cardiac disease. *Lancet*, 1970, 2, 590–591.

103. Moir, D. C. Tricyclic antidepressants and cardiac disease. *Am. Heart J.*, 1973, 86, 841–842.

104. Norman, T. R., and Burrows, G. D. Plasma levels of psychotropic drugs and clinical response. In: *Advances in Human Psychopharmacology*, edited by G. D. Burrows and J. Werry. JAI Press, Connecticut, Vol. 1, 1980, p. 103–140.

105. Freyschuss, U., Sjoqvist, F., Tuck, D., and Asberg, M. Circulatory effects in man of nortriptyline, a tricyclic antidepressant drug. *Pharmacol. Clin.*, 1970, 2, 68–71.

106. Burrows, G. D., Vohra, J., Dumovic, P., Maguire, K., Scoggins, B. A., and Davies, B. Tricyclic antidepressant drugs and cardiac conduction. *Prog. Neuropsychopharmacol.*, 1977, 1, 329–334.

107. Vohra, J., Burrows, G. D., Hunt, D., and Sloman, G. The effect of toxic and therapeutic doses of tricyclic antidepressant drugs on intracardiac conduction. *Eur. J. Cardiol.*, 1975, 3, 219–227.

108. Ziegler, V. E., Co, B. T., and Biggs, J. T. Plasma nortriptyline and ECG findings. *Am. J. Psychiatry*, 1977, 134, 441–443.

109. Ziegler, V. E., Co, B. T., and Biggs, J. T. Electrocardiographic findings in patients undergoing amitriptyline treatment. *Dis. Nerv. Syst.*, 1977, 38, 697–699.

110. Kantor, S. J., Bigger, T., Glassman, A. H., Macken, D. L., and Perel, J. M. Imipramine induced heart block: A longitudinal case study. *JAMA*, 1975, 231, 1364–1366.

111. Kantor, S. J., Glassman, A. H., Bigger, T., Perel, J. M., and Giardina, E. V. The cardiac effects of therapeutic plasma concentrations of imipramine. *Am. J. Psychiatry*, 1978, 135, 534–538.

112. Michon, P., Larcan, Huriet, C., Beaudouin, D., and Berthier, X. Intoxication volontaire mortelle par imipramine. *Bull. Soc. Med. Hosp. (Paris)*, 1959, 75, 989–992.

113. Kuhn, R. The treatment of depressive states with G22355 (imipramine hydrochloride). *Am. J. Psychiatry*, 1958, 115, 459–464.

114. Bickel, M. H. Poisoning by tricyclic antidepressants. *Int. J. Clin. Pharmacol. Biopharm.*, 1975, 11, 145–176.

115. Vohra, J., and Burrows, G. D. Cardiovascular complications of tricyclic antidepressant overdosage. *Drugs*, 1974, 8, 432–437.

116. Vohra, J., Hunt, D., Burrows, G. D., and Sloman, G. Intracardiac conduction defects following overdose of tricyclic antidepressant drugs. *Eur. J. Cardiol.,* 1975, 2, 453–458.
117. Maguire, K. P. Studies on the interaction and relationship between clinical response and plasma levels of psychotropic drugs. Doctoral dissertation, University of Melbourne, 1977.
118. Spiker, D. G., Weiss, A. N., Chang, S. S., Ruwitch, J. F., and Biggs, J. T. Tricyclic antidepressant overdose: Clinical presentation and plasma levels. *Clin. Pharmacol. Ther.,* 1975, 18, 539–546.
119. Petit, J. M., Spiker, D. G., and Biggs, J. T. Psychiatric diagnosis and tricyclic plasma levels in 36 hospitalised overdosed patients. *J. Nerv. Ment. Dis.,* 1976, 163, 289–293.
120. Spiker, D. G., and Biggs, J. T. Tricyclic antidepressants: Prolonged plasma levels after overdose. *JAMA,* 1976, 236, 1711–1712.
121. Hallstrom, C., and Gifford, L. Antidepressant blood levels in acute overdose. *Postgrad. Med. J.,* 1976, 52, 687–688.
122. Hunt, P., Kannengiesser, M. H., and Raynaud, J. P. Nomifensine: A new potent inhibitor of dopamine uptake into synaptosomes from rat brain corpus striatum. *J. Pharm. Pharmacol.,* 1974, 26, 370–371.
123. Schacht, U., and Heptner, W. Effect of nomifensine (Hoe 984), a new antidepressant, on uptake of noradrenaline and serotonin and on release of noradrenaline in rat brain synaptosomes. *Biochem. Pharmacol.,* 1974, 23, 3413–3422.
124. Samanin, R., Bernasconi, S., and Garattini, S. The effect of nomifensine on the depletion of brain serotonin and catecholamines induced respectively by fenfluramine and 6-hydroxy-dopamine in rats. *Eur. J. Pharmacol.,* 1975, 34, 377–380.
125. Tuomisto, J. Nomifensine and its derivatives as possible tools for studying amine uptake. *Eur. J. Pharmacol.,* 1977, 42, 101–106.
126. Heptner, W., Hornke, I., Cavagna, F., Fehlhaber, H., Rupp, W., and Neubauer, H. P. Metabolism of nomifensine in man and animal species. *Arzneim. Forsch.,* 1977, 28, 58–64.
127. Acebal, E., Subira, S., Spatz, J., Faleni, R., Merzbacher, B., Gales, A., and Moizeszowicz, J. A double blind comparative trial of nomifensin and desipramine in depression. *Eur. J. Clin. Pharmacol.,* 1976, 10, 109–113.
128. Angst, J., Koukkou, M., Bleuler-Herzog, M., and Martens, H. Ergebnisse eines offenen und eines Doppelblind versuches von Nomifensin im Vergleich zu Impramin. *Arch. Psychiatr. Nervenkr.,* 1974, 219, 265–276.
129. Madalena, J. C., De Azevedo, O. F., Morais, M. L. S., Santana, R. L., Rzezinsky, P. C., De Almeida, M. J., and Lovenkron, T. S. A new antidepressant psychotropic drug: Nomifensin. First clinical trials. *Rev. Bras. Clin. Terap.,* 1973, 2, 311–316.
130. Moizeszowicz, J., and Subira, S. Controlled trial of nomifensin (Hoe 984) and viloxazine in the treatment of depression in the elderly. *J. Clin. Pharmacol.,* 1977, 17, 81–83.
131. Burrows, G. D., Vohra, J., Dumovic, P., Scoggins, B. A., and Davies, B. M. Cardiological effects of nomifensine, a new antidepressant. *Med. J. Aust.,* 1978, 1, 341–343.
132. Montgomery, S., Crome, P., and Braithwaite, R. Nomifensine overdosage. 1978, *Lancet,* 2, 828–829.
133. Vohra, J., Burrows, G. D., McIntyre, I., and Davies, B. Cardiovascular effects of nomifensine. *Lancet,* 1978, 2, 902–903.
134. Dawling, S., Braithwaite, R., and Crome, P. Nomifensine overdose and plasma drug concentration. 1979, *Lancet,* 1, 56.
135. Brogden, R. N., Heel, R. C., Speight, T. M., and Avery, G. S. Mianserin: A review of its pharmacological properties and therapeutic efficacy in depressive illness. *Drugs,* 1978, 16, 273–301.
136. Fell, P. J., Quantock, D. C., and Van Derburg, W. J. The human pharmacology of GB-94—a new psychotropic agent. *Eur. J. Clin. Pharmacol.,* 1973, 5, 166–173.
137. Peet, M., Tienari, P., and Jaskari, M. O. A comparison of the cardiac effects of mianserin and amitriptyline in man. *Pharmakopsychiatrie,* 1977, 10, 309.
138. Burgess, C. D., Turner, P., and Wadsworth, J. Cardiovascular responses to mianserin hydrochloride: A comparison with tricyclic antidepressant drugs. *Br. J. Clin. Pharmacol. [Suppl. I],* 1978, 5, 21S–28S.
139. Burckhardt, D., Raeder, E., Muller, V., Imhof, P., and Neubauer, H. Cardiovascular effects of tricyclic and tetracyclic antidepressants. *JAMA,* 1978, 239, 213–216.
140. Kopera, H., and Schenk, H. Poisoning with antidepressants. *Br. Med. J.,* 1977, 2, 773.

141. Burrows, G. D., Davies, B., Hamer, A., and Vohra, J. Effect of Mianserin on cardiac conduction. *Med. J. Aust.,* 1979, 2, 97–98.
142. Crome, P., Braithwaite, R. A., Newman, B., and Montgomery, S. A. Choosing an antidepressant. *Br. Med. J.,* 1978, 1, 859.
143. Jansen, H., Drykoningden, G., and De Ridder, J. J. Poisoning with antidepressants. *Br. Med. J.,* 1977, 2, 896.
144. Green, S. D. R., and Kendall-Taylor, P. Heart block in mianserin hydrochloride overdose. *Br. Med. J.,* 1977, 2, 1190.
145. Montgomery, S., McAuley, R., and Montgomery, D. B. Relationship between mianserin plasma levels and antidepressant effect in a double-blind trial comparing single nighttime and divided daily dose regimens. *Br. J. Clin. Pharmacol.,* 1978, 5, 71S–76S.
146. Coppen A. et al. Mianserin hydrochloride: A novel antidepressant. *Br. J. Psychiatry,* 1976, 129, 342.
147. Crome, P., and Newman, B. Poisoning with maprotiline and mianserin. *Br. Med. J.,* 1977, 2, 260.
148. Benkert, O., Laakmann, G., Ott, L., Strauss, A., and Zimmer, R. Effect of Zimelidine (H102/ 09) in depressive patients. *Arzneim. Forsch.,* 1977, 27, 2421–2423.
149. Coppen, A., Rama Rao, V. A., Swade, C., and Wood, K. Zimelidine: A therapeutic and pharmacokinetic study in depression. *Psychopharmacology,* 1979, 63, 199–202.
150. Burgess, C. D., Montgomery, S., and Wadsworth, J. Cardiovascular effects of amitriptyline, mianserin and zimelidine in depressed patients. Abstr. 2569, 7th IUPHAR Congress, Paris, 1978.
151. Astra Pty. Ltd. Unpublished data, 1978.
152. Hollister, L. E. Psychiatric disorders. In: *Drug Treatment,* edited by G. S. Avery. Adis Press, Sydney, 1976.
153. Tilkian, A. G., Schroeder, J. S., Kao, J. J., and Hultgren, H. N. The cardiovascular effects of lithium in man. A review of the literature. *Am. J. Med.,* 1976, 61, 665–670.
154. Schou, M. Electrocardiographic changes during treatment with lithium and with drugs of the imipramine type. *Acta Psychiatr. Scand.,* 1962, 38, 331–336.
155. Hansen, H. E., and Amdisen, A. Lithium intoxication (report of 23 cases and review of 100 cases from the literature. *Q. J. Med.,* 1978, 47, 123–144.
156. Wilson, J. R., Kraus, E. S., Bailis, M. M., and Rakita, L. Reversible sinus-node abnormalities due to lithium carbonate therapy. *N. Engl. J. Med.,* 1976, 294, 1223–1224.
157. Tseng, H. L. Interstitial myocarditis probably related to lithium carbonate intoxication. *Arch. Pathol. Lab. Med.,* 1971, 92, 444–448.
158. Jaffe, C. M. First degree atrioventricular block during lithium carbonate treatment. *Am. J. Psychiatry,* 1977, 134, 88–89.
159. Swedberg, K., and Winblad, B. Heart failure as complication of lithium treatment. *Acta Med. Scand.,* 1974, 196, 279–280.
160. Dumovic, P., Burrows, G. D., Chamberlain, K., Vohra, J., Fuller, J., and Sloman, J. G. Effect of therapeutic dosage of lithium on the heart. *Br. J. Clin. Pharmacol.* 1980, *in press.*
161. Burrows, G. D., Davies, B. M., and Kincaid-Smith, P. Unique tubular lesion after lithium. *Lancet,* 1978, I, 1310.
162. Hullin, R. P., Coley, V. P., Birch, N. S., Thomas, T. H., and Morgan, D. B. Renal function after long term treatment with lithium. *Br. Med. J.,* 1979, 1, 1457–1459.
163. Muller, O. F., Goodman, N., and Bellet, S. The hypotensive effect of imipramine hydrochloride in patients with cardiovascular disease. *Clin. Pharmacol. Ther.,* 1961, 2, 300–307.
164. Rasmussen, E. B., and Kristjansen, P. ECG changes during amitriptyline treatment. *Am. J. Psychiatry,* 1963, 119, 781–782.
165. Ayd, F. J. Long term administration of doxepin (Sinequan). *Dis. Nerv. Syst.,* 1971, 32, 617–622.
166. Martin, G. I., and Zaug, P. J. ECG monitoring of enuretic children given imipramine. *JAMA,* 1973, 224, 902–903.
167. Muller, R., and Burckhardt, D. Effect of tricyclic and tetracyclic antidepressant drugs on heart and circulation. *Schweiz. Med. Wochenschr.,* 1974, 104, 1911–1913.
168. Martin, G. I., and Zaug, P. J. ECG monitoring of enuretic children receiving therapeutic doses of imipramine. *Am. J. Psychiatry,* 1975, 132, 540–542.

169. Winsberg, B. G., Goldstein, S., Yepes, L. E., and Perel, J. M. Imipramine and ECG abnormalities in hyperactive children. *Am. J. Psychiatry*, 1975, 132, 542–545.
170. Shader, R. I. Cardiac effects of imipramine hydrochloride in the elderly. *Psychopharmacol. Bull.*, 1975, 11, 15–16.
171. Burckhardt, D., Fleischhauer, H. J., Muller, V., and Neubauer, H. W. Beitrag zur Wirkung tri- und tetrazyklischer Antidepressiva auf Herz und Kreislaug. *Schweiz. Med. Wochenschr.*, 1976, 106, 1896–1903.
172. Brorson, L., and Wennerblom, B. Electrophysiological methods in assessing cardiac effects of the tricyclic antidepressant imipramine. *Acta Med. Scand.*, 1978, 203, 429–432.
173. Arneson, G. A. A near fatal case of imipramine overdosage. *Am. J. Psychiatry*, 1961, 117, 934–936.
174. Davies, D. M., and Allaye, R. Amitriptyline poisoning. *Lancet*, 1963, 2, 643.
175. Prout, B. J., Young, J., and Goddard, P. Imipramine poisoning in childhood and suggested treatment. *Br. Med. J.*, 1965, 1, 972.
176. Tchen, P., Weatherhead, A. D., and Richards, N. G. Acute intoxication with desipramine. *N. Engl. J. Med.*, 1966, 274, 1197.
177. Bickel, M. H., Brochon, R., Friolet, B., Herrmann, B., and Stoffer, A. R. Clinical and biochemical results of a fatal case of desipramine intoxication. *Psychopharmacologia*, 1967, 10, 431–436.
178. Brackenridge, R. G., Peters, T. J., and Watson, J. M. Myocardial damage in amitriptyline and nortriptyline poisoning. *Scot. Med. J.*, 1968, 13, 208–210.
179. Rosenberg, D., Monnet, P., David, L., Fayard, C., and Robin, J. Y. L'intoxication par l'imipramine et ses devives en pediatrie. *Presse Med.*, 1969, 77, 1383–1384.
180. Williams, R. B., and Sherter, C. Cardiac complications of tricyclic antidepressant therapy. *Ann. Intern. Med.*, 1971, 74, 395–398.
181. Slovis, T. L., Ott, J. E., Teitelbaum, D. T., and Lipscomb, W. Physostigmine therapy in acute tricyclic antidepressant poisoning. *Clin. Toxicol.*, 1971, 4, 451–459.
182. Brown, T. C. K., Barker, C. A., Dunlop, M. E., and Loughnan, P. M. The use of sodium bicarbonate in the treatment of tricyclic antidepressant-induced arrhythmias. *Anaesth. Int. Care*, 1973, 1, 203–210.
183. Thorstrand, C. Cardiovascular effects of poisoning with tricyclic antidepressants. *Acta Med. Scand.*, 1974, 195, 505–514.
184. Goel, K. M., and Shanks, R. A. Amitriptyline and imipramine poisoning in children. *Br. Med. J.*, 1974, 1, 261–263.
185. Tobias, J., and Das, B. N. Cardiac complications in amitriptyline poisoning. *JAMA*, 1976, 235, 1474–1476.
186. O'Brien, J. P. A study of low-dose amitriptyline overdoses. *Am. J. Psychiatry*, 1977, 134, 66–68.
187. Giller, E. L., Bialos, D. S., Docherty, J. P., Jatlow, P. L., and Harkness, L. Chronic amitriptyline toxicity. *Am. J. Psychiatry*, 1979, 136, 458–459.

Stress and the Heart, edited by D. Wheatley,
Raven Press, New York © 1981.

Cardiovascular Effects of Antidepressants: Clinical Implications

Carl Burgess and Paul Turner

As the authors of the previous chapter comment, although the advent of antidepressant drug therapy has revolutionized the treatment of depression, the incidence of cardiovascular complications has proved distressing. Antidepressants may affect the cardiovascular system (CVS) either directly or through drug interactions, causing arrhythmias and affecting the inotropic state of the heart and blood pressure. Abnormalities may occur within the therapeutic dosage range. Because of these side effects, their use is limited.

Clinically, the depressive illnesses can be classified into uni- or bipolar, retarded or agitated. Unfortunately, clinical classification does not result in an understanding of the basic metabolic errors in these disorders; therefore, a rational approach to therapy is lacking. In 1965, Schildkraut (1) proposed the catecholamine hypothesis as the main cause of depression. This postulated that in some depressive illnesses "there was an absolute or relative deficiency of catecholamines, particularly noradrenaline (NA), at functionally important adrenergic receptor sites in the brain." Since 1965, other amines besides norepinephrine (NE) have assumed greater importance, e.g., 5-hydroxytryptamine (5-HT) and dopamine (DA). In addition, changes in cyclic adenosine monophosphate (AMP) have also been suggested as a cause for depression. As this compound is involved in so many other reactions in the body, however, it is difficult to assess its relevance in the etiology of depression (2). At present, it is believed that depression may not be only by altered transmitter availability but also by altered postsynaptic receptor sensitivity. All the biogenic amines probably are involved to a greater or lesser extent and probably in some interrelated fashion rather than acting independently (3).

The development of new drugs has tended to be concentrated into a search for compounds that modify either production or uptake of the biogenic amines. Because the biogenic amines involved (namely, 5-HT, NE, and DA) all have potent effects on the CVS, it is not surprising that drugs interfering with their metabolism should also have effects on the CVS.

It is conventional to classify the antidepressant drugs according to their chemical structure or mode of action, as shown in Table 10.1.

Although all the above compounds act on the biogenic amines, they do so in different ways; thus complications occurring in one group may not occur with others.

173

TABLE 10.1. *Classification of antidepressant drugs*[a]

Class	Example
Bicyclic compounds	Zimelidine
	Viloxazine
Tricyclic compounds	Amitriptyline
	Imipramine
	Clomipramine
	Doxepin
	Nortriptyline
Tetracyclic compounds	Maprotiline
	Mianserin
MAO inhibitors	Phenelzine
	Tranylcypromine
	Pargyline
Others	Lithium carbonate
	Tryptophan
	Nomifensine

[a] This list is not intended to be exhaustive but rather to contain the popular antidepressant drugs in use.

TRICYCLIC AND BICYCLIC ANTIDEPRESSANTS

If one is to understand the cardiovascular effects of these agents, a basic understanding of their pharmacology is required.

For normal affective function of the individual, the biosynthesis of all three amines, NE, 5-HT, and DA, is required. The formation of these compounds is shown in Fig. 10.1.

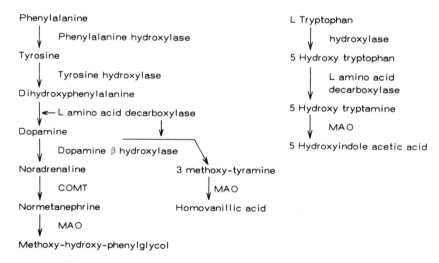

FIG. 10.1. Metabolic pathways of NE (noradrenaline), DA, and 5-HT.

Both dopa and dopamine are synthesized in the cell cytoplasm, the latter entering storage vesicles where it is converted to NE. The NE is then released into the synaptic cleft where it acts on its receptor, the action being terminated by reuptake. It is then stored for further release. Located in intraneural mitochondria, the enzyme monoamine oxidase (MAO) inactivates that portion of NE that leaks from the storage vesicle or that portion that is not taken up after termination of action.

In the brain, 5-HT is synthesized from tryptophan and released in a bound form; it then acts and is taken up in a similar fashion to NE (4,5). Drugs, such as reserpine, effect rapid release of 5-HT. After release, it is metabolized by MAO to 5-hydroxyindole acetic acid, which is then excreted (6).

Tricyclics act within these systems; it is thought that they prevent reuptake of the biogenic amines. Thus either NE or 5-HT, or both, will remain longer at its site of action, that is, in the synaptic cleft; probably in this way they bring about their antidepressant effect. However, different tricyclics and bicyclic agents may affect these systems differently; for example, zimelidine is a potent inhibitor of 5-HT reuptake but has little effect on NE (7), whereas nomifensine appears to act particularly on dopaminergic systems (8).

ETIOLOGY OF CARDIOVASCULAR EFFECTS

Table 10.2 shows the pharmacologic activity of the tricyclic antidepressants and their effects on the CVS (9–12). From this table, it can be seen why so much difficulty has arisen in attempting to define the cause of the individual abnormalities produced.

The quinidine-like effect can be seen after therapeutic dosage or after overdos-

TABLE 10.2. *Pharmacologic actions and cardiovascular effects of tricyclic antidepressants*

Action	Effect on CVS
Anticholinergic (9)	Sinus bradycardia then sinus tachycardia
	AV junctional rhythm
	PR interval may be normal
Norepinephrine reuptake blockade (10)	Sinus bradycardia
	PR interval prolonged
	AV junctional rhythm and AV dissociation
	Ventricular arrythmias
	Hypertension
5-HT reuptake blockade (11)	Hypertension
	Sinus bradycardia, sinus tachycardia
	PR interval prolonged
	AV junctional tachycardia
Quinidine-like (12)	Prolonged QRS time
	Prolonged Q-Tc interval
	Decreased contractility

age and is thought to be due to a direct action on the myocardium. It is known that these drugs have a high affinity for myocardium (13); it is not surprising that after overdosage, this effect dominates. This action probably is due to the local anesthetic activity (cocaine-like) of these agents (14). Quinidine is a class 1 antiarrhythmic agent that acts by affecting the action potential; it decreases the rate of rise of the action potential (phase 0), thereby prolonging the effective refractory period; and it delays conduction, as evidenced by prolongation of the QRS, QT, and PR intervals on the electrocardiogram (EKG) (12). It also depresses contractility, especially in doses above the therapeutic range and in patients with prior cardiac disease (15). These effects are brought about by interfering with the fast initial inward current of sodium ions (16). The tricyclics are also known to have adrenolytic activity (17,18), but this effect may be masked in those agents that block reuptake of NE.

For convenience, we may consider the effects of these drugs on the CVS in four categories: effect on (a) conduction, (b) hemodynamics, (c) blood pressure, and (d) drug interactions.

Effect on Conduction

The first report of EKG changes in man was by Kristjansen (19), who described ST-T segment changes and hypotension occurring following exercise in depressed patients who were taking imipramine. To recapitulate, since then, various abnormalities have been described, including sinus tachycardia, T wave changes, complete heart block, atrial fibrillation, P-R interval prolongation, and sudden death. Following overdosage, additional abnormalities, including supraventricular tachycardia, ventricular arrhythmias, torsade de pointes, and asystole, have been described.

From the clinical point of view, some of these claims of abnormality due to tricyclics merit further comment. In the two retrospective studies reporting sudden death and described in the previous chapter (20,21), death occurred only in patients who were known to have prior cardiac disease (ischemic heart disease, IHD). The deaths were thought to be arrhythmic deaths, although the precise cause is unknown; it is known, however, that in IHD, catecholamine levels are higher than normal in the myocardium (22). Thus medication with an agent that allowed catecholamines to remain at their site of action for a longer period of time might result in arrhythmias becoming more common. Catecholamines are also increased in the blood after administration of tricyclics. Furthermore, the histologic appearance of the myocardium of patients who died suddenly after taking tricyclics resembles that of patients who died from pheochromocytoma (23). On the other hand, as described in the last chapter, the Boston Survey of 1972 (24) could not demonstrate increased risk of sudden death. The patient described by Ramanarthan et al. (25), in whom atrial fibrillation developed upon exposure to imipramine, was also taking thyroxine, which sensitizes tissues to circulating catecholamines. In another study by Muller and

Burckhardt (26), two of 30 patients developed first degree heart block. The authors compared trimipramine, maprotiline, amitriptyline, mianserin, and imipramine. Unfortunately, it is not noted in which group these disturbances occurred.

The studies undertaken by Burrows and his colleagues in Australia (27,28) on EKG effects of various tricyclics are fully described in the previous chapter. In Great Britain, we have shown that the QT interval was prolonged after 6 weeks of therapy with amitriptyline and tended to be prolonged after treatment with the new bicyclic agent zimelidine (29), although the PR and QRS intervals were not prolonged by either drug. All patients had normal plasma levels in this study. In addition, amitriptyline caused significant tachycardia, whereas zimelidine tended to slow the heart. Undoubtedly, the tachycardia produced by tricyclics is due to the anticholinergic action of these drugs. It has also been shown to occur with nortriptyline (30) and clomipramine (31), together with prolongation of the PR, QRS, and QT intervals. Conversely, in a double-blind study in volunteers (31), we demonstrated that after a single dose of amitriptyline (50 mg), there was slowing of the heart rate, although plasma levels were subtherapeutic, which probably explains this phenomenon. In low doses, anticholinergic drugs cause bradycardia before causing tachycardia (9); thus if plasma levels are subtherapeutic, one would expect the anticholinergic effect to be reduced and a bradycardia to occur.

Because of this quinidine-like activity, Bigger et al. (32) treated two depressed patients, who had both atrial and ventricular premature beats, with imipramine. Each patient showed a significant decrease in both atrial and ventricular premature beats, and the PR, QRS, and QT intervals were all significantly prolonged. In this case, the drug behaved as an antiarrhythmic agent. It must be remembered, however, that all antiarrhythmic agents are also potentially arryhthmogenic. This study is of importance as it draws attention to the problem of treating patients with tricyclics and using other class 1 antiarrhythmics (e.g., quinidine, procainamide, disopyramide) concurrently. Often, however, patients who have arrhythmias have compromised left ventricular function and are taking diuretics, a situation that may cause urinary problems. Thus the routine use of drugs with potent anticholinergic activity in the treatment of arrhythmias is not advisable.

Finally, the newer drugs of this type do not give rise to the frequent problems found with the older compounds. Doxepin is relatively safe even in patients with cardiovascular disease (33), and dothiepin has been studied in a group of 25 geriatric patients (34). Of these, one developed tachycardia, one ventricular extrasystoles, and one ST depression. However, no data are available on the different EKG intervals in the study.

After overdosage, tricyclics are often lethal. The main EKG and other changes are outlined in the previous chapter, but further comment is appropriate. In the studies by Spiker and his colleagues (35–37), it was observed that the QRS duration was greater than or equal to 100 msec when plasma levels exceeded

1,000 ng/ml; the normal QRS duration varies and may be normal up to a duration of 100 msec. In addition, patients with bundle-branch block have a QRS duration of 110 msec or longer (38), thus stressing the need for a predose EKG.

Other studies have shown similar results. Thorstrand (39,40) analyzed 153 cases of tricyclic overdosage (mainly amitriptyline) and found that the QRS interval was greater than 110 msec in 42%, that 49% showed QT interval prolongation, and 28% PQ prolongation. Unlike the QT interval, QRS width was not related to heart rate. Thorstrand concluded that the QRS complex duration was probably the best indicator of severity of poisoning. Coma correlated well with this parameter. Although the QT interval was prolonged in 49% of cases, the author did not find it as good an indicator as QRS width, because at normal EKG speed, the QT interval is difficult to measure accurately. It may not be easy to delineate a change from the end of the T wave to the U wave or to differentiate between the T wave and P wave in tachycardia.

More severe changes have been noted by other investigators. Rose (41) noted that after moderate or severe overdosage in 53 patients, 12 developed ST-T wave abnormalities, 10 sinus or supraventricular tachycardia, six first degree heart block, five ventricular arrhythmias, and one died in asystole. Similarly, Robinson and Barker (42) agree that arrhythmias tend to be dose related after overdosage, but they do not stress the duration of the QRS interval. On the other hand, Brubakk and Kalager (43) concluded that arrhythmias were uncommon after overdosage, but the degree of poisoning is difficult to assess in their 21 patients, since nine took more than one drug.

In contrast to the conclusions of Burrows et al. (28) concerning the lack of EKG changes with doxepin (see Chapter 9), Williams (44) found that several arrhythmias could occur following overdosage with this tricyclic; furthermore, respiratory depression occurred. Although there are no published reports of dothiepin overdosage and cardiac complication, the drug has been known to cause death and abnormal cardiac rhythms after overdosage (Boots Co. Ltd, *personal communication*).

The bicyclic agents viloxazine and zimelidine have not yet been incriminated as causing arrhythmias, but these drugs are relatively new, and further reports are awaited.

Effect on Hemodynamics

Most research into the hemodynamic effects of antidepressants has been performed on animal models (see Chapter 9) and is not mentioned further here.

Because cardiac catheterization has a definite risk of morbidity and mortality (45), and because studies must be repeated in patients to observe long-term effects on the circulation, we are dependent on noninvasive studies to assess the hemodynamic effects of antidepressants. Most studies have used systolic time intervals (STI), which provide a reliable and repeatable means of assessing the inotropic state of the left ventricle, provided that conditions in the laboratory are carefully controlled (46).

We have shown in volunteers (31) that amitriptyline depresses cardiac contractility after a single 50-mg dose. A similar effect occurs after 6 weeks of treatment with amitriptyline (150 mg/day) (29); in our studies, zimelidine did not affect the STI and would seem to be a safer drug. Burckhardt et al. (47) showed that tricyclics depressed cardiac contractility. This effect could last as long as the drug was prescribed, but cardiac function returned to normal on withdrawal. Similar effects have been shown after treatment with nortriptyline; cardiac function seems to deteriorate as the plasma levels rise (48).

The negative inotropic effect of these drugs is probably caused by the accumulation of these agents in cardiac tissue and their local anesthetic effects on myocardium. As early as 1959, it was known that these agents could precipitate heart failure even in therapeutic doses (49).

After overdosage, Thorstrand (39) showed that cardiac output was increased, arterial venous oxygen difference was decreased, and pulmonary artery diastolic pressure was normal, while pulse rate was increased. He surmised that after overdosage, the patients developed a hyperkinetic circulation; probably due to an adrenergic stimulatory effect on the circulation. Stroke volume, however, was not increased, which would be unusual if there were high levels of circulating catecholamines; this finding could be explained by the fact that tricyclics have an adrenolytic effect (17,18). Thus alpha-blockade would cause tachycardia and a reflex increase in cardiac output. Unfortunately, it is not clear how severe the poisonings were in his study, as it is known from animal data (see Chapter 9) that cardiac function deteriorates as the tricyclic levels rise. Contrary to Thorstrand's findings (39), Brubakk and Kalager (43) noted similar findings after overdosage as are found after therapeutic dosage (i.e., decreased contractility).

Effect on Blood Pressure

Both hypertension and hypotension have been reported to occur with the tricyclic antidepressants. Hessov (50) reported hypertension in three patients who were treated with clomipramine, while postural hypotension occurs commonly with their use, especially in the first 14 days of therapy (51). In a comparison of previous studies, Hattab (52) found the incidence of postural hypotension to be 10% with imipramine, 8.6% with amitriptyline, and 2.6% with doxepin. The cause of either hypertension or hypotension is unclear, although the adrenolytic activity of these drugs probably accounts for hypotension. Hypertension is thought to be due to the blockade of adrenergic neuron uptake, which potentiates the pressor effect of NE.

The problems with postural hypotension are particularly troublesome in the elderly and in those patients with poor cardiac reserve. In a recent publication, Glassman et al. (53) showed that the incidence of this complication was not related to age or dose (all their patients were taking imipramine) but rather to the degree of orthostatic drop in pressure before treatment. They concede, however, that the repercussions of postural hypotension (e.g., cerebrovascular accidents) are more likely to increase with increasing degrees of cardiovascular disease or advancing age. It would thus seem prudent to use these drugs carefully, if at all, in the elderly.

DRUG INTERACTIONS

Because of their mode of action, these agents interact with direct- and indirect-acting sympathomimetics. Boakes et al. (54) investigated the interaction between sympathomimetic amines and different antidepressants in man, finding that imipramine potentiated the pressor effects of phenylephrine (two- to threefold), NE (four- to eightfold), and epinephrine (two- to fourfold). Dysrhythmias occurred with epinephrine. Because of the ability of antidepressants to block the uptake of catecholamines, Freyschuss et al. (55) devised a test to assess the pressor response to tyramine (an indirect acting sympathomimetic) alone and after antidepressant drugs. It can be shown that after tricyclics, more tyramine is needed to gain the same pressor response. Thus patients taking drugs that contain indirect-acting sympathomimetic amines (e.g., antitussives and some bronchodilator remedies) would not benefit from the effect of these medications if tricyclics were added to their regimen. This stresses the need to ask patients about their other medication before prescribing these agents.

In addition, the adrenergic-blocking agents guanethidine, debrisoquine, and bethanidine are taken up in a similar fashion to NE. Tricyclics prevent the uptake of these agents, with consequent hypertension (56,57). They also interact with the antihypertensive action of clonidine, possibly by increasing levels of circulating catecholamines (58). As has been pointed out earlier, many of these drugs have a quinidine-like action and would potentiate the action of class I antiarrhythmic agents, which also have a myocardial depressant action (e.g., quinidine and procainamide).

Although it has been conventional to suppose that tricyclic antidepressants should not be used with MAO inhibitors, Schukit et al. (59), after reviewing the literature, concluded that adverse reactions were probably no more common with combined therapy than with either drug alone. Finally, some drugs may cause depression (e.g., methyldopa, reserpine, and steroids); in this case, although the tricyclics are not known to interact with these agents, it would be advisable to change the original drug rather than treat such an iatrogenic effect with a potentially harmful drug.

TREATMENT OF CARDIOTOXICITY

As the mechanism of production of cardiac arrhythmias is complex, it follows that definitive therapy is not really satisfactory.

In the case of either arrhythmias or heart failure occurring while the patient is taking therapeutic doses of these drugs, the best form of treatment is immediate withdrawal of the drug and observation. Symptomatic treatment may be required (see below). Tricyclic compounds have long half-lives and tend to accumulate in tissues; observation over a number of days is preferable.

After overdosage, basic methods of treatment must be followed, e.g., maintenance of airway, gastric lavage, and an adequate fluid intake. Activated charcoal should be given (41), and the patients must be monitored for EKG abnormalities (60). There is no specific antidote.

Specific Measures for Tricyclics

There is no place for forced diuresis or dialysis (61,62). In cases where the anticholinergic phenomena are dominant or where coma has supervened, physostigmine has been used with good effect (63). Dosage should be 2 mg i.v.; if the state of coma decreases, an infusion of 2.5 mg/hr may be given. After severe overdosage, however, caution should be exercised, as physostigmine has been shown to increase the likelihood of precipitating seizures. This seems especially important with imipramine (64). Probanthine should be given to block the peripheral cholinergic effects.

The main problem in treating the arrhythmias that occur is that they may change rapidly from one variety to another; in this case, treatment may prove hazardous. A variety of agents have been used, e.g. phenytoin (39,62), which is also useful in treating tricyclic-induced seizures. Although phenytoin is a class I antiarrhythmic agent, it decreases auriculoventricular (AV) conduction time and does not have the negative inotropic effects of the conventional class I agents. However, it must not be used in supraventricular arrhythmias. The beta-adrenergic blocking agents practolol and propranolol have been used (39,65), but they may cause hypotension and must be used with great care. Thorstrand (39) found that propranolol did not shorten the QRS complex, whereas Brown's experiments in dogs (65) did show shortening of the QRS complex with practolol. The probable reason for this difference in effect is that practolol, unlike propranolol, does not have any class I antiarrhythmic activity.

The major problem arising from overdosage is with ventricular arrhythmias if they occur, especially if the abnormality is ventricular tachycardia (VT) or fibrillation (VF). These drugs have been implicated in causing the syndrome of *torsade de pointes* (66), in addition to conventional VT or VF. In the case of *torsade de pointes,* defibrillation or intravenous isoprenaline should be given to shorten repolarization time. A clue to this diagnosis is that the Q-T interval is often prolonged prior to the onset of VT or VF, the bouts of arrhythmia may initially occur in short bursts, and the axis of the arrhythmia often changes during a single bout. Class I antiarrhythmic agents must not be used in this condition. In any variety of ventricular arrhythmia, the use of quinidine or procainamide can only be mentioned to be condemned. Not only do they cause similar changes to the action potential as the tricyclics, but they also possess anticholinergic activity. In the case of isolated ventricular ectopic beats, propranolol is the drug of choice.

In the case of supraventricular arrhythmias, isolated ectopic beats should not be treated. In supraventricular tachycardia (SVT), treatment is needed if there is cardiac failure or if the bout is prolonged. Digoxin may be tried, as long as the physician is aware that its use may prove hazardous. Practolol or propranolol are probably safer agents; if heart failure is present, a diuretic should be added. Other drugs used for SVT may prove dangerous, e.g., verapamil, which increases the P-R interval (often prolonged after tricyclic poisoning). When bradyarrhythmias occur, e.g., heart block, an intravenous pacemaker would be the best method of treatment. Atropine should not be used.

Some studies have shown that correcting acid-base balance is of importance (65). Others disagree (39), and at present this question remains unanswered. In a recent study, Sutherland et al. (67) reported that patients in coma following tricyclic overdosage frequently suffered from a mixed metabolic and respiratory acidosis. None had cardiac arrhythmias. Thus the importance of these abnormalities is doubtful. Theoretically, correction of acid-base status and hypoxia would seem logical, as both these phenomena may be associated with cardiac arrhythmia.

TETRACYCLIC ANTIDEPRESSANTS

Maprotiline

Maprotiline hydrochloride has a similar action to the tricyclics, although it does not block reuptake of 5-HT. It also possesses anticholinergic activity, blocks the reuptake of NE as assessed by the tyramine pressor response, and has been shown to antagonize the effects of adrenergic neuron blocking agents (68). EKG abnormalities have been described with large doses of maprotiline (> 300 mg), and Jukes (69) has shown that the drug may cause arrhythmias after overdosage, especially if a combination of drugs is taken (e.g., alcohol, chlorpromazine, catecholamines, MAO inhibitors, or other tricyclics). In a further survey, Crome and Newman (70) found that after overdosage in 41 patients, tachycardia occurred in five, bradycardia in three, cardiac arrest in three, hypotension in two, and hypertension in one.

The drug is known to cause tachycardia and postural hypotension in therapeutic dosage, the incidence being much lower than with conventional tricyclics; Hattab (52) showed that postural hypotension occurred in 1.6% of cases and tachycardia in 4.2% following therapeutic dosage. Hemodynamically, Reale and Motolese (71) showed that after a single dose of 50 mg i.v., left ventricular stroke work index increased, left ventricular end-diastolic pressure decreased, and myocardial oxygen consumption was unaltered. Systemic arterial resistance decreased. The authors suggested that these results may indicate vasodilation in certain vascular beds. Cardiac index and stroke volume index tended to increase; it would seem that left ventricular function improved. The changes occurring in this study can be explained by the fact that the drug was producing an adrenolytic action (by blocking reuptake of NE). Hypotension did not occur, but the patients were lying down throughout the study. In a further study, Selvini et al. (72) compared maprotiline (25 mg) with diazepam (5 mg) both being given twice daily following myocardial infarction, in 126 patients. In their study, which lasted an average of 2 weeks, there were no cardiotoxic effects from maprotiline; however, the dosage was subtherapeutic.

Although maprotiline is probably safer than the other tricyclics, it has the potential to be cardiotoxic, especially after overdosage.

Mianserin

Mianserin is a new antidepressant agent that does not have anticholinergic activity, nor does it prevent reuptake of NE in man (73). In animal studies, it does not cause the serious cardiac side effects that are associated with the tricyclics (see Chapter 9). It is believed to increase production of NE centrally (74) and antagonize the venoconstrictor response to 5-HT (75).

Few studies have been performed in man after therapeutic dosage. We (31) showed that acute administration of 20 mg in healthy volunteers prolonged the QT interval after 150 min. An initial study in two depressed patients showed prolongation of the QT interval at 1 week, but this returned to normal after 2 weeks of therapy. There were no changes in the STI in these studies. We (29) then investigated the changes on the EKG and STI after 6 weeks of treatment with mianserin in eight depressed patients. There were no changes in the EKG, and heart rate was unaltered. Changes in the STI were seen but probably reflected the peripheral effects of the drug. Left ventricular ejection time (LVET) and QS2 interval were decreased, but the ratio of the preejection period (PEP) to the LVET was increased. As shortening of the QS_2 interval implies a positive inotropic effect, and PEP/LVET ratio increase implies a negative inotropic effect, it is unlikely that these effects were due to direct actions on the heart. Robson et al. (76) have shown that mianserin resembles the classic presynaptic alpha-adrenoceptor antagonists piperoxan and yohimbine. Furthermore, Baumann and Maitre (77) have demonstrated that clonidine stimulation of presynaptic alpha-adrenoceptors is antagonized by mianserin, in the same manner as by phentolamine and phenoxybenzamine. This adrenolytic activity, by causing peripheral dilatation, may reflexly increase cardiac output and shorten the QS_2 interval. Perhaps stroke volume is decreased due to antagonism of the venoconstrictor response to 5-HT, with reduction of preload, which in turn would tend to increase the PEP/LVET ratio.

Further evidence of the benign effect of this agent on the CVS is demonstrated by studies that have shown that it does not antagonize the antihypertensive effects of propranolol, propranolol and hydralazine, guanethidine, or bethanidine

(31). Its safety in depressed patients with cardiac disorders is demonstrated in the next chapter.

Following overdosage, one case of first degree heart block has been reported (78), while in 20 cases of overdosage, Crome and Newman (70) found that there were no arrhythmias, but two patients developed sinus tachycardia, three hypertension, and one hypotension. At present, the reason for these abnormalities is unclear.

In summary, mianserin hydrochloride appears to be a safer drug than the tricyclic antidepressants, as it does not have the same cardiodepressant effects; nor does it have the same propensity to cause lethal arrhythmias, even following overdosage.

MAO Inhibitors

The MAO inhibitors may be seen as the second line of treatment for depression, although interest in them has been revived recently (79). In general, they are less effective than the tricyclics, and their use has been limited because they are associated with unfortunate reactions, which may be fatal. Many of these reactions have been blamed on flimsy evidence and have been uncritically perpetuated.

Their main action is on the metabolism of tryptophan (see Fig. 10.1), where 5-HT will accumulate. They also affect the metabolism of NE, since the NE that does not undergo reuptake into the vesicles is metabolized by MAO (80). The main complication with MAO inhibitors consists of hypertensive reactions with other drugs or foodstuffs. On their own, some of the MAO inhibitors have been used as antihypertensive agents, e.g., pargyline. This effect may be due to reduced NE release in response to preganglionic stimulation. Pargyline has its major effect in the erect posture, which indicates interference with sympathetic venoconstriction. It is reported to reduce transmission through sympathetic, but not parasympathetic, ganglia (81). Hemodynamic studies have shown pargyline to decrease peripheral resistance and cardiac output (82,83). The hypertensive reaction of MAO inhibitors results from interaction with indirect sympathomimetic amines, e.g., amphetamine and tyramine.

Elis et al. (84) investigated the interactions of MAO inhibitors with the sympathomimetic agents NE, ephedrine, and phenylephrine. They found that NE was not importantly inactivated by MAO and was not potentiated. Similar findings with epinephrine and isoprenaline were demonstrated by Boakes et al. (54).

Ephedrine is an indirect-acting sympathomimetic; i.e., it acts by discharging NE from its stores at nerve endings. It is unaffected by MAO. In the presence of an MAO inhibitor, however, more NE would be available for release, thus potentiating the effect of ephedrine, which these studies demonstrated as being fourfold. Because it is not metabolized by MAO, the potentiation was the same whether it was given orally or intravenously.

Phenylephrine acts almost entirely directly on adrenergic receptors, with little indirect effect. It is a substrate for MAO, however, and MAO is present in large amounts in the intestine and liver. Thus if a patient is taking a MAO inhibitor, more drug would be available for activity, and its effect would be potentiated. This was confirmed by Elis et al. (84) since, in most of their experiments, the studies had to be terminated because of hypertensive reactions. After intravenous dosage, phenylephrine was potentiated and blood pressure increased 2 to 2.5 times.

The major problem of MAO inhibitors has been with foodstuffs that release tyramine. Foodstuffs to be avoided to prevent hypertensive reactions are: matured cheese, marmite, bovril, chianti wine, broad bean pods, banana skins, and pickled herrings. Patients should eat only fresh or freshly prepared food (85). As for the interaction between drugs, the following are contraindicated: methyldopa, indirect-acting sympathomimetic amines, antihistamines, sedatives, narcotics, and levodopa (86).

Should a hypertensive crisis ensue, the best treatment is with an alpha-adrenoceptor blocking agent, such as phentolamine.

OTHER ANTIDEPRESSANTS

Lithium

Lithium carbonate has been used for some years in the affective disorders, mainly for the prophylactic treatment of recurrent unipolar or bipolar affective illness and for the acute treatment of mania. In a recent study, lithium was found to be superior to maprotiline in the prophylactic treatment of recurrent affective disorders (87).

It is still unclear how lithium acts. Many theories have been advanced, but the most likely are the ones put forward by Singer and Rothenberg (88).

Ion Transport Mechanism

Lithium is a cation that may act as an imperfect substitute for other cations (predominantly sodium and potassium) that normally participate in processes of ionic transfer or distribution to produce and maintain the proper electrochemical gradients or osmotic steady state.

Cellular microenvironment

Lithium may act as a critical member of the cellular microenvironment that determines the basic spatial structure, energy supply, or time course of cellular processes. It is thought that it thus interferes with the production of cyclic AMP.

In the central nervous system, lithium accelerates presynaptic destruction of NE, inhibits the neuronal release of NE and 5-HT, and increases uptake of NE. It may be through these mechanisms that lithium exerts its main effects, which are described in the previous chapter.

Tryptophan

Tryptophan has been recently introduced for the treatment of depression. Its action is thought to increase brain 5-HT, which may be decreased in depression (89). We know of no cardiovascular abnormalities that have been described with its use.

Nomifensine

Nomifensine is a new antidepressant with a tetrahydroquinoline structure. Animal studies show that it differs from the more conventional drugs in that it is a potent inhibitor of DA and NE uptake in the brain (90).

As this is a new agent, few human studies have been performed. The studies by Burrows and his colleagues (91) are described in the previous chapter. In another study in three patients, no change was seen on the STI, but the drug depressed T wave heights in all three patients (Burgess, *unpublished observations*). At present, there is little evidence of cardiotoxicity in man, but it is too early to come to a final conclusion about this agent. It will be interesting to see if this drug affects the CVS after overdosage, and if the effect differs from the tricyclics, because of its DA uptake blocking action.

CONCLUSIONS

Although the tricyclic compounds are the most frequently used drugs for the treatment of depression, they are probably also the most cardiotoxic. Following overdosage, they may be lethal; indeed, in the United Kingdom, they are the most common cause of fatal poisoning in children under the age of 5 years (92).

After therapeutic dosage, serious cardiovascular complications do not occur frequently, although postural hypotension has been known to occur in up to 20% of patients treated with imipramine (53). The more serious complications are more likely to occur in the aged and in those with cardiovascular disease. A thorough history and cardiovascular examination should be made before prescribing these drugs. An EKG should be performed before treatment is begun, about 10 to 14 days later, and at regular intervals thereafter. A knowledge of other drugs that the patient is taking simultaneously is mandatory to prevent needless drug interactions.

At present, the safest drugs for the treatment of depression are probably mianserin, nomifensine, and perhaps maprotiline, followed by the newer tricyclics doxepin and dothiepin; maprotiline, doxepin, and dothiepin, however, may be lethal after overdosage. We suggest that these drugs be the first line of treatment, rather than the older compounds amitriptyline and imipramine, in those patients with heart disease in whom drugs are indicated for the treatment of depression. In the relapsing type of depression, lithium is probably the most effective drug, provided its use is monitored carefully.

REFERENCES

1. Schildkraut, J. J. The catecholamine hypothesis of affective disorders. A review of supporting evidence. *Am. J. Psychiatry,* 1965, 24, 509.
2. Editorial. Cyclic AMP and depressive illness. *Lancet,* 1975, 1, 559.
3. Ridges, A. P. The potential value of biochemical parameters in the diagnosis and medication of affective disorders. *Postgrad. Med. J. [Suppl. 3],* 1976, 9.
4. Coppen, A. J. The chemical pathology of the affective disorders. *J. Int. Med. Res. [Suppl. 3],* 1975, 3, 52.
5. Shaw, D. M. Tricyclic antidepressants, tryptophan and affective disorders. *Postgrad. Med. J. [Suppl. 3]* 1976, 52, 47.
6. Harper, H. A. *Review of Physiological Chemistry.* Lange Publications, Los Altos, California, 1965.
7. Siwers, B., Ringberger, V., Tuck, J. R., and Sjoquist, F. Initial clinical trial based on biochemical methodology of zimelidine (a serotonin uptake inhibitor) in depressed patients. *Clin. Pharmacol. Ther.,* 1977, 21, 194.
8. Schacht, J., Leven, M., and Backer, G. Studies on brain metabolism of biogenic amines. *Br. J. Clin. Pharmacol. [Suppl. 2], 1977, 4,* 775.
9. Gravenstein, J. S., Ariet, M., and Thornby, J. I. Atropine on the electrocardiogram. *Clin. Pharmacol. Ther.,* 1969, 10, 660.
10. Innes, I. R., and Nickerson, M. Norepinephrine, epinephrine and the sympathomimetic amines. In: *Pharmacological Basis of Therapeutics,* edited by L. S. Goodman and A. Gilman, p. 491, 1975. Macmillan, New York.
11. James, T. N., Isobe, J. H., and Urthaler, F. Analysis of components in a cardiogenic hypertensive reflex. *Circulation,* 1975, 52, 179.
12. Heisenbuttel, R. H., and Bigger, J. T. The effect of quinidine on intraventricular conduction in man. Correlation of plasma quinidine with changes in QRS duration. *Am. Heart J.,* 1970, 80, 453.
13. Cassano, G. B., Sjastrond, S. E., and Hansson, E. Distribution and fate of C^{14}-amitriptyline in mice and rats. *Psychopharmacologia,* 1965, 8, 1.
14. Axelrod, J., and Weinshilbaum, R. Catecholamines. *N. Engl. J. Med.,* 1972, 287, 237.
15. Moe, G. K., and Abildskov, J. A. Anti-arrhythmic drugs. In: *Pharmacological Basis of Therapeutics,* edited by L. S. Goodman and A. Gilman, p. 682, 1975. Macmillan, New York.
16. Morgan, P. H., and Mathison, I. W. Arrhythmias and anti-arrhythmic drugs: Mechanism of action and structure-activity relationships II. *J. Pharm. Sci.,* 1976, 65, 635.
17. Sigg, E. B., Osborne, M., and Korol, B. Cardiovascular effects of imipramine. *J. Pharmacol. Exp. Ther.,* 1963, 141, 237.
18. Cairncross, K. D. On the peripheral pharmacology of amitriptyline. *Arch. Int. Pharm.,* 1965, 154, 438.
19. Kristjansen, E. S. Cardiac complications during treatment with imipramine (tofranil). *Acta Psychiatr. Neurol.,* 1961, 36, 427.
20. Coull, D. C., Crookes, J., Dingwall-Fordyce, I., Scott, A., and Weir, R. D. Amitriptyline and cardiac disease. Risk of sudden death identified by monitoring system. *Lancet,* 1970, 2, 590.
21. Moir, D. C., Crooks, J., Cornwell, W. B., O'Malley, M., Dingwall-Fordyce, I., Turnbull, M. J., and Weir, R. D. Cardiotoxicity of amitriptyline. *Lancet,* 1972, 2, 561.
22. Pentillä, O., Menkallio, E., Pispa, J., Klinge, E., Saltanen, P., and Kyösola, K. Auricular tyrosine hydroxylase and dopamine beta hydroxylase activities and noradrenaline content in ischaemic heart disease. *Acta Med. Scand.,* 1978, 203, 161.

23. Alexander, C. S., and Niño, A. Cardiovascular complications in young patients taking psychotropic drugs. *Am. Heart J.,* 1969, 78, 757.
24. Boston Collaborative Drug Surveillance Program Report. Adverse reactions to the tricyclic anti-depressant drugs. *Lancet,* 1972, 1, 529.
25. Ramanarthan, K. B., and Davidson, C. Cardiac arrhythmia and imipramine therapy. *Br. Med. J.,* 1975, 1, 661.
26. Muller, V., and Burckhardt, D. Effects of tri and tetracyclic antidepressants on the cardiovascular system. *Schweiz Med. Wochenschr.,* 1974, 104, 1911.
27. Vohra, S., Burrows, G. D., and Sloman, J. G. Assessment of cardiovascular side effects of therapeutic doses of tricyclic antidepressant drugs. *Aust. N.Z. Med. J.,* 1975, 5, 7.
28. Burrows, G. D., Vohra, J., Hunt, D., Sloman, J. G., Scoggins, B. A., and Davies, B. Cardiac effects of different tricyclic anti-depressant drugs. *Br. J. Psychiatry,* 1976, 129, 335.
29. Burgess, C. D., Montgomery, S. A., and Wadsworth, J., and Turner, P. Cardiovascular effects of amitriptyline, mianserin, zimelidine and nomifersine in depressed patients. *Postgrad. Med. J.,* 1979, 55, 704.
30. Ziegler, V. E., Co, B. T., and Biggs, S. T. Plasma nortriptyline levels and ECG findings. *Am. J. Psychiatry,* 1977, 134, 141.
31. Burgess, C. D., Turner, P., and Wadsworth, J. Cardiovascular responses to mianserin hydrochloride—A comparison with tricyclic antidepressant drugs. *Br. J. Clin. Pharmacol. [Suppl. 1],* 1978, 5, 21S.
32. Bigger, J. T., Giardina, E. G. C., Kantor, S. J., and Glassman, A. H. Cardiac anti-arrhythmic effect of imipramine hydrochloride. *N. Engl. J. Med.,* 1977, 296, 206.
33. Pinder, R. M., Brogden, R. N., Speight, T. M., and Avery, G. S. Doxepin up to date. *Drugs,* 1977, 13, 161.
34. Khan, A. U. A study of dothiepin hydrochloride in elderly patients, with special reference to the cardiovascular system. *Mod. Geriatr.,* 1975, 5, 26.
35. Spiker, D. G., Weiss, A. N., and Chang, S. S. Tricyclic antidepressant overdose, clinical presentation and plasma levels. *Clin. Pharmacol. Ther.,* 1975, 18, 539.
36. Spiker, D. G., and Biggs, J. T. Tricyclic antidepressants. *JAMA,* 1976, 236, 1711.
37. Petit, J. M., Spiker, D. G., Ruwitch, J. F., Ziegler, V. E., Weiss, A. N., and Biggs, J. T. Tricyclic anti-depressant plasma levels and adverse effects after overdosage. *Clin. Pharmacol. Ther.,* 1977, 21, 47.
38. Schamroth, L. *An Introduction to Electrocardiography.* Blackwell, Oxford, 1973.
39. Thorstrand, C. Cardiovascular effects of poisonings with tricyclic antidepressants. *Acta Med. Scand.,* 1974, 195, 505.
40. Thorstrand, C. Clinical features in poisonings by tricyclic antidepressants with special reference to the ECG. *Acta Med. Scand.,* 1976, 199, 337.
41. Rose, J. B. Tricyclic antidepressant toxicity. *Clin. Toxicol.,* 1977, 11, 391.
42. Robinson, D. S., and Barker, E. Tricyclic antidepressant cardiotoxicity. *JAMA,* 1976, 236, 2089.
43. Brubakk, O., and Kalager, T. Non invasive assessment of cardiac function in poisoning with drugs. *Acta. Med. Scand.,* 1978, 204, 39.
44. Williams, J. O. Respiratory depression in tricyclic antidepressant overdosage. *Br. Med. J.,* 1972, 1, 631.
45. Beckmann, C. H., and Dooley, B. Complications of left heart angiography: A study of 1000 consecutive cases. *Circulation,* 1970, 41, 825.
46. Lewis, R. P., Rittgers, S. E., Forester, W. F., and Boudoulas, H. A critical review of the systolic time intervals. *Circulation,* 1977, 56, 146.
47. Burckhardt, D., Raeder, E., Muller, V., Imhof, P., and Neubauer, H. Cardiovascular effects of tricyclic and tetracyclic antidepressants. *JAMA,* 1978, 239, 213.
48. Taylor, D. J. E., and Braithwaite, R. A. Cardiac effects of tricyclic antidepressant medication. A preliminary study of nortriptyline. *Br. Heart J.,* 1978, 40, 1005.
49. Mann, A., Catterson, A., and Macpherson, A. Toxicity of imipramine: Reports of serious side effects and massive overdose. *Can. Med. Assoc. J.,* 1959, 81, 23.
50. Hessov, I. Hypertension during chlorimipramine therapy. *Br. Med. J.,* 1971, 3, 743.
51. Hayes, J. R., Born, G. F., and Rosenbaum, A. H. Incidence of orthostatic hypertension in patients with primary affective disorders treated with tricyclic antidepressants. *Mayo Clin. Proc.,* 1977, 52, 502.

52. Hattab, J. R. The cardiovascular effects of Ludiomil in comparison with those of some tricyclic antidepressants. Ludiomil Symposium, Malta, 1977.
53. Glassmann, A. H., Giardina, E. V., Perel, J. M., Bigger, J. T., Kantor, S. J., and Davies, M. Clinical characteristics of imipramine-induced orthostatic hypotension. *Lancet,* 1979, 1, 468.
54. Boakes, A. J., Lawrence, D. R., Teoh, P. C., Barar, F. S. K., Benedicter, L. T. D., and Prichard, B. N. C. Interactions between sympathomimetic amines and antidepressants in man. *Br. Med. J.,* 1973, 1, 311.
55. Freyschuss, U., Sjoquist, R., and Tuck, D. Tyramine pressor response effects in man before and during treatment with nortriptyline or E.C.T. *Pharmacol. Clin.,* 1970, 2, 72.
56. Skinner, C., Coull, D. C., and Johnson, A. W. Antagonism of the hypertension of bethanidine and debrisoquine by tricyclic antidepressants. *Lancet,* 1969, 2, 564.
57. Meyer, J. F., McAllister, C. K., and Goldberg, L. I. Insidious and prolonged antagonism of guanethidine by amitriptyline. *JAMA,* 1970, 213, 1487.
58. Briant, R. H., Reid, J. L., and Dollery, C. T. Interaction between clonidine and desipramine in man. *Br. Med. J.,* 1973, 1, 522.
59. Schukit, M., Robins, E., and Feighner, J. Monoamine oxidase inhibitors combined therapy in the treatment of depression. *Arch. Gen. Psychiatry,* 1971, 24, 509.
60. Wood, C. A., Brown, J. R., Coleman, J. H., and Evans, W. E. Management of tricyclic antidepressant toxicities. *Dis. Nerv. Syst.,* 1976, 37, 459.
61. Noble, J., and Matthew, H. Acute poisoning by tricyclic antidepressants. Clinical factors and management of 100 patients. *Clin. Toxicol.,* 1969, 2, 403.
62. Davis, J. M. Overdose of psychotropic drugs—tricyclic antidepressants. *Psychiatr. Ann.,* 1973, 3, 6.
63. Aquilonius, S. M., and Hedstand, U. The use of physostigmine as an antidote in tricyclic antidepressant atoxicity by physostigmine in mice. *Clin. Toxicol.,* 1977, 11, 413.
64. Vance, M. A., Ross, S. M., Millington, W. R., and Blumberg, J. B. Potentiation of tricyclic antidepressant atoxicity by physostigmine in mice. *Clin. Toxicol.,* 1977, 11, 413.
65. Brown, T. C. K. Sodium bicarbonate treatment for tricyclic antidepressant arrhythmia in children. *Med. J. Aust.,* 1976, 2, 380.
66. Krikler, D. M., and Curry, P. V. L. Torsade de pointes, an atypical ventricular tachycardia. *Br. Heart J.,* 1976, 38, 117.
67. Sutherland, G. R., Park, J., and Proudfoot, A. T. Ventilation and acid-base changes in deep coma due to barbiturate or tricyclic antidepressant poisoning. *Clin. Toxicol.,* 1977, 11, 403.
68. Briant, R. H., and George, C. F. The assessment of potential drug interactions with a new tricyclic antidepressant drug. *Br. J. Clin. Pharmacol.,* 1974, 1, 113.
69. Jukes, A. M. Maprotiline (Ludiomil). Side effects and overdosage. *J. Int. Med. Res. [Suppl. 2],* 1975, 3, 126.
70. Crome, P., and Newman, B. Poisoning with maprotiline and mianserin. *Br. Med. J.,* 1977, 2, 260.
71. Reale, A., and Motolese, M. *Depressive illness: An International Symposium, St. Moritz.* Hans Huber, Bern, Switzerland.
72. Selvini, A., Rossi, C., Belli, C., Corallo, S., and Lucarelli, P. E. Antidepressant treatment with maprotiline in the management of emotional disturbances in patients with acute myocardial infarction. A controlled study. *J. Int. Med. Res.,* 1976, 4, 42.
73. Ghose, K., Coppen, A., and Turner, P. Autonomic actions and interactions of mianserin hydrochloride (Org. G.B. 94) and amitriptyline in patients with depressive illness. *Psychopharmacology,* 1976, 49, 201.
74. Leonard, B. E. Some effects of mianserin on monoamine metabolism in the rat brain. *Br. J. Clin. Pharmacol. [Suppl. 1],* 1977, 5, 11.
75. Saxena, P. R., Houwelingen, P., and Van Barta, I. L. The effects of mianserin hydrochloride on the vascular responses evoked by 5 hydroxy tryptamine and vasoactive substances. *Eur. J. Pharmacol.,* 1971, 13, 295.
76. Robson, R. D., Antonaccio, M. J., Saelens, J. K., and Liebman, J. Antagonism by mianserin and classical alpha adrenoreceptor blocking drugs of some cardiovascular and behavioral effects of clonidine. *Eur. J. Pharmacol.,* 1978, 47, 431.
77. Baumann, P. A., and Maitre, L. Effect of mianserin on noradrenaline uptake and release. *NauynSchmiedebergs Arch. Pharmacolo.,* 1977, 300, 31.

78. Green, S. D. R., and Kendall-Taylor, P. Heart block in mianserin hydrochloride overdosage. *Br. Med. J.,* 1977, 4, 1190.
79. Editorial. New look at monoamine oxidase inhibitors. *Br. Med. J.,* 1976, 2, 69.
80. Berger, F. M. Depression and antidepressant drugs. *Clin. Pharmacol. Ther.,* 1975, 18, 241.
81. Puig, M., Wakade, A. R., and Kirkpekar, S. M. Effect on the sympathetic nervous system of chronic treatment with paragyline and L-Dopa. *J. Pharmacol. Exp. Ther.,* 1972, 182, 130.
82. Onesti, G., Novak, P., Ramiraz, O., Brest, A. N., and Mayer, J. H. Haemodynamic effects of pargyline in hypertensive patients. *Circulation,* 1964, 30, 830.
83. Sannerstedt, R. Haemodynamic effects of pargyline hydrochloride at rest and during exercise in hypertension. *Acta Med. Scand.,* 1967, 181, 699.
84. Elis, J., Laurence, D. R., Mattie, H., and Prichard, B. N. C. Modification by monoamine oxidase inhibitors of the effect of some sympathomimetics on blood pressure. *Br. Med. J.,* 1967, 2, 75.
85. Massey-Stewart, M. M.A.O.I.s and food—fact and fiction. *Adverse Drug React. Bul.,* 1976, 58, 200.
86. Goldberg, L. I. M.A.O.I. Adverse reactions and possible mechanisms. *JAMA* 1964, 190, 456.
87. Coppen, A. J., Montgomery, S. A. Gupta, R. K., and Bailey, J. E. A double blind comparison of lithium carbonate and maprotiline in the prophylaxis of the effective disorders. *Br. J. Psychiatry,* 1976, 128, 479.
88. Singer, I., and Rothenberg, D. Mechanisms of lithium action. *N. Engl. J. Med.,* 1973, 289, 254.
89. Editorial. Tryptophan and depression. *Br. Med. J.,* 1976, 1, 242.
90. Spencer, P. S. J. Review of the pharmacology of existing antidepressants. *Br. J. Clin. Pharmacol. [Suppl. 2],* 1977, 4, 57.
91. Dumovic, P., Burrows, G. D., Vohra, J., and Freeman, S. E. Cardiological studies with nomifensine. IUPHAR 7th International Congress of Pharmacology, Abstr. p. 830, 1978.
92. Office of Population Censuses and Surveys. *Deaths by Accidental Poisonings 1962–1976.* H.M.S.O., London, 1978.

Stress and the Heart, edited by D. Wheatley,
Raven Press, New York © 1981.

Antidepressants in Cardiac Patients

Hans Kopera

The popularity of antidepressant drugs has increased enormously in recent years. One of the main reasons is the growing awareness that depression is an illness that merits the serious attention of the physician. There has been a consequent intensification of efforts to find new effective compounds and a remarkable number of substances have been synthesized, tested in animals, and tried in the human. The efficacy of many of these is not in doubt, but the value of a drug is determined also by its quality and, above all, safety. With a number of compounds available for equivalent efficacy, the focus of attention has become concentrated on safety. In the treatment of depression, cardiotoxic effects of the therapeutic agents employed have emerged as the most deadly drawback to their widespread use for all cases. Nowhere is this more important than when considering the use of these drugs in patients who are suffering from cardiac conditions.

As with all chronic disabling illnesses, depression is an ineradicable component of the common psychosomatic manifestations so commonly encountered with the cardiac case. As seen in the preceding chapters, the effects of many different antidepressant drugs have been studied in both animals and man, but it is important to know what may be expected with these drugs when given to patients suffering from a known cardiac complaint. It is of paramount importance to the clinician to be provided with information concerning the relative safety of different compounds. This can only be provided by controlled studies in cardiac patients.

THE MAGNITUDE OF THE PROBLEM

Within the last years, a new generation of antidepressant drugs has been developed with structures that differ from the traditional tricyclic configuration. Thus we have the bicyclics (viloxazine, zimelidine), "bridged" tricyclics (maprotiline), tetracyclics (mianserin), and others (nomifensine, trazodone). These new compounds differ from the tricyclics in various respects, not the least of these being their actions on the heart.

Untoward influences on cardiac function are among the important side effects of monoamine oxidase inhibitors and the drugs most frequently used for depression at present, the tricyclic antidepressants. They have been reported since shortly after these compounds became available for therapeutic use (1–6). Cardiac effects have been observed not only in children, in cases of accidental and intentional overdose but also with therapeutic doses. Depending on a multitude of factors, including the intrinsic differences of the various compounds, the dose, the premorbid condition of the patient, and eventual drug-drug interactions, they can occur unpredictably in any subject treated. A dose-effect relationship is not always present, although some electrocardiographic (EKG) abnormalities tend to occur in a dose-dependent fashion (7–12) (see Chapter 10).

Fortunately, these effects are infrequent, and many are subtle and transient despite continued therapy (13). Some cardiac complications, however, are distressing, and a few are dramatic and life-threatening. Congestive heart failure, myocardial infarction, and an increased incidence of sudden deaths, probably due to cardiogenic shock and cardiac arrest, have been associated with the use of some tricyclic antidepressants (14–16).

More important than the occasional severe cardiac effects of therapeutic doses is the fact that EKG abnormalities have been observed in 70 to 90% of patients with acute poisoning (17,18), and that effects on cardiac function are a major component of the toxicity of most tricyclic overdoses (19). Since suicidal behavior is so often a feature of depressive illness, the patient is often presented with the means of accomplishing this in the very remedy prescribed for his disease. As seen in the previous chapter, tricyclic antidepressants account for about 10% of deaths from drug poisoning (20). Furthermore, it is estimated that in 1974 there were at least 20 deaths per million prescriptions of tricyclic antidepressants in Great Britain; and, if all suicidal, accidental, and undetermined deaths involving tricyclics are included, this number is doubled (21).

In most instances, the mechanism of action responsible for these cardiac effects is obscure. Factors such as disturbance of the electrolyte balance (22), disturbance of membrane permeability for sodium-potassium, disturbance of cell metabolism, energy production, membrane stabilization, inhibition of ATP hydroxylase and other enzymes, and production of focal ischemia are thought to be involved. Two influences on the autonomic nervous system are of particular importance for many of the cardiac and cardiotoxic effects: a block of the reuptake of norepinephrine at the cell membrane of both central and peripheral adrenergic neurons, producing increased levels of norepinephrine at the receptor site with the consequent potentiation of transmittor action, and the atropine-like anticholinergic properties of many antidepressants. Both actions cause an autonomic nervous system imbalance in favor of sympathetic dominance. Other effects, such as direct myocardial depression, negative inotropism, orthostatic hypotension, and reduction in coronary flow (23,24), are fully discussed in the previous chapter.

Unquestionably, many details of the cardiovascular actions of tricyclic antidepressants are still ill-defined and incompletely understood, but it is encouraging that some compounds of the new generation of antidepressants are evidently less cardiotoxic than their predecessors.

STUDIES WITH MIANSERIN

The tetracyclic piperazinoazepine compound mianserin has a particularly interesting pharmacologic profile. It differs considerably from other antidepressants in regard to its mechanism of action. Mianserin blocks presynaptic α-adrenoceptor activity, lacks anticholinergic effects, shows many differences to tricyclics in classic animal tests for antidepressants based on amine reuptake inhibition, increases the turnover of norepinephrine without affecting the turnover of dopamine and 5-hydroxytryptamine (25,26), and does not inhibit peripheral norepinephrine uptake in man (27,28). The finding that mianserin is decidedly less cardiotoxic in animals in *in vitro* and *in vivo* experiments (see Chapter 10) stimulated us to undertake similar investigations in the human.

We decided to study the cardiac effects of mianserin in healthy volunteers, in nondepressed cardiac patients, and in depressed noncardiac patients.

Healthy Subjects

The study was a double-blind, randomized, between-group comparison of mianserin, amitriptyline, and placebo, treatments being randomly allocated for both female and male subjects (29). Patients with increased intraocular pressure were excluded. Eighteen healthy volunteers, nine nonpregnant females and nine males (age range 18 to 35 years), completed the study. The subjects were drug-free for at least 7 days before the trial and did not take any but the test medication during the investigation period.

Groups of three females and three males were treated with amitriptyline, mianserin, or placebo tablets; all tablets were identical in appearance. Dosage was gradually increased from 1 tablet daily (amitriptyline, 25 mg; mianserin, 10 mg) to 6 tablets daily by trial day 6. The highest dose (150 mg amitriptyline, 60 mg mianserin, or six placebo tablets per day, respectively) was maintained until trial day 8 (end of the treatment period).

The following parameters relevant for cardiac function and performance were monitored:

1. EKG with determination of the variables: heart rate/min, P-R interval/ sec, QRS-time/sec, QT-time/sec, QT_c/% (QT-time corrected for frequency), T-amplitude/cm, R-amplitude/cm. These measurements were made at rest and after standardized exercise. With respect to the latter, the variables were recorded before and 1, 3, 5, 10, and 15 min after a rectangular exercise test with maximal load of 6 min (30).

2. Systolic time intervals (STI) with the variables: left ventricular ejection time (LVET) and preejection period (PEP). Both were corrected for heart rate using the regression equations of Weissler (31). In addition, the uncorrected PEP/LVET ratio was determined.

3. Echocardiography with the variables: end-diastolic diameter (EDD), end-

systolic diameter (ESD), left ventricular end-diastolic volume (LVEDV), left ventricular end-systolic volume (LVESV), stroke volume (SV), ejection fraction (EF), and velocity of circumferential fiber shortening (VCF).

All parameters were assessed before the first medication and on trial day 8. In addition, blood pressure, EKG at rest, and STI were also recorded on trial day 4. The different variables were statistically analyzed by a two-way analysis of covariance or, when not applicable, by a two-way analysis of variance.

Results in Healthy Subjects

The EKGs at rest as well as before and after standardized exercise, did not show significant drug effects due to the test preparations on any variable with the exception of heart rate, which increased significantly in the amitriptyline-treated volunteers. No significant differences between treatment groups could be demonstrated with the raw data for both PEP and LVET after 4 and 8 days of treatment, but some became evident when the data were corrected for heart rate. Analysis showed a significant difference between mianserin and amitriptyline for the ΔPEP values of the males; ΔPEP in the amitriptyline group was increased. There was also an increase in the latter group in the PEP/LVET ratio, but this between-drug difference was not sex-linked. There were no other differences between the treatment groups (Table 11.1).

Analysis of the echocardiography variables resulted in only one significant difference. The mean value of the left ventricular end-systolic volume in the mianserin-treated subjects was smaller than the mean in the placebo group (Table 11.2).

Cardiac Patients

This part of the investigation was performed as a double-blind, group-comparative trial. It was not primarily intended to study cardiotoxic effects but rather to investigate a possible interaction between mianserin and a coumarin derivative (32,33).

Sixty inpatients of either sex, between the ages of 25 and 79 years, participated in this investigation. Their clinical condition necessitated anticoagulant therapy because of diseases such as myocardial or pulmonary infarction, coronary heart disease, stroke, and arterial or deep venous thrombosis. Additional medication was restricted during the trial period to the absolute minimum, and drugs were avoided which are claimed to interact with anticoagulants of the coumarin type.

The daily dose of phenprocoumon was continuously adjusted to keep the prothrombin activity reduced to 15 to 25%. After an initial control period of 1 week with the required reduced prothrombin activity, each subject was randomly allocated to one of three treatment groups, while phenprocoumon therapy continued. One group was treated with 5-mg tablets of mianserin, the second

TABLE 11.1. *Estimated difference in mean variable value between treatment groups on trial day 8 (after correction for pretreatment differences between groups and regression) and the corresponding 95% confidence interval*

Variable	Mianserin as compared with	Estimated corrected difference		95% Confidence interval
ΔPEP	Amitriptyline	Male	−30.4[a]	−49.1 to −11.6
		Female	− 1.5	−27.2 to 24.2
	Placebo	Male	− 2.2	−21.1 to 16.7
		Female	6.2	−17.3 to 29.8
PEP/LVET	Amitriptyline		− 0.07[a]	−0.14 to 0.00
	Placebo		0.00	−0.07 to 0.07

[a] Significant ($p \leq 0.05$).

with 10-mg tablets, and the third with placebo tablets. In all groups, the number of tablets taken was uniformly increased during the first 6 days to the maximum of six tablets, i.e. 30 or 60 mg mianserin or six placebo tablets per day. This dose was maintained for the subsequent 14 days. Treatment was given on a double-blind basis and lasted for 3 consecutive weeks, followed by an additional week without administration of mianserin or placebo.

The same EKG variables as in the first trial were recorded. At the end of the investigation, sufficient EKG data were available on 50 of the subjects for statistical analysis (Table 11.3).

None of the mean values of the EKG variables showed any drug effect in any of the three treatment groups. The same holds true for the differences in mean values between the mianserin-treated patients and those receiving the placebo (Table 11.4).

TABLE 11.2. *Estimated difference in left ventricular end-systolic volume between two treatment groups on trial day 8 (after correction for pretreatment differences between groups and regression) and the corresponding 95% confidence interval*

Mianserin as compared with	Estimated corrected difference[a]	95% Confidence interval
Amitriptyline	− 4.2	−22.9 to 14.5
Placebo	−18.3[b]	−36.2 to −0.4

[a] The negative difference means that the mean value in the mianserin group was lower than in the comparative group.
[b] Significant at 5% level.

TABLE 11.3. *Patients with cardiac diseases under treatment with phenprocoumon concomitantly receiving mianserin or placebo*

		Treatment	
		Mianserin max. daily dose	
Diagnosis	Placebo	30 mg	60 mg
Myocardial infarction	9	12	7
Status postmyocardial infarction	4	2	1
Cardiac failure	1	4	4
CHD and other circulatory diseases	2	2	2
	16	20	14

Depressed Patients

The third trial is still in progress. The trial design is a double-blind comparative study on 12 male, noncardiac, depressed patients. The parameters under study include all those described in the trial conducted on healthy volunteers, with the addition of 12-hr heart rate recordings for rhythm analysis before as well as 7 and 28 days after treatment. The patients are randomly allocated to treatment with either amitriptyline or mianserin for a minimum of 4 weeks.

PRACTICAL INFERENCES

There is abundant evidence from animal experiments (26,34,35) and clinical observations (4,36) that tricyclic antidepressants can cause untoward cardiovas-

TABLE 11.4. *Differences in mean values between mianserin- and placebo-treated groups after correction for possible differences in mean values at baseline, and the corresponding 95% confidence intervals*

Variable	Mianserin 30 mg— placebo	Mianserin 60 mg— placebo
Heart rate freq/min	5 (−1 to 11)[a]	0 (−6 to 6)
P-R/sec	0.009 (−0.003 to 0.021)	0.004 (−0.008 to 0.017)
QRS/sec	−0.001 (−0.008 to 0.006)	0 (−0.008 to 0.008)
QT/sec	−0.003 (−0.020 to 0.014)	−0.002 (−0.020 to 0.016)
QT_c/%	1.6 (−3.7 to 6.9)	−1.0 (−6.8 to 4.8)
T/cm	0.05 (−0.04 to 0.14)	−0.05 (−0.15 to 0.05)
R/cm	0.16 (−0.08 to 0.40)	0.13 (−0.13 to 0.39)
BP (mm Hg)		
Systolic	1 (−4 to 6)	−5 (−11 to 1)
Diastolic	0.9 (−2.7 to 4.5)	−0.5 (−4.5 to 3.5)

[a]Corresponding 95% confidence intervals in parentheses.

cular effects. The results of our study in healthy subjects are compatible with these observations in that the STI variables indicate a negative inotropic influence with amitriptyline due to a decrease in myocardial contractility. Thus after 8 days of treatment, amitriptyline prolonged the ΔPEP in the male volunteers and increased the PEP/LVET ratio in both males and females.

This is in agreement with the reports of previous investigations, which showed not only acute impairment of myocardial function, such as increased PEP index and PEP/LVET ratio (12,37–39), but also a persisting impairment (40); normal cardiac function was restored only after discontinuation of the tricyclic. No such cardiac effects were seen by us with the tetracyclic compound mianserin, which is basically consistent with the observations reported by others (38,39,41). These other investigators observed a seemingly paradoxical effect of mianserin on the heart of depressed patients; they found an increase in the PEP/LVET ratio, indicating a decrease in contractility, and a shortening of the LVET and the QS_2 interval, the latter assumed to be the most sensitive indicator of a positive inotropic effect. These changes are probably not the result of a direct effect on the heart but rather of effects on the peripheral circulation. These would take the form of a decrease of pre- and afterload, both of which affect the STI in opposite directions (39,41).

Cardiac performance was unaffected by amitriptyline in our healthy volunteers. However, the significantly smaller left ventricular end-systolic volume after 8 days of mianserin treatment suggests a favorable effect of mianserin on cardiac performance, possibly resulting from an increase in ejection fraction.

Increased susceptibility of particular individuals to undesirable heart effects of tricyclic antidepressants has not been established with certainty (42), although patients with cardiovascular disease and aged persons, who are thought to develop higher plasma levels (43), might be at greater risk (1,2,15,16,37,44). The results of our study in 50 cardiac patients who were not suffering from depression showed no unexpected deterioration in any case. There was also no effect on the various EKG parameters of two therapeutic doses of mianserin, 30 or 60 mg/day, respectively, given during 3 consecutive weeks and compared with a placebo. This indicates that mianserin did not affect cardiac function in any of the 34 heart patients, some of whom were suffering from conditions as severe as myocardial infarction. Our findings, in agreement with those of others (45), suggest that mianserin probably will be without harm for patients with cardiovascular diseases.

Other studies with mianserin in noncardiac, depressed patients revealed no untoward effects on heart rate and EKG (38,46–53). In healthy subjects, only a transient prolongation of the corrected Q-T interval was observed (38). In contrast, the tricyclic antidepressants produce a much more pronounced effect on this, i.e., shortening of the frequency-corrected Q-T interval, prolongation of the P-R interval and the QRS duration, decrease of T-wave height, and, in therapeutic doses, an increase in heart rate (4,11,38,47–49,53).

Using His bundle cardiography, Hamer et al. (54) found no significant effect of mianserin on heart rate or conduction in 10 noncardiac, depressed patients, either before or after 3 weeks of treatment with 60 mg/day mianserin. This is in contradistinction to experience with tricyclic antidepressants (4,55). The suggestion of Burckhardt et al. (13,56) that the cardiac effects of tricyclics and mianserin would not differ does not seem valid, since their data do not permit a distinction between the two types of drug with respect to the observed cardiac effects (57,58).

All clinical reports (59) strongly support the assumption derived from animal experiments (35) that therapeutic doses of mianserin will not prove to be cardiotoxic. This is supported by the data concerning 50 patients who have taken excessive doses of mianserin with suicidal intention and who have shown no or only few and transient cardiotoxic symptoms (60–64).

DRUG INTERACTIONS WITH MIANSERIN

Animal experiments are of rather limited predictive value concerning drug interactions, as they are no substitute for clinical pharmacologic studies. The latter should approximate as closely as possible the therapeutic situation (65,66). The practice of polypharmacy is widespread (67) and thought to be at its zenith in psychiatric medicine (65). Thus antidepressants are often taken together with other medicines.

Drug interactions of monoamine oxidase inhibitors and tricyclic antidepressants (65,68–71) are described in the preceding chapter, but less is known of interactions with the antidepressants of the new generation, which have not yet been used long enough. The available data concerning mianserin, however, are quite encouraging.

Sympathomimetic Amines

The mode of action of tricyclic-catecholamine interaction is described in the previous chapter. In contrast, mianserin does not affect the norepinephrine uptake pump and thus does not alter the norepinephrine-dose/pressor or the tyramine-dose/pressor response; nor does it inhibit the mydriatic effect of tyramine or hydroxyamphetamine (72–75).

Anticholinergics

Obviously, the atropine-like effect of tricyclic antidepressants is increased when given together with anticholinergic drugs (e.g., with medicaments for peptic ulcer therapy, antiparkinsonian drugs, and some antihistamines). No such interference is to be expected from mianserin, which has practically no anticholinergic properties (76).

Antihypertensives

The interactions of tricyclic antidepressants with adrenergic neuron blocking antihypertensive drugs are also described in the previous chapter. The resultant loss of blood pressure control can constitute a serious clinical problem (77,78,79). Preliminary investigations, which require confirmation in more extensive trials, indicate that mianserin apparently does not interact substantially with the hypotensive effect of bethanidine or guanethidine or with the β-adrenergic blocking agent propranolol (38,80).

Anticoagulants

Antidepressants can interfere with the anticoagulant action of coumarin-type drugs by various mechanisms. We investigated the possible interaction between mianserin and the coumarin derivative phenprocoumon (33).

The design of the trial has already been described. Of the 60 patients treated, 21 received the maximum dose of 30 mg mianserin daily; 20 were treated with 60 mg daily; and 19 received a placebo. The variables employed to measure the anticipated effects were: (a) daily dosage of phenprocoumon necessary to reduce prothrombin activity to 15 to 25%, (b) prothrombin time, (c) bleeding time, (d) whole blood coagulation time, determined at least twice a week, and (e) plasma γ-glutamyltransferase activity, measured at least once a week (Table 11.5).

Statistical evaluation of the results showed that neither the dosage of phenprocoumon nor the prothrombin, bleeding, or coagulation times were significantly affected by either of the two different doses of mianserin, administered during 3 weeks, in comparison to placebo. It can be concluded that there is no clinically important interaction between antidepressant doses of mianserin and anticoagulant doses of phenprocoumon. As the pharmacologic properties of coumarin-type anticoagulants do not differ greatly, it is unlikely that other coumarin anticoagulants will interact with mianserin.

Alcohol

Tricyclic antidepressants and mianserin seem to interact additively with alcohol. In healthy subjects, mianserin together with alcohol was found to affect some tests for coordinative and reactive skills, as well as attention. This interaction of mianserin was restricted to the first day and was clearly less pronounced than that of amitriptyline, which lasted up to 7 days. In contradistinction to amitriptyline, mianserin did not interact with alcohol with respect to learning and memory (71,81). No studies have yet been undertaken on possible interactions between mianserin and alcohol in depressed patients.

TABLE 11.5. *Mean phenprocoumon consumption in tablets daily in patients requiring anticoagulants treated with two mianserin dosages in comparison to placebo*

Test preparation	Maximum dose (mg)	No. of subjects	Pretreatment period	Treatment period			Posttreatment period
				Week 1	Week 2	Week 3	
Mianserin	60	20	0.79	0.79	0.80	0.77	0.76
Mianserin	30	21	0.77	0.81	0.79	0.75	0.76
Placebo		19	0.85	0.83	0.81	0.86	0.84

CONCLUSIONS

There is no doubt that monoamine oxidase inhibitors and tricyclic antidepressants can cause untoward effects on the cardiovascular system. The risk of cardiac morbidity and mortality during treatment with these antidepressants is low. However, cardiotoxicity can occur unpredictably in any subject treated, with a possible preference for the older generation and for heart patients.

Although reported experiences with the tetracyclic antidepressant mianserin are considerably fewer than with the older antidepressants, which have been in use for more than 20 years, it is remarkable how few untoward cardiovascular effects of mianserin have been reported. This is in agreement with animal experiments, which have shown the drug to have a much weaker cardiotoxic effect than the tricyclic antidepressants.

Confirmation of this low cardiotoxicity with mianserin is provided by our pharmacologic studies made in healthy subjects, in noncardiac, depressed patients, and in patients with preexisting cardiac diseases. In none of these were any cardiodepressant effects of therapeutic doses of mianserin observed. These findings are compatible with reports of patients who have taken excessive doses of mianserin, in all of whom no or minimal cardiotoxic effects were recorded.

Severely disturbed cardiac function is one of the major causes of death by tricyclic antidepressant overdoses. Therefore, an antidepressant with low cardiotoxicity is a less suitable tool for suicidal acts. In effect, mianserin reduces the danger of successful misuse by depressives of the prescribed medication for suicidal acts. In addition, mianserin has been found to be more effective on suicidal ideation and dysphoric mood than amitriptyline in depressed patients (82), thus diminishing suicidal intention.

Mianserin is practically free from interactions with other drugs. This has been established for direct-acting sympathomimetics, such as norepinephrine, indirect-acting sympathomimetic amines, such as tyramine, and coumarin-type anticoagulants. There are good reasons for assuming lack of interaction with anticholinergics; it is likely that this is true for antihypertensive drugs as well.

All available data on mianserin indicate that this compound is not only effective but also a remarkably safe antidepressant, particularly suitable for psychiatric outpatients, for medication in general practice, and as a drug of choice for elderly and cardiac patients.

REFERENCES

1. Kristiansen, E. S. Cardiac complications during treatment with imipramine (Tofranil). *Acta Psychiatr. Neurol.*, 1961, 36, 427.
2. Moccetti, T., Lichtlen, P., Albert, H., Meier, E., and Imbach, P. Kardiotoxizität der trizyklischen Antidepressiva. *Schweiz. Med. Wochenschr.*, 1971, 101, 1.
3. Jefferson, J. W. A review of the cardiovascular effects and toxicity of tricyclic antidepressants. *Psychosom. Med.*, 1975, 37, 160.
4. Burrows, G. C., Vohra, J., Hunt, D., Sloman, J. G., Scoggins, B. A., and Davies, B. Cardiac effects of different tricyclic antidepressant drugs. *Br. J. Psychiatry*, 1976, 129, 335.

5. Moccetti, T. *Kardiotoxische Medikamente unter besonderer Berücksichtigung der Phenothiazine und Imipraminderivate.* Huber, Bern, 1976.

6. Bigger, J. T., Jr., Kantor, S. J., Glassman, A. H., and Perel, J. M. Cardiovascular effects of tricyclic antidepressant drugs. In: *Psychopharmacology: A Generation of Progress,* edited by M. A. Lipton, A. DiMascio, and K. F. Killam, p. 1033, Raven Press, New York, 1978.

7. Spiker, D. G., Weiss, A. N., Sidney, S. C., Ruwitch, J. F., and Biggs, J. T. Tricyclic antidepressant overdose: Clinical presentation and plasma levels. *Clin. Pharmacol. Ther.,* 1975, 18, 539.

8. Vohra, J., Hunt, D., Burrows, G. C., and Sloman, G. Intracardiac conduction defects following overdose of tricyclic antidepressant drugs. *Eur. J. Cardiol.,* 1975, 2, 453.

9. Biggs, J. T., Spiker, D. G., Petit, J. M., and Ziegler, V. E. Tricyclic antidepressant overdose. Incidence of symptoms. *JAMA,* 1977, 238, 135.

10. Petit, J. M., Spiker, D. G., Ruwitch, J. F., Ziegler, V. E., Weiss, A. N., and Biggs, J. T. Tricyclic anti-depressant plasma levels and adverse effects after overdosage. *Clin. Pharmacol. Ther.,* 1977, 21, 47.

11. Ziegler, V. E., Co, B. T., and Biggs, J. T. Plasma nortriptyline levels and ECG findings. *Am. J. Psychiatry,* 1977, 134, 441.

12. Taylor, D. J. E., and Braithwaite, R. A. Cardiac effects of tricyclic antidepressant medication. A preliminary study on nortriptyline. *Br. Heart J.,* 1978, 40, 1005.

13. Burckhardt, D., Raeder, E., Müller, V., Imhof, P., and Neubauer, H. Cardiovascular effects of tricyclic and tetracyclic antidepressants. *JAMA,* 1978, 239, 213.

14. Mann, A., Catterson, A., and MacPherson, A. Toxicity of imipramine: Reports of serious side effects and massive overdose. *Can. Med. Assoc. J.,* 1959, 81, 23.

15. Coull, D. C., Crooks, J., Dingwall-Fordyce, I., Scott, A. M., and Weir, R. D. Amitriptyline and cardiac disease. *Lancet,* 1970, 2, 590.

16. Moir, D. C., Crooks, J., Cornwell, W. B., O'Malley, K., Dingwall-Fordyce, I., Turnbull, M. J., and Weir, R. D. Cardiotoxicity of amitriptyline. *Lancet,* 1972, 2, 561.

17. Serafimowski, N., Thorball, N., Asmussen, I., and Lunding, M. Forgiftning med tricykliske antidepressiva specialt med henblik på den kardiale påvirkning. *Ugeskr. Laeger,* 1975, 137, 1389.

18. Thorstrand, C. Clinical features in poisonings by tricyclic antidepressants with special reference to the ECG. *Acta Med. Scand.* 1976, 199, 337.

19. Williams, R. B., and Sherter, M. D. Cardiac complications of tricyclic antidepressant therapy. *Ann. Int. Med.* 1971, 74, 395.

20. Office of Population Censuses and Surveys. Mortality Statistics, HMSO, London, 1977.

21. Brewer, C. Risks of tricyclic antidepressants. *Br. J. Psychiatry,* 1978, 132, 107.

22. Wheatley, D. Antidepressants, EKG changes, and plasma potassium levels. In: *Stress and the Heart,* edited by D. Wheatley. Raven Press, New York, 1977.

23. Barth, N., and Muscholl, E. Die Rolle adrenerger Mechanismen bei der Entstehung von Arrhythmien nach Einnahme trizyklischer Antidepressiva. *Dtsch. Med. Wochenschr.,* 1976, 101, 88.

24. Bonaccorsi, A., and Garattini, S. Cardiac effects of nortriptyline and other tricyclic antidepressant drugs. *Gen. Pharmacol.,* 1978, 9, 81.

25. Leonard, B. E. Mianserin, an antidepressant with a unique neuropharmacological profile. *Acta Psychiatr. Belg.,* 1978, 78, 770.

26. van Riezen, H., and van der Burg, W. J. The pharmacology of mianserin (Org GB 94) Lerivon®, a really different antidepressant. *Acta Psychiatr. Belg.,* 1978, 78, 756.

27. Leonard, B. E., and Kafoe, W. F. Comparison of effects of Org GB 94 with some tricyclic antidepressants on brain monoamine metabolism in the rat. *J. Pharmacol.,* 1974, 5, 59.

28. Peet, M., and Turner, P. (Eds.): Proceedings of a symposium on mianserin. *Br. J. Clin. Pharmacol. [Suppl.],* 1978, 5.

29. Kopera, H., Fluch, N., Harpf, H., Klein, W. W., and Stulemeijer, S. Cardiovascular effects of mianserin, a comparative study with amitriptyline and a placebo in healthy subjects. *Int. J. Clin. Pharmacol. Biopharm. Ther. Toxicol.* 1980, 18, 104.

30. Kaltenbach, M. *Die Belastungsuntersuchung von Herzkranken.* Kardiologische Diagnostik, Boehringer Mannheim, 1975.

31. Weissler, A. M., Harris, W. S., and Schoenfeld, C. D. Bedside technics for the evaluation of ventricular function in man. *Am. J. Cardiol.,* 1969, 23, 577.

32. Kopera, H., and Schenk, H. Antidepressiva und Kardiotoxizität. Beobachtungen mit Mianserin. *Dtsch. Med. Wochenschr.,* 1978, 103, 1373.

33. Kopera, H., Schenk, H., and Stulemeijer, S. Phenprocoumon requirement, whole blood coagulation time, bleeding time and plasma γ-GT in patients receiving mianserin. *Eur. J. Clin. Pharmacol.*, 1978, 13, 351.

34. Harper, B., and Hughes, I. E. A comparison in rabbit isolated hearts of the dysrhythmogenic potential of amitriptyline, maprotiline and mianserin in relation to their ability to block noradrenaline uptake. *Br. J. Pharmacol.*, 1977, 59, 651.

35. Hughes, I. E., and Radwan, S. The relative toxicity of amitriptyline, imipramine, maprotiline and mianserin in rabbits in vivo. *Br. J. Pharmacol.*, 1979, 65, 331.

36. Kopera, H. Die Herz- und Kreislaufwirkungen der Antidepressiva. *Med. Klin.*, 1979, 74, 1339.

37. Müller, V., and Burckhardt, D. Die Wirkung tri- und tetrazyklischer Antidepressiva auf Herz and Kreislauf. *Schweiz. Med. Wochenschr.*, 1974, 104, 1911.

38. Burgess, C. D., Turner, P., and Wadsworth, J. Cardiovascular responses to mianserin hydrochloride: A comparison with tricyclic antidepressant drugs. *Br. J. Clin. Pharmacol.* [*Suppl. 1*], 1978, 5, 21.

39. Burgess, C. D., Wadsworth, J., Montgomery, S., and Turner, P. Cardiovascular effects of amitriptyline, mianserin, zimelidine and nomifensine in depressed patients. *Postgrad. Med. J.*, 1979, 55, 704.

40. Raeder, E. A., Burckhardt, D., Neubauer, H., Walter, R., and Gastpar, M. Long-term tri- and tetracyclic antidepressants, myocardial contractility, and cardiac rhythm. *Br. Med. J.*, 1978, 2, 666.

41. Montgomery, S. A., Burgess, C. D., and Montgomery, D. B. Clinical and cardiac effects of mianserin and amitriptyline in depressed patients. In: *Progress in the Pharmacotherapy of Depression: Mianserin HCl*, edited by G. Drykoningen, W. Linford Rees, and C. Ruiz Ogara, p. 60. Excerpta Medica, Amsterdam, 1979.

42. Jick, H. et al. Adverse reactions to the tricyclic antidepressant drugs. *Lancet*, 1972, 1, 529.

43. Carr, A. C., and Hobson, R. P. High serum concentrations of antidepressants in elderly patients. *Br. Med. J.*, 1977, 2, 1151.

44. Kantor, S. J., Glassman, A. H., Bigger, J. T., Perel, J. M., and Giardina, E. V. The cardiac effects of therapeutic plasma concentrations of imipramine. *Am. J. Psychiatry*, 1978, 135, 534.

45. Amdisen, A. Workshop on the clinical pharmacology and efficacy of mianserin. *Br. J. Clin. Pharmacol.* [*Suppl. 1*], 1978, 5, 94.

46. Bohacek, N., Mihovilovic, M., and Bakran, I. Therapeutic efficacy and side-effects of tricyclic and tetracyclic antidepressive drugs. A comparative double-blind trial of amitriptyline and mianserin (Org GB 94). *Acta Med. Iug.*, 1976, 30, 425.

47. Jaskari, M. O., Ahlfors, U. G., Ginman, L., Lydecken, K., and Tienari, P. Three double-blind comparative trials of mianserin (Org GB 94) and amitriptyline in the treatment of depressive illness. *Pharmakopsych. Neuropsychopharmacol.*, 1977, 10, 101.

48. Peet, M., Tienari, P., and Jaskari, M. O. A comparison of the cardiac effects of mianserin and amitriptyline in man. *Pharmakopsychiatrie*, 1977, 10, 309.

49. Hoc, J. Etude clinique comparative en double insu de la mianserine et de la nortriptyline. *Acta Psychiatr. Belg.*, 1978, 78, 833.

50. Conti, L., Cassano, G. B., and Sarteschi, P. Clinical experiences with mianserin. In: *Progress in the Pharmacotherapy of Depression: Mianserin HCl*, edited by G. Drykoningen, W. Linford Rees, and C. Ruiz Ogara, p. 65. Excerpta Medica, Amsterdam, 1979.

51. Saldana-Hernández, O. H., Oliva-Ruiz, H., Arriaga-Garcia, J. J., Alcántar, A., Camacho, R., Castaneda, C., Corral, J. B., and Pinzón, A. Mianserin, a new medication for the treatment of depression. In: *Progress in the Pharmacotherapy of Depression: Mianserin HCl*, edited by G. Drykoningen, W. Linford Rees, and C. Ruiz Ogara, p. 26. Excerpta Medica, Amsterdam, 1979.

52. Songar, A. Cardiovascular side-effects of mianserin. In: *Progress in the Pharmacotherapy of Depression: Mianserin HCl*, edited by G. Drykoningen, W. Linford Rees, and C. Ruiz Ogara, p. 56. Excerpta Medica, Amsterdam, 1979.

53. Tienari, P. A tripartite double-blind comparative trial of mianserin and amitriptyline in the treatment of depressive illness. In: *Progress in the Pharmacotherapy of Depression: Mianserin HCl*, edited by G. Drykoningen, W. Linford Rees, and C. Ruiz Ogara, p. 40. Excerpta Medica, Amsterdam, 1979.

54. Hamer, A. W. F., Vohra, J. K., Sloman, J. G., Burrows, G. D., and Davies, B. M. Mianserin

and intracardiac conduction. *IRCS Med. Sci.: Cardiovasc. Syst.; Clin. Med. Clin. Pharmacol. Ther.; Drug Metab. Toxicol.; Psychol. Psychiatry,* 1979, 7, 220.

55. Brorson, L., and Wennerblom, B. Electrophysiological methods in assessing cardiac effects of the tricyclic antidepressant imipramine. *Acta Med. Scand.,* 1978, 203, 429.
56. Burckhardt, D., Fleischhauer, H.-J., Müller, V., and Neubauer, H. W. Beitrag zur Wirkung tri- und tetrazyklischer Antidepressiva auf Herz und Kreislauf. *Schweiz. Med. Wochenschr.,* 1976, 106, 1896.
57. Peet, M., and Jansen, F. H. J. Briefe an die Redaktion. *Schweiz. Med. Wochenschr.,* 1977, 107, 1238.
58. Jansen, F. H. J. Mianserin differentiated from tricyclic antidepressants. *JAMA,* 1978, 240, 1339.
59. Brogden, R. N., Heel, R. C., Speight, T. M., and Avery, G. S. Mianserin: A review of its pharmacological properties and therapeutic efficacy in depressive illness. *Drugs,* 1978, 16, 273.
60. Crome, P., and Newman, B. Poisoning with maprotiline and mianserin. *Br. Med. J.,* 1977, 2, 260.
61. Green, S. D. R., and Kendall-Taylor, P. Heart block in mianserin hydrochloride overdose. *Br. Med. J.,* 1977, 2, 1190.
62. Jansen, F. H. J., Drykoningen, G., and de Ridder, J. J. Poisoning with antidepressants. *Br. Med. J.,* 1977, 2, 896.
63. Crome, P., Braithwaite, R., Newman, B., and Montgomery, S. Choosing an antidepressant. *Br. Med. J.,* 1978, 1, 859.
64. Drykoningen, G. J., Pinder, R. M., and de Ridder, J. J. Review of mianserin overdose cases. In: *Progress in the Pharmacotherapy of Depression: Mianserin HCl,* edited by G. Drykoningen, W. Linford Rees, and C. Ruiz Ogara, p. 74. Excerpta Medica, Amsterdam, 1979.
65. Braithwaite, R. A. The significance of drug interactions in the evaluation of psychotropic drugs. *Br. J. Clin. Pharmacol. [Suppl. 1],* 1976, 3, 29.
66. Kopera, H. Wechselwirkungen von Arzneimitteln. *Pharm. Acta Helv.,* 1977, 52, 79.
67. Prescott, L. F. Clinically important drug interactions. *Drugs,* 1973, 5, 161.
68. Boakes, A. J., Laurence, D. R., Teoh, P. C., Barar, F. S. K., Benedikter, L. T., and Prichard, B. N. C. Interactions between sympathomimetic amines and antidepressant agents in man. *Br. Med. J.,* 1973, 1, 311.
69. Hartshorn, E. A. Interactions of CNS drugs psychotherapeutic agents—antidepressants. *Drug. Intell. Clin. Pharm.,* 1974, 8, 591.
70. Cocco, G., and Agué, C. Interactions between cardioactive drugs and antidepressants. *Eur. J. Clin. Pharmacol.,* 1977, 11, 389.
71. Seppälä, T. Psychomotor skills during acute and two-week treatment with mianserin (Org GB 94) and amitriptyline, and their combined effects with alcohol. *Ann. Clin. Res.,* 1977, 9, 66.
72. Coppen, A. J., and Ghose, K. Clinical and pharmacological effects of treatment with a new antidepressant. *Arzneim. Forsch. Drug Res.,* 1976, 26, 1166.
73. Ghose, K. Correlation of pupil reactivity to tyramine or hydroxyamphetamine and tyramine pressor responses in patients treated with amitriptyline or mianserin. *Br. J. Clin. Pharmacol.,* 1976, 3, 666.
74. Ghose, K., Coppen, A., and Turner, P. Autonomic actions and interactions of mianserin hydrochloride (Org. GB 94) and amitriptyline in patients with depressive illness. *Psychopharmacology,* 1976, 49, 201.
75. Ghose, K. Studies on the interaction between mianserin and noradrenaline in patients suffering from depressive illness. *Br. J. Clin. Pharmacol.,* 1977, 4, 712.
76. Kopera, H. Anticholinergic and blood pressure effects of mianserin, amitriptyline and placebo. *Br. J. Clin. Pharmacol. [Suppl. 1],* 1978, 5, 29.
77. Avery, G. S. (Ed.) *Drug Treatment,* p. 824, Adis Press, Sydney, 1976.
78. Skinner, C., Coull, D. C., and Johnston, A. W. Antagonism of the hypotensive action of bethanidine and debrisoquine by tricyclic antidepressants. *Lancet,* 1969, 2, 564.
79. Briant, R. H., Reid, J. L., and Dollery, C. T. Interaction between clonidine and desipramine in man. *Br. Med. J.,* 1973, 1, 522.
80. Coppen, A., Ghose, K., Swade, C., and Wood, K. Effect of mianserin hydrochloride on peripheral uptake mechanisms for noradrenaline and 5-hydroxytryptamine in man. *Br. J. Clin. Pharmacol. [Suppl. 1],* 1978, 5, 13.

81. Mattila, M. J., Liljequist, R., and Seppälä, T. Effects of amitriptyline and mianserin on psychomotor skills and memory in man. *Br. J. Clin. Pharmacol.* [*Suppl. 1*], 1978, 5, 53.
82. Montgomery, S., Cronholm, B., Åsberg, M., and Montgomery, D. B. Differential effects on suicidal ideation of mianserin, maprotiline and amitriptyline. *Br. J. Clin. Pharmacol.* [*Suppl. 1*], 1978, 5, 77.

Prologue: Stress Factors in Hypertension

The etiology of hypertension remains an enigma, despite the wealth of research that has been undertaken, both experimentally and clinically. There may be a connection between development of abnormally high blood pressure and external stresses of various kinds, since temporary blood pressure elevation is a normal physiologic response to such stimuli. However, the theory that continued external stress may result in permanently elevated blood pressure in susceptible individuals has never been proved.

The first chapter in this section surveys the many experimental procedures which have been undertaken in the laboratory to investigate the importance of stress factors in hypertension. As Friedman points out, it is relatively easy to produce elevation of blood pressure in experimental animals under various conditions of physical and behavioral stress; it is much more difficult to produce a condition of sustained hypertension comparable to the human disease of hypertension. A number of other factors are involved, not least of which is the influence of genetics. It is interesting to speculate as to why this should be so, but environmental factors may be of importance in this context. Animals in the wild are constantly assaulted by major stresses of a life-threatening nature. They are constantly alert to stressful encounters; in consequence, adaptation may have occurred so that the cardiovascular responses do not produce permanent physiologic changes. In contrast, the relative security of the human environment may possibly render a person more susceptible to the sustained effects of stress when this is encountered, and particularly when it is prolonged.

The chapter by Marwood and Lockett carries this basic research a step further. The authors have been able to demonstrate that stresses of a "negative" nature (i.e., sound withdrawal) will also produce elevation of blood pressure in experimental animals. Even more important, within the context of the human situation, is that sound-withdrawal hypertension, once induced, may become permanent. Confirmation of the applicability of these experimental procedures to the human model is provided by two recent studies. In the first of these, Jonsson and Hansson (1) demonstrated that 44 male industrial workers with a noise-induced auditory impairment had significantly higher systolic and diastolic blood pressures than 74 males of the same age with normal hearing. Moreover, significantly more individuals with hypertension were found in the group with noise-induced loss of hearing. In the second study, Lynch and Convey (2) reviewed the evidence linking human loneliness, or a sense of separateness, to disease and premature death. Among a number of examples, these authors noted a much higher mortality rate due to hypertensive disease in those who were widowed or divorced, as compared to married and single subjects. For example, quoting the mortality per 100,000 for the United States from 1959 to 1961, there were 110 such deaths in divorced white males, 103 in widowed white males, 90 in single white males, and only 55 in married white males. Similar figures were quoted for the incidence of coronary heart disease.

From this description of experimental procedures, it is clear that stress and emotion may be intimately involved in the development of hypertension, although not necessarily as basic causes. This important experimental work provides sufficient evidence to justify investigating the association between emotional and physical stress and hypertension in humans.

Behavioral factors may not only contribute to the development of hypertension, they may be used in treatment, as outlined in the next chapter by Patel. She demonstrates how meditational and relaxational techniques, together with biofeedback procedures, can enable some patients to control their own blood pressure and to "will" it down in cases of hypertension. Such techniques, however, are time-consuming for both patient and physician or instructor. It may also be difficult to achieve sustained normotension by behavioral techniques, as has been demonstrated by Pollack et al. (3). These workers studied 20 hypertensive patients over a 6-month period of sessions of transcendental meditation but failed to demonstrate any permanent reduction in either systolic or diastolic blood pressure.

The alternative to physical behavioral techniques is to use psychotropic agents, which may achieve the same effect. The last chapter in this section is concerned with studies undertaken by the General Practitioner Research Group in England to assess the importance of anxiety factors in hypertension and the possibilities of using antianxiety drugs in the long-term management of hypertension.

REFERENCES

1. Jonsson, A., and Hansson, L. Prolonged exposure to a stressful stimulus (noise) as a cause of raised blood-pressure in man. *Lancet,* 1977, i, 86.
2. Lynch, J. J., and Convey, W. H. Loneliness, disease, and death: Alternative approaches. *Psychosomatics,* 1979, 20, 702.
3. Pollack, A. A., Weber, M. A., Case, D. B., and Laragh, J. H. Limitations of transcendental meditations in the treatment of essential hypertension.*Lancet,* 1977, i, 71.

Stress and the Heart, edited by D. Wheatley,
Raven Press, New York © 1981.

Experimental Psychogenic Hypertension

Richard Friedman

To state that stressful stimuli can cause profound transient cardiovascular responses is almost trivial and hardly needs documentation in scientific circles. The special concern of this chapter is the relevance of these stimuli in the pathogenesis of chronic hypertension.

As early as 1929, Cannon (1) demonstrated that cats exposed to barking dogs exhibited increased autonomic activity and subsequent acute elevations in blood pressure. Significantly, Cannon also demonstrated that initially neutral stimuli, when temporally paired with noxious events, acquired the ability to elevate blood pressure. The types of stimuli that have been demonstrated to acutely elevate blood pressure via autonomic activation have been greatly expanded since Cannon's early studies (2). These experimental results, coupled with clinical observations, have led psychosomatic researchers to hypothesize that repeated or prolonged exposure to stimuli that produce acute blood pressure elevations might eventually result in chronic hypertension, persisting even after the initiating stimuli were removed (3). Confirmation of this hypothesis, however, has not been unequivocal. Studies designed to examine the psychogenic development of hypertension have varied the qualitative and quantitative aspects of the stressful stimuli, as well as the environmental and genetic predisposition of the exposed organism.

The goal of this chapter is to present a fairly comprehensive and cohesive review of the studies that have attempted to confirm or refute the hypothesis stated above. The organization of the chapter revolves around the two broad classes of independent variables used in these studies: (a) the nature of the stressful stimuli, and (b) the characteristics of the exposed organism. Although they are discussed sequentially, there is obvious overlap. Where relevant, the attempts at correlating stress-induced anatomical, behavioral, biochemical, and physiologic changes with changes in blood pressure are discussed. The voluminous literature comprised of observational and correlational data derived from clinical experience, demographic, and/or epidemiologic studies, which has such an important historic role in this line of inquiry, is not extensively examined. Rather, the emphasis is on well-controlled laboratory investigations, which necessarily weights the discussion toward animal models.

QUALITATIVE AND QUANTITATIVE ASPECTS OF STRESS

Recently, Cohen and Obrist (4) emphasized the need to classify the experimental procedures that have been used to investigate behavioral-cardiovascular interactions. Their classification schema is simply a restatement of the distinction made by Cannon (1) in the previously mentioned studies. For cats, exposure to a barking dog is a stimulus that automatically, i.e., reflexively, results in acute blood pressure elevations. On the other hand, the sight of the experimenter, inter alia, which did not initially result in an acute blood pressure elevation, does elicit that response after the experimenter has repeatedly led the barking dog into the cat's presence. The dog, in Pavlovian terminology, is an unconditioned stimulus, while the experimenter becomes a conditioned stimulus, for acute blood pressure elevations. Situations in which the former category of stimuli serve as the stressor have been labeled reflex behavior or, simply, reflex models. Situations involving the second category have been labeled learning behavior or learning models. This second class also includes studies in which the noxious or nociceptive stimuli are presented contingent on the organism's behavior (4). Both types of studies have tried to determine whether exposure to these stimuli results in sustained blood pressure elevations, but the experimental procedures are quite different.

Reflex Models

Medoff and Bongiovanni (5) exposed rats to aversive auditory stimulation for five to 10 min each day for more than 10 months. Of the 31 rats exposed, 17 exhibited at least one systolic elevation above 180 mmHg. No data concerning the development or maintenance of the elevations were presented, nor was any reference made to blood pressure levels after the auditory stimulation was discontinued. In a later study (6), rats were first tested for emotionality using an open field and then exposed to loud noise. After presentation of a minimum of 167 auditory stimuli, 10 of 12 experimental subjects exhibited blood pressure elevations above 160 mmHg. Additionally, the subjects that exhibited the highest blood pressures had scored highest in emotionality. The finding of a relationship between emotionality and stress-induced blood pressure elevations experimentally supports an important component of the psychosomatic explanation of hypertension (3). The suggestion that behavioral characteristics may somehow be predictive of an organism's predisposition to hypertension, although often clinically suggested, has only recently (7) been experimentally pursued in a systematic way using animal models.

The subsequent use of intensive auditory stimulation to produce hypertension has resulted in both positive and negative reports. Whereas one group (8) failed to observe any hypertension in Glaxo laboratory rats following 12 months of intense stimulation, another (9) reported modest increases, i.e., 20 to 30 mmHg above baseline, which tended to peak and eventually decline to baseline even though the stimulation continued to be presented. With respect to chronic hypertension, the above studies were unimpressive for three reasons. First, the elevations in blood pressure were modest compared to levels typically exhibited by human essential hypertensives. Second, there was no evidence that once the noxious stimulation was discontinued, the blood pressures remained elevated; i.e., the hypertension was "time locked" to stimulus presentation. In fact, there was some indication that habituation to the stimuli occurred, and that the stimuli became less hypertensinogenic with repeated exposure. It is important to emphasize that a genuine example of psychogenic hypertension would require chronic elevations in blood pressure which persist even after the initiating stimulus is removed. The third unimpressive aspect of the above studies is the absence of any physical evidence that chronic hypertension had been produced. None of the animals was reported to have developed the arterial lesions which characterize hypertensive vascular disease. In several more recent studies, rats repeatedly exposed to both auditory and visual stimulation exhibited not only modest elevations in blood pressure (152 mmHg) compared to controls (134 mmHg) (10) but also accompanying left ventricular hypertrophy and vacuolization of all three zones of the adrenal cortex (11). Although the physiologic manifestations may indicate chronic hypertension, no poststimulation recovery period was allowed. Hence, it could not be determined if the elevations in blood pressure would have been maintained following termination of the aversive stimulation.

The technique of producing transient and modest elevations in blood pressure by exposing rats to intense lights and sounds appears to be reliable and has been incorporated into pharmacologic research concerning the testing of antihypertensive drugs (12). Lockett and Marwood (13), however, in a reversal of conditions, have reported hypertension in rats resulting from chronic sound deprivation and, as was the case with audiogenic hypertension, the blood pressure of the sound-deprived rats reached a modest mean peak value (170 mmHg) in 4 weeks. Thereafter, although the conditions did not change, the pressures declined but still remained above baseline. This work is fully described in the next chapter. It appears that, for rats at least, chronic exposure to too much or too little auditory stimulation can bring about modest and somewhat persistent blood pressure changes.

Although most research on reflex behavioral models has used noise and/or lights, Schunk (14) followed Cannon's lead and repeatedly exposed cats to aggressive dogs. He reported that half of the subjects exhibited increased blood pressure throughout the exposure period but did not allow any postexposure recovery period. Rather, the cats were sacrificed, and those that had exhibited the increases in blood pressure also showed slightly increased heart weights and some renal damage.

There have been several other attempts to produce chronic hypertension by simply repeatedly exposing animals to nociceptive or noxious stimuli. These studies, however, involved organisms with special genetically or environmentally determined sensitivities and are discussed later.

Learning Models

In contrast to reflex models, the situations used in learning models involve stimuli that acquire the capacity to alter blood pressure as a function of training. For present purposes, learning models can be further divided into classic (Pavlovian) and instrumental (operant) conditioning paradigms.

Classic Conditioning Paradigms

The essential characteristic of classic conditioning is that initially neutral stimuli, by virtue of their temporal or spatial proximity with noxious or nociceptive stimuli, can bring about responses similar (but not necessarily identical) to the responses which automatically are elicited by the noxious or nociceptive stimuli themselves.

This paradigm has not frequently been used to test the psychogenic hypertension hypothesis.[1] A review of the Russian literature, however, revealed several demonstrations of severe acute blood pressure elevations in dogs upon presentation of electric shock or stimuli classically conditioned to electric shocks. The conditioning procedures were often maintained for many months, but in no case were the blood pressure elevations maintained in the absence of the conditioned or unconditioned stimuli. As might be expected, if the conditioned stimulus was repeatedly presented without the unconditioned stimulus, the ability of the conditioned stimulus to elicit acute elevations diminished (16). Dykman and Gantt (17) reported that a stimulus that produced an elevation in blood pressure in dogs after it had been paired with electric shock could still do so after a 13-month period. Since no measurements of blood pressure were made outside the environment in which the conditioning took place, it could not be concluded that hypertension was present outside the experimental milieu. This result is notable, however, since it is apparently the only reported study in which the effects of classic conditioning on blood pressure have been examined over an extended period of time. The studies simply demonstrated that the acute rises in blood pressure, which apparently automatically attend electric shock, can be classically conditioned. The conditioned blood pressure response extinguishes if the conditioned stimulus is no longer paired with the unconditioned stimulus. The demonstration that the conditioned response occurred after 13 months merely suggests that the persistence of classically conditioned responses may be great but says nothing about the development of hypertension. In a series of studies designed to specifically test the chronic effects of aversive classic conditioning on blood pressure, Shapiro and his co-workers (18–21) failed

---

[1] In contrast, researchers interested in acute cardiovascular changes, especially heart rate, often use this experimental procedure. The advantage of the arrangement is the ability to study the anticipatory cardiovascular changes which occur in the interval between presentation of the conditioned and unconditioned stimuli (15).

to produce any significant long-term changes in cats (18) and rats (19–21) after exposures of up to 12 weeks.

Instrumental Conditioning Paradigms

In the instrumental conditioning paradigm, a stimulus or a collection of stimuli are paired with a nociceptive or noxious stimulus, and conditioning proceeds in the same manner as in classic conditioning. The essential distinction is that in classic conditioning, the experimenter imposes the noxious stimulation on the subject, regardless of that subject's behavior. In instrumental conditioning, the noxious stimulation is contingent on some aspect of the subject's behavior.

Instrumental paradigms have been used by cardiovascular researchers in two ways. First, attempts have been made to directly reinforce or punish cardiovascular responses themselves. This line of experimental endeavor, which addresses the basic question of whether cardiovascular responses can be learned using instrumental techniques, has received considerable attention both inside and outside the scientific community (22). Furthermore, the seminal animal studies have led to the development of clinical strategies incorporating biofeedback training as a treatment modality for human essential hypertension (23; see also Chapter 14). Irrespective of the veracity and ultimate utility of these procedures, a point of considerable controversy (22), they have been generally considered to be of no significance in testing the psychogenic hypertension hypothesis. If organisms develop hypertension as a result of exposure to stress, it is not reasonable to suggest that this occurs because they have been reinforced for blood pressure elevations and hence emit the response in order to obtain additional reinforcement. However, a recent report suggests exactly this possibility (24).

It had been suggested that decreased baroreceptor stimulation increases behavioral reactivity (25), while increased baroreceptor stimulation decreases reactivity (26,27). Hence, it was hypothesized that acute elevations in blood pressure and ensuing increases in stimulation would not only bring about reflex cardiovascular adjustments but also reduce behavioral reactivity, probably by stimulation of the brainstem reticular formation. To test the hypothesis, rats were required to run on a treadwheel to terminate or avoid noxious stimuli. When blood pressure was acutely raised by phenylephrine infusion, escape and avoidance responding decreased, suggesting that the elevated blood pressure reduced reactivity to the stimulation. This reduced reactivity, however, was not seen in rats with denervated baroreceptors. This indicated that the rise in blood pressure and subsequent baroreceptor stimulation could have motivational consequences. The authors went on to state: "some hypertension may begin as an instrumentally learned blood pressure response for which the reward is a baroreceptor-mediated reduction in anxiety or in the aversiveness of ambient noxious stimulation" (24).

Support for this hypothesis can be obtained from several quarters. First, hypertensive rats do appear to have a higher pain threshold (28). Furthermore, the results of studies of clonidine, which apparently increases baroreceptor activity (29) while reducing the behavioral response to aversive stimulation (30), are consistent with the hypothesis. Hence, the demonstration that animals (31,32) and man (33,34) can learn sustained increases in blood pressure in the laboratory by appropriate manipulation of reinforcement may have been an experimental analog of a more naturally occurring situation. However, the recent *New York Times* headline asking "Hypertension: Is it too pleasant to give up?" (35) suggests rather incautious haste in accepting a phenomenon on the basis of initial laboratory investigations. Nonetheless, the possibility that stress-induced blood pressure elevations may have behavioral and psychologic utility is certain to be incorporated into our future conception of the psychogenic hypothesis.

The second way researchers have used instrumental conditioning paradigms to study cardiovascular disease involves conditioning of overt somatomotor responses with concomitant measurement of cardiovascular changes. In much the same way that one can suggest that repeated or prolonged exposure to noxious or nociceptive stimuli could chronically elevate blood pressure, it can be hypothesized that constant exposure to a situation that requires active behavioral responding might be hypertensinogenic. A basic point must be addressed in this regard. Obviously, an investigator interested in psychogenic hypertension is not most directly concerned with the effects of skeletal-muscular activity on blood pressure. Exercise is not the type of "stress" dealt with in this volume. Rather, the psychologic components of the behavioral demand are most interesting; involving specifically the stress of deciding what response to make and when to make it, and the anticipation of the consequences of the response.

RELEVANT EXPERIMENTAL MODELS

Aceto et al. (36) were the first to report the use of an instrumental conditioning paradigm to study elevations in blood pressure; they exposed rats to a pole jumping avoidance task. Subjects were given three brief sessions per week, and rapid elevations ensued; systolic pressures rose from an average of 114 mmHg to an average of 145 mmHg in only 4 weeks. By the 27th week of conditioning, which represents almost 25% of the rat's lifespan, the average pressures had reached a peak at 160 mmHg and thereafter actually declined to the 140 to 150 mmHg range, although the weekly avoidance sessions were maintained.

A follow-up study (37) exposed rats to this avoidance task in conjunction with passive exposure to intense auditory and visual stimulation. In this study, the blood pressures reached a peak at about the same level, namely, 163 mmHg, but at week 11 rather than week 27. Again, despite continued stimulation, the pressures gradually decreased to an average of 154 mmHg by week 27. An unfortunate aspect of the above studies was the absence of unstimulated controls, since the studies were intended to examine drug effects and hence were not adequately designed to specifically test the psychogenic hypothesis. More serious, however, is the absence of any posttraining blood pressure data.

As was the case for passive noxious stimulation, it cannot be determined if chronic hypertension would have been manifested after the rats were allowed a recovery period. Since a downward trend in the mean blood pressures occurred in both studies, it is reasonable to suggest that a stress-free recovery period would have produced baseline pressures.

Studies With Primates

More recent studies using primates have also employed various avoidance conditioning procedures. In contrast to the studies discussed above, the blood pressures in these experiments were obtained directly using intra-arterial cannulae. This allows more precise examination of the relationship between exposure to aversive stimulation and the temporal characteristics of the cardiovascular response. Exposing monkeys to a fixed-ratio avoidance task for between 4 and 11 months resulted in blood pressure elevations during avoidance conditioning session but not outside the testing situation (38). If a fixed-interval avoidance task was used, however, the elevations in blood pressure tended to persist even between the testing sessions. This indicates that the behavioral demands and stimulus characteristics of the aversive conditioning schedule determine the hypertensive potency.

Benson and his colleagues (39) have also reported behaviorally induced elevations in blood pressure in monkeys using a fixed-ratio shock avoidance schedule. In this case, the rapid response rates resulted in quite severe blood pressure elevations, which were diminished after termination of the schedule yet remained above preexposure levels. Essentially similar findings were obtained in another study with a longer (4-month) exposure period (40). In this study, the contribution of vasomotor and cardiac factors to the stress-induced blood pressure elevations was assessed by administration of either an α- or a β-adrenergic blocking agent, or the combination of both. The results suggested that both vasomotor and cardiac factors were responsible for the elevations in blood pressure, and that compensation of one mechanism took place when the other was compromised by pharmacologic blockage (41). Using baboons, Brady et al. (42) have confirmed that exposure to a fixed-ratio avoidance schedule elevates the blood pressure, at least during the avoidance task proper.

Using the free-operant avoidance paradigm, Forsyth (43) demonstrated that after initial increases in blood pressure, continued exposure to the schedule for 16 hr/day for 15 days actually did not produce any further elevations in blood pressure, unless the demands on the subjects (monkeys) were such that continuous responding was required. Despite the demand characteristics of the schedule, however, no generalizations to the nonavoidance conditions occurred. Forsyth (44) then subjected rhesus monkeys to a Sidman shock-avoidance schedule, which required the subjects to press a lever at least once every 20 sec in order to avoid electric shock. The response requirement was in effect 12 hr each day from 7 to 14 months. While these monkeys exhibited average blood pressure elevations of approximately 160 mmHg, only one subject was reported to have maintained the hypertension after the avoidance schedule was discontinued. This subject's blood pressure remained higher than base level for 2 months, namely, 152 mmHg as compared to 136 mmHg, although it was lower than it had been during the last month of conditioning (163 mmHg). As Forsyth pointed out, there was no evidence that a "fixed" hypertension had been produced. Following this 2-month rest period, conditioning was resumed, which eventually reelevated the blood pressure.

During the course of these studies, an interesting observation was made. The hypertensive effect of exposure to the free-operant schedule was compared to the effects of exposing monkeys to a snake (45). Although both situations increased blood pressure, heart rate, cardiac output, and stroke volume and decreased peripheral resistance, the blood pressure response to the avoidance schedule was greater. Forsyth (46) has determined that during the avoidance sessions, for the first few hours, increased heart rate and cardiac output predominated, followed by increased cardiac output and increased peripheral resistance at 24 hr. If conditioning is continued up to 72 hr, only increased peripheral resistance persists. Another significant observation to emerge from these studies is that the exposed monkeys exhibited increased irritability to neutral stimuli during conditioning.

Conflict and Hypertension

Minisnoshvilli (47) used a different type of instrumental conditioning paradigm. He required monkeys to cross an electrified grid in order to receive either food or the company of a sexual partner. This type of approach-avoidance conflict differs in some important ways from the active avoidance procedure described above. In avoidance conditioning, after sufficient training, the subject, by responding correctly, can entirely eliminate aversive stimulation; thus an appropriate coping response is made available. In approach-avoidance conflict, responding has positive consequences, such as food or sex. Failure to respond results in the avoidance of shock but also the avoidance of positive contingencies. The behavioral consequences of exposure to approach-avoidance situations have received a great deal of attention by experimental psychologists (48). The present concern, however, is whether exposure to such conflict is hypertensinogenic; in this context, the Minisnoshvilli study was not particularly rigorous. The monkeys were intermittently exposed to the conflict over a 2-year period; two of the subjects exhibited no blood pressure elevations; one died during the second year after blood pressure rose above 180 mmHg; and the remaining two showed persistent elevations between 180 and 200 mmHg throughout the 2-year period. Although no data concerning the maintenance of hypertension following this period were reported, the results suggest that conflict may be a fairly potent stimulus for blood pressure elevations.

Another attempt to use conflict to elevate blood pressure has been made by

Henry and his colleagues (49). They produced long-term elevations in blood pressure in mice as a result of "psychosocial" stimulation, such as forced competition for food or females. Although these elevations in systolic pressure were maintained for months, when repeated stimulation was discontinued, pressures often returned to or toward normal values. There was, however, some indication that a few animals, after many months of intense social conflict, maintained elevated blood pressures even after they had been placed in a competition-free situation. These persistent blood pressure changes are of particular importance, since the mice were reported to have an increased incidence of acute and chronic interstitial nephritis, glomerular mesangial changes, myocardial fibrosis, and arteriosclerotic degeneration of the intramural coronary vessels (50).

Henry's work is particularly supportive of the psychogenic hypothesis of hypertension. Rodents were placed in an environment which required conflict-laden behavioral adjustments for a significant portion of their life spans. With sufficiently prolonged exposure, cardiovascular changes occurred, including hypertension, which persisted even when the conflict was removed. (Henry's work is discussed again below with respect to environmental predisposition.) The same psychosocial stress procedures have also been used with rats but with relatively poor results. Neither the severity of the elevations (rarely above 170 mmHg) nor the percentage of affected subjects (approximately 33%) was impressive (51).

In summary, passive exposure to noxious stimulation, which reflexively brings about acute elevations in blood pressure, or to classic conditioning situations, in which the unconditioned stimulus is nociceptive or noxious, does not result in chronic hypertension. In fact, much of the evidence suggests that with repeated or prolonged stimulation, habituation occurs, and the severity of the stress-induced blood pressure elevations decreases. Aversive instrumental conditioning procedures are more potent as well as more heuristic. Those situations in which aversive stimulation was contingent on the subject's behavior appear to be more hypertensinogenic than situations in which behavioral adjustments are neither required nor allowed.

It is appropriate to briefly mention the relationship between behavioral control and disease onset as it applies to another putative psychosomatic disease. In a series of elegant studies conducted by Weiss (52–54), it was demonstrated that rats allowed to avoid electric shocks developed less gastric ulceration than rats that were passively exposed to electric shocks irrespective of their behaviors. Hence, in this case, the ability to control the application of the nociceptive stimulation reduced the severity of the pathology. If the situation was slightly changed, however, so that the successful avoidance response was now also punished with a brief electric shock, the subjects given behavioral control developed more gastric ulceration than the rats passively exposed to shock. In certain circumstances, behavioral control can be more pathogenic.

The key variable appears to be conflict. If an effective coping mechanism is available, as is the case in avoidance conditioning, then learning, and using, this coping response is effective in reducing the severity of stress-related pathology. If the coping response brings about negative as well as positive consequences, however, pathology is increased above that which would have occurred if no behavioral control were possible. The situation for gastric ulceration may be true for hypertension as well. The avoidance conditioning procedures applied are often so rigorous as to require continuous behavioral adjustment on the subject's part. When the response demands of the schedule are severe, a genuine conflict arises. On the one hand, responding allows shock avoidance; on the other, almost continuous vigilance to the schedule requirements prevents any relaxation. Additionally, the most impressive results obtained with respect to chronic hypertension are those of Henry et al. (49). The mice in his study were continually faced with approach-avoidance conflicts, being required to traverse a narrow runway to obtain food, a task which surely has reinforcing properties. Entering the runway, however, was likely to result in confronting a conspecific with similar intentions, which would lead to fighting. Throughout the day, the mouse was constantly confronted by these choices.

Direct comparisons between the hypertensive effect of conflict exposure and other types of aversive conditioning have recently been reported. In one study, reported as an abstract, Long-Evans rats exposed to avoidance-avoidance conflict exhibited greater elevations in blood pressure than physically restrained rats. Rats passively exposed to electric shocks, however, also developed elevations in blood pressure comparable to conflict-exposed subjects. In both groups, the modest elevations were maintained hours after the experimental sessions ended (55). Other studies, reported in more detail, have examined the relative hypertensive potency of conflict in animal models with specific genetically determined predispositions to hypertension. These studies are discussed below.

GENETIC AND ENVIRONMENTAL PREDISPOSITION

Psychologic stress does not act in a vacuum. In many experiments, stress has been treated as a rather global concept, which has been putatively linked to hypertension as if it were a single cause rather than one factor that interacts with other factors in the complex physiology of high blood pressure. In several of the studies discussed above, considerable variability among subjects was reported. For example, when Schunk (14) exposed cats to aggressive dogs, only half exhibited sustained blood pressure increases. Similarly, some monkeys exposed to conflict exhibited rather dramatic increases in blood pressure, while in others, no hypertension developed (47). Possible reasons for this variability may be the genetic predisposition of the organism or environmentally acquired factors, such as diet or injury.

Environmental Predisposition and Psychogenic Hypertension

Relatively few studies have examined the way psychologic stress interacts with other environmental factors in the production of hypertension. In a series of studies previously discussed, Shapiro and his co-workers (18–21) failed to observe hypertension in cats or rats following classic conditioning or fixed-interval avoidance procedures. The major positive results of their studies, however, concern the interaction of other factors with aversive conditioning. Although incapable of initiating the disease, classic and instrumental training did accelerate the onset of hypertension in response to renal insults. Subsequently (56), it was demonstrated that pyelonephritis induced by *proteus mirabilis* but not *E. coli,* predisposed rats to develop classically conditioned blood pressure elevations. Hence, the precise nature of environmentally produced predispositions determines the efficacy of conditioned blood pressure elevations.

In addition to renal injury or disease, another environmental factor examined has been early rearing experience. In the psychosocial conflict paradigm of Henry (49), several experimental manipulations have been performed. Significantly, Henry and his colleagues (57) have emphasized that the only mice in which psychosocial conflict resulted in "fixed" hypertension were those with a history of social deprivation prior to stimulation.

These demonstrations suggest that environmental conditions can increase the sensitivity of subjects to stress-induced blood pressure elevations. It is almost tautologic to state that two putative hypertensinogenic agents acting in concert would have more pronounced cardiovascular effects than either one alone. However, the nature of the interactive effects of, for example, renal artery stenosis and stress or high sodium chloride ingestion and stress have not been adequately studied. Furthermore, the demonstration that early social experiences determine the cardiovascular response to stress is of great practical and theoretical interest. This line of inquiry has not been experimentally pursued.

Genetic Predisposition and Psychogenic Hypertension

Careful experiments have established beyond a doubt that a predisposition to hypertension may be selectively bred in rat strains. Smirk and Hall (58), Dahl and his colleagues (59), Okamoto and Aoki (60), and Ben-Ishay and his co-workers (61) have all successfully developed rat models that evince genetically determined predispositions to hypertension. The specific characteristics of these models, however, are quite different. Schlager (62) has similarly developed a genetically hypertensive mouse strain. Attempts to investigate the interaction of psychic and genetic factors using these models have been relatively neglected until recently.

The first experimental suggestion that genetic factors determine blood pressure responsiveness to stress was in the study by Rothlin et al. (8), discussed above. After failing to produce any hypertension in Glaxo laboratory rats following 12 months of intense auditory and visual stimulation, cross-breeding with wild rats was initiated. When the progeny of this cross-breeding were exposed to auditory stimulation, elevations in blood pressure ensued. Generally, noxious stimulation has a much greater cardiotoxic effect on wild than on domesticated animals (63).

Several studies using the selected animal models mentioned above and which only indirectly relate to the psychogenic hypothesis of hypertension have been completed. Using Smirk's New Zealand strain of genetically hypertensive rat (58), it has been demonstrated that the acute blood pressure response to sympathetic nervous system stimulation is augmented, compared to unselected subjects (64). Furthermore, peripheral sympathectomy due to repeated neonatal injections of 6-hydroxydopamine prevented the development of hypertension in the genetically hypertensive rat (65). No chronic studies concerning sympathetic stimulation and none involving psychologic factors using this strain have been reported. The Hebrew University strains developed by Ben-Ishay et al. (61) have not been used in psychologic stress studies. The genetically hypertensive mice developed by Schlager (62) behave differently than their low blood pressure controls. The association between behavioral differences and blood pressure could not be attributed to genetic linkage, pleiotropy, or a direct causal relationship between blood pressure extremes and behavior (66). These mice have not been used in psychologic stress studies.

The remaining two animal models, the spontaneously hypertensive rat (SHR) of Okamoto and Aoki (60) and the Dahl salt-sensitive (DS) and salt-resistant (DR) model (59), have been used more directly in testing the psychogenic hypothesis. The SHR rat is the most widely used experimental model for the study of genetic factors in hypertension, although it is beyond the scope of this chapter to delineate what is known about these rats. Briefly, SHR rats spontaneously exhibit significant blood pressure elevations beginning at 4 to 5 weeks of age. The pathogenesis of the disease is not completely understood, although the weight of evidence suggests that the sympathetic nervous system plays an important role. Renal and adrenal factors have been implicated as playing some part in the development of hypertension in these rats as well but probably not a primary one. Two volumes, devoted exclusively to the characteristics of SHR, are currently available (67,68).

The Dahl model differs from the SHR model in several important ways. The DS rats predictably develop severe, often fatal, hypertension upon exposure to a variety of putative hypertensionogenic stimuli. In contrast to the SHR, DS rats remain normotensive if not exposed to a hypertensinogenic stimulus. Equally important is the availability of the DR rat which, upon exposure to the same stimuli, shows no elevations in blood pressure (69). Renal homograft transplantation and parabiosis studies have indicated that a considerable part of the difference in sensitivity is due to differences in kidney function (70,71). More recently, however, studies have implicated central (72) and peripheral (73) nervous system factors as being partially responsible for differences between the DS and DR rats.

SPONTANEOUSLY HYPERTENSIVE RATS

A direct test of the psychogenic hypothesis of hypertension using SHR as subjects is not possible, since these rats develop serious elevations in blood pressure spontaneously. It is possible to examine only the exacerbational influences of stressors in the development of hypertension, not to investigate their etiologic significance. Results from such studies should be interpreted with this caveat in mind. It has been demonstrated that the blood pressures of these animals (SHR) can be potentiated by chronic, passive exposure to aversive conditions, such as combined visual, auditory, and electrical stimulation, as well as physical restraint and cold temperatures (74). Similarly, acute blood pressure elevations in response to stimuli which would activate the sympathoadrenomedullary system, such as flashing lights, loud noises, or vibration, were significantly higher in SHR than in normotensive controls (75).

Subsequently, Hallbäck (76) hypothesized that the ultimate development of hypertension in the SHR might be due to the hyperreactivity of these rats to environmental stimulation. In an important study, she tested the hypothesis by socially isolating SHR at weaning until they were 7 months of age. The isolation procedure was an attempt to reduce the environmental influences which ordinarily induce psychologic activation. When compared to group-reared SHR, the social isolates exhibited significantly lower baseline blood pressures. However, the cardiovascular responses of these isolated rats to acute aversive stimulation were equal to the group-reared rats. The Hallbäck study is notable on several points. First, it is the only demonstration reported in the literature whereby an environmental manipulation that might be considered psychologic had a salubrious effect on blood pressure. Second, it strongly suggests that stimuli affecting the higher portions of the central nervous system play a role in the pathogenesis of spontaneous hypertension in these rats. Furthermore, the study emphasizes the need to investigate the interaction of both environmental and genetic predisposition in the development of hypertension.

Relationship With the Sympathetic System

Recently, a series of studies have been reported concerning the relationship between acute exposure to aversive stimulation and sympathoadrenomedullary activation in the SHR. McCarty and his colleagues (77) have demonstrated that SHR exhibit excessive and prolonged discharge of catecholamines into the circulatory system during and following periods of forced immobilization. Similarly, SHR also exhibited greater adrenergic reactivity in anticipation of footshock than normotensive controls (78). Furthermore, the anticipation of footshock resulted in greater increases in heart rate and mean arterial blood pressure in the SHR than in controls. The actual application of electric shocks, however, resulted in decreases in mean arterial blood pressures but increase in heart rate, while controls developed shock-induced increases in both arterial pressure and heart rate (79). The findings that rats with a genetic predisposition to spontaneous hypertension exhibit adrenergic hyperresponsivity to forced immobilization and anticipation of footshock suggest that excessive discharge of norepinephrine and epinephrine into plasma during stress may contribute to the development and maintenance of high blood pressure in the SHR model.

Behavioral Influences

The relationship of behavior to the development of spontaneous hypertension has also been examined using the SHR. The only consistent finding appears to be a greater level of locomotor activity exhibited in SHR compared to Wistar-Kyoto normotensive controls (80). This difference emerged even at a very early age, before hypertension had developed (81); these behavioral differences may be due to differences in forebrain catecholamine activity (82). It is not clear, however, that these differences are meaningfully related to the genetic predisposition to hypertension. Correlations between characteristics, such as behavioral measures and blood pressure elevations, in genetically selected populations such as SHR may be fortuitous. Since appropriate genetic analyses concerning the relationship between behavioral characteristics and spontaneous hypertension have not been reported, it is not possible to make any firm conclusions concerning their association. Despite the differences in locomotor activity, the anticipation of footshock resulted in similar behavioral responses in SHR and controls, while the cardiovascular and adrenergic responses were dramatically different (83). Hence, at least in this situation, behavioral reactivity was not predictive of cardiovascular reactivity.

Exposure to aversive stimulation can exacerbate the development of spontaneous hypertension, while isolation from environmental stimulation can ameliorate its development. The SHR model is characterized by cardiovascular and adrenergic hyperactivity to psychologic stimulation, which may play a role in the pathogenesis of its hypertension. These facts must be incorporated into the psychogenic hypothesis of hypertension. As stated above, however, because the development of hypertension is spontaneous in these rats, it is difficult to assess the etiologic significance of stress. Furthermore, it is not clear that the SHR represents the most appropriate animal experimental analog of human essential hypertension (68).

Lawler and his colleagues (84) have noted the limited utility of the SHR model for studying the relevance of psychologic inputs to the production of hypertension. To reduce the spontaneous development of hypertension which confounds the interpretation of the etiologic significance of stress, they cross-bred SHR and normotensive Kyoto-Wistar rats. The resulting offspring had systolic blood pressures between 140–160 mmHg prior to conditioning; these pressures were significantly lower than those of SHR but significantly above those of Kyoto-Wistars. After 12 weeks of avoidance-avoidance conflict similar to that used by Weiss (54), the cross-bred rats had an average systolic blood pressure of 186 mmHg, compared to the cross-bred control average of 150 mmHg. Significantly, cross-bred animals that were restrained but not shocked did not develop sustained blood pressure elevations. Lawler *(personal communication)* indicated that heart weight/body weight ratios were greater in the conflict-exposed rats, and that despite a poststress recovery period of 10 weeks, the conflict-induced blood pressures did not return to control levels. This study represents a direct verification of the psychogenic hypothesis and strongly emphasizes the hypertensinogenic potency of conflict paradigms. It must be noted, however, that the cross-bred rats began with borderline hypertension.

Etiologic Significance of Stress

Studies examining the etiologic significance of stress in the development of hypertension using the Dahl model began in 1968 (85). Dahl failed to observe any elevations in blood pressure in DS rats following repeated passive exposure to electric shocks, overcrowding, or cold temperatures. There was some indication that salt-induced hypertension was aggravated by the shock exposure. Dahl reasoned that since the DS rat was so sensitive to other putative hypertensinogenic stimuli, the inability of stress to elevate blood pressure independently in these rats was strong negative evidence against the psychogenic hypothesis (86). The subsequent accumulation of evidence that instrumental conditioning paradigms were more hypertensinogenic resulted in a new series of studies.

Friedman and Dahl (87) directly compared the effects of chronic approach-avoidance conflict with the effects of passive exposure to aversive stimulation. Throughout the 13-week study, conflict-exposed DS rats consistently exhibited higher blood pressures than DS rats passively exposed to precisely the same aversive events. The mean blood pressure of the conflict-exposed DS rats (166 mmHg) was statistically higher than the unstimulated DS control mean (140 mmHg). Hence, although these results do support the notion that conflict is a more hypertensinogenic stimulus than passive stimulation, the absolute blood pressure levels evinced were not impressive. Furthermore, a 13-week poststress recovery period resulted in a gradual but consistent reduction to control blood pressure levels.

In a subsequent study, a modest amount of sodium chloride was added to the diet of conflict-exposed DS rats, thereby combining genetic and environmental (dietary) predisposition (88). The results of this study were somewhat more impressive. The absolute magnitude of the blood pressures evinced was only slightly higher than previously noted, but following the 13-week conditioning period, when the DS rats were no longer exposed to conflict and were placed on a low-salt diet, the blood pressures did not, in all cases, return to baseline. Furthermore, the conflict procedure which resulted in moderate and sustained elevations in blood pressure in the DS rats was completely ineffective in producing any elevations in DR rats (89). This particular result reinforces the paramount importance of considering genetic predisposition in assessing the importance of psychologic stimuli in the development of hypertension.

CONCLUSIONS

Clearly, exposure to aversive conditioning procedures can result in rather impressive elevations in blood pressure. There is compelling evidence that activation of the sympathoadrenomedullary system is the underlying physiologic mechanism for this process. In situations that require continuous behavioral adjustment, blood pressures often remain elevated for as long as the behavioral adjustments are required; when the aversive schedules are discontinued, however, the blood pressures return to or toward normal values.

Confirmation of the psychogenic hypothesis requires stress-induced blood pressure elevations that are self-sustaining following removal of the initiating stimulus. This is not an excessive requirement for other forms of experimental hypertension, e.g., desoxycorticosterone plus saline administration. With sufficient exposure, the elevations in blood pressure are indeed not reversed when treatment is discontinued. The relative lack of success, however, in using psychologic stimuli is probably due to the relatively subtle effect of these stimuli on the cardiovascular system, as well as the ability of experimental subjects to habituate to passive aversive stimulation or to develop effective coping responses in instrumental conditioning situations. Simply stated, the magnitude of stress-induced elevations is not large enough to eventuate the pathophysiologic changes which would cause sustained elevations.

Two strategies have evolved in response to this lack of experimental success. The first is the use of conditioning procedures that prevent effective coping; and the second is the use of animals with genetic and/or environmental sensitivity to hypertension. Both these strategies have resulted in greater experimental verification of the psychogenic hypothesis. The sum of the experimental evidence to date suggests that the conflict procedures are the most hypertensinogenic paradigms. Furthermore, stress can exacerbate genetically related spontaneous, borderline, or salt-induced hypertension. Equally important, environmental experiences or genetic factors can ameliorate or completely prevent the development of stress-induced hypertension.

With respect to human essential hypertension, it must be concluded that psychologic factors probably play a relatively minor role. Extraordinary procedures must be experimentally employed to bring about even modest elevations in blood pressure. An aversive paradigm must be designed which prevents effective coping; and it must be applied for a substantial portion of the organism's lifespan. Furthermore, even these procedures are only modestly hypertensinogenic in organisms with genetic or environmental predispostions to hypertension. Whether this represents an appropriate experimental analog to the human condition is debatable.

A few years ago, Dahl, an eminent hypertensinologist, reviewed the experimental literature concerning psychogenic hypertension. He then interpreted the results from the perspective of a clinician concerned with the treatment of essential hypertension. The studies conducted since his review only substantiate these observations. Hence, it is appropriate to conclude this review with a restatement of Dahl's comments (90):

> I have no doubt that stress can raise the blood pressure transiently in virtually all people under some circumstances. I suspect that it can play an etiological role in

the individual who is genetically predisposed to develop hypertension. I do not doubt that it can exacerbate preexisting hypertension. Because I believe hypertension to be a multigenic, multifactorial disease, I would be prepared to accept stress in an accessory etiological role in conjunction with more effective agents, but I doubt that it plays the primary etiological role in most human cases. Consequently, it behooves the physician to become cognizant of any significant stress which might adversely affect his hypertensive patients. However, the acknowledgement of stress as a potential hypertensinogenic factor should not cause one to abandon traditional therapeutic procedures in favor of hypertensive therapies which assume a psychic etiology. The evidence which would justify such a shift simply does not exist.

ACKNOWLEDGMENTS

The author currently holds a Research Career Development Award from the National Heart, Lung and Blood Institute. The author wishes to thank Dr. Sonja B. Haber for her helpful comments concerning the preparation of this manuscript.

REFERENCES

1. Cannon, W. B. *Bodily Changes in Pain, Fear, Hunger and Rage.* Appleton, New York, 1929.
2. Wolf, S., Cardon, P. V., Shepard, E. M., and Wolff, H. G. *Life Stress and Essential Hypertension.* Williams & Wilkins, Baltimore, 1955.
3. Weiner, H. *Psychobiology and Human Disease.* Elsevier, New York, 1977.
4. Cohen, D. H., and Obrist, P. A. Interactions between behavior and the cardiovascular system. *Circ. Res.,* 1975, 37, 693.
5. Medoff, H. S., and Bongiovanni, A. M. Blood pressure in rats subjected to audiogenic stimulation. *Am. J. Physiol.,* 1945, 143, 300.
6. Farris, E. J., Yeakel, E. H., and Medoff, H. Development of hypertension in emotional gray Norway rats after air blasting. *Am. J. Physiol.,* 1945, 144, 331.
7. Friedman, R., Haber, S. B., and Iwai, J. Behavioral correlates of genetic predisposition to experimental hypertension. *Behav. Genet.,* 1978, 8, 92.
8. Rothlin, E., Cerletti, A., and Emmenegger, H. Experimental psychoneurogenic hypertension and its treatment with hydrogenated ergot alkaloids (hydergine). *Acta. Med. Scand.* [*Suppl.*], 1956, 312, 27.
9. Hudak, W. J., and Buckley, J. P. Production of hypertensive rats by experimental stress. *J. Pharm. Sci.,* 1961, 50, 263.
10. Smookler, H. H., Goebel, K. H., Siegel, M. I., and Clark, D. E. Hypertensive effects of prolonged auditory, visual, and motion stimulation. *Fed. Proc.,* 1973, 32, 3105.
11. Buckley, J. P., and Smookler, H. H. Cardiovascular and biochemical effects of chronic intermittent neurogenic stimulation. In: *Physiological Effects of Noise,* edited by B. L. Welch and A. S. Welch. Plenum, New York, 1970.
12. Perhach, J. L., Ferguson, H. C., and McKinney, G. R. Elevation of antihypertensive agents in the stress-induced hypertensive rats. *Life Sci.,* 1976, 16, 1731.
13. Lockett, M. F., and Marwood, J. F. Sound deprivation causes hypertension in rats. *Fed. Proc.,* 1973, 32, 2111.
14. Schunk, J. Emotionale faktoren in der pathogenese der essentiellen hypertonie. *Z. Klin. Med.,* 1954, 152, 251.
15. Obrist, P. A., Black, A. H., Brener, J., and DiCara, L. V. *Cardiovascular Psychophysiology.* Aldine, Chicago, 1974.
16. Simonson, E., and Brozek, J. Russian search on arterial hypertension. *Ann. Int. Med.,* 1959, 50, 129.
17. Dykman, R., and Gantt, W. A. Experimental psychogenic hypertension: Blood pressure changes conditioned to painful stimuli. *Bull. Johns Hopkins Hosp.,* 1960, 107, 72.

18. Shapiro, A. P., and Horn, P. W. Blood pressure, plasma pepsinogen and behavior in cats subjected to experimental production of anxiety. *J. Nerv. Ment. Dis.,* 1955, 122, 222.
19. Belkin, G. A., and Shapiro, A. P. Behavioral disturbances in animals. Effects on blood pressure, pepsinogen and adrenal weight in rats. *Tex. Rep. Biol. Med.,* 1956, 14, 415.
20. Shapiro, A. P., and Melhado, J. Factors affecting the development of hypertensive vascular disease in rats after renal injury. *Proc. Soc. Exp. Biol. Med.,* 1957, 96, 619.
21. Shapiro, A. P., and Melhado, J. Observations on blood pressure and other physiologic and biochemical mechanisms in rats with behavioral disturbances. *Psychosom. Med.,* 1958, 20, 303.
22. Miller, N. E., and Dworkin, B. R. Visceral learning: Recent difficulties with curarized rats and significant problems for human research. In: *Cardiovascular Psychophysiology,* edited by P. A. Obrist, A. H. Black, J. Brener, and L. V. DiCara, p. 312. Aldine, Chicago, 1974.
23. Blanchard, E. B., and Young, L. D. Self-control of cardiac functioning: A promise as yet unfulfilled. *Psychol. Bull.,* 1973, 79, 145.
24. Dworkin, B. R., Filewich, R. J., Miller, N. E., Craigmyle, N., and Pickering, T. G. Baroreceptor activation reduces reactivity to noxious stimulation: Implications for hypertension. *Science,* 1979, 205, 1299.
25. Bartorelli, C., Bizzi, E., Libretti, A., and Zanchett, A. Inhibitory control of sino-carotid pressoceptive afferents on hypothalamic autonomic activity and sham rage behavior. *Arch. Ital. Biol.,* 1960, 98, 308.
26. Lacey, J. I., Kagan, J., Lacey, B. C., and Moss, H. A. The visceral level: Situational determinants and behavioral correlates of autonomic response patterns. In: *Expression of the Emotions in Man,* edited by P. H. Knapp, p. 161. Academic Press, New York, 1960.
27. Lacey, B. C., and Lacey, J. I. Studies of heart rate and other bodily processes in sensorimotor behavior. In: *Cardiovascular Psychophysiology,* edited by P. A. Obrist, A. H. Black, J. Brener, and L. V. DiCara, p. 538. Aldine, Chicago, 1974.
28. Zamir, N., and Segal, M. Hypertension-induced analgesia: Changes in pain sensitivity in experimental hypertensive rats. *Brain Res.,* 1979, 160, 170.
29. Sleight, P., West, M. J., Koner, P. I., Chalmer, J. P., and Robinson, J. L. The action of clonidine on the baroreflex control of heart rate in conscious animals and man and on single aortic baroreceptor discharge in the rabbit. *Arch. Int. Pharmacodyn. Ther.,* 1975, 214, 4.
30. Laverty, R., and Taylor, K. M. Behavioral and biochemical effects of 2-(2,6)-dichlorophenyl-amino-2-imidazoline hydrochloride (ST 155) on the central nervous system. *Br. J. Pharmacol.,* 1969, 35, 253.
31. Benson, H., Herd, J. A., Morse, W. H., and Kelleher, R. T. Behavioral induction of arterial hypertension and its reversal. *Am. J. Physiol.,* 1969, 217, 30.
32. Harris, A. H., Gilliam, W. J., Findley, J. D., and Brady, J. V. Instrumental conditioning of large-magnitude, daily, 12-hour blood pressure elevations in the baboon. *Science,* 1973, 182, 175.
33. Krist, D. A., and Engel, B. T. Learned control of blood pressure in patients with high blood pressure. *Circulation,* 1975, 51, 370.
34. Elder, S. T., Welsh, D. M., Longacre, A., and McAfee, R. Acquisition discriminative stimulus control, and retention of increases/decreases in blood pressure in normotensive human subjects. *J. Appl. Behav. Anal.,* 1977, 10, 381.
35. Schmeck, H. M. Hypertension: Is it too pleasant to give up? *New York Times,* Section C, p. 1. September 25, 1979.
36. Aceto, M. D. G., Kinnard, W. J., and Buckley, J. P. Effects of compounds on blood pressure and behavioral responses of rats chronically subjected to an avoidance-escape situation. *Arch. Int. Pharmacodyn. Ther.,* 1963, 144, 214.
37. Buckley, J. P., Kato, H., Kinnard, W. J., Aceto, M. D. G., and Estevez, J. M. Effects of reserpine and chlorpromazine on rats subjected to experimental mental stress. *Psychopharmacologia,* 1964, 6, 87.
38. Herd, J. A., Morse, W. H., Kelleher, R. T., and Jones, L. G. Arterial hypertension in the squirrel monkey during behaviorial experiments. *Am. J. Physiol.,* 1969, 217, 24.
39. Benson, H., Herd, J. A., Morse, W. H., and Kelleher, R. T. Behaviorally induced hypertension in the squirrel monkey. *Circ. Res. [Suppl.],* 1970, 26, 181.
40. Grace, S. A., Herd, J. A., Morse, W. H., and Kelleher, R. T. Behavioral hypertension in the squirrel monkey. *Fed. Proc.,* 1971, 30, 549.
41. Kelleher, R. T., Morse, W. H., and Herd, J. A. Effects of propranolol, phentolamine and

methylatropine on cardiovascular function in the squirrel monkey during behavorial experiments. *J. Pharmacol. Exp. Ther.,* 1972, 182, 204.

42. Brady, J. V., Findley, J. D., and Harris, A. Experimental psychopathology and the psychophysiology of emotion. *J. Exp. Psychopathol.,* 1971, 119.

43. Forsyth, R. P. Blood pressure and avoidance conditioning. A study of 15-day trials in the rhesus monkey. *Psychosom. Med.,* 1968, 30, 125.

44. Forsyth, R. P. Blood pressure responses to long-term avoidance schedules in the restrained rhesus monkey. *Psychosom. Med.,* 1969, 31, 300.

45. Forsyth, R. P., and Harris, R. E. Circulatory changes during stressful stimuli in rhesus monkeys. *Circ. Res. [Suppl. I],* 1970, 36, 113.

46. Forsyth, R. P. Regional blood flow changes during 72-hour avoidance schedules in the monkey. *Science,* 1971, 173, 546.

47. Minisnoshvilli, D. I. Experimental neurosis in monkeys. In: *Theoretical and Practical Problems of Medicine and Biology in Experiments on Monkeys,* p. 53. Pergamon, New York, 1960.

48. Lazarus, R. S. *Patterns of Adjustment.* McGraw-Hill, New York, 1976.

49. Henry, J. P., Meehan, J. P., and Stephens, P. M. The use of psychosocial stimuli to induce prolonged systolic hypertension in mice. *Psychosom. Med.,* 1967, 29, 408.

50. Henry, J. P., Ely, D. L., Stephens, P. M., Ratcliffe, H. L., Santisteban, G. A., and Shapiro, A. P. The role of psychosocial factors in the development of arteriosclerosis in CBA mice: Observations on the heart, kidney, and aorta. *Atherosclerosis,* 1971, 14, 203.

51. Alexander, N. Psychosocial hypertension in members of a Wistar rat colony. *Proc. Soc. Exp. Biol. Med.,* 1974, 146, 163.

52. Weiss, J. M. Effects of coping responses on stress. *J. Comp. Physiol. Psychol.,* 1968, 65, 251.

53. Weiss, J. M. Effects of coping behavior in different warning signal conditions on stress pathology in rats. *J. Comp. Physiol. Psychol.,* 1971, 77, 1.

54. Weiss, J. M. Effects of punishing the coping response (conflict) on stress pathology in rats. *J. Comp. Physiol. Psychol.,* 1971, 77, 14.

55. Buchholz, R. A., Lawler, J. E., and Barker, G. F. The effects of short vs. long term psychological stress on the blood pressure of rats. *Physiologist,* 1979, 22, 16.

56. Lipman, R. L., and Shapiro, A. P. Effects of a behavioral stimulus on blood pressure of rats with experimental pyelonephritis. *Psychosom. Med.,* 1967, 29, 612.

57. Henry, J. P., Ely, D. L., and Stephens, P. M. Changes in catecholamine controlling enzymes in response to psychosocial activation of defense and alarm reactions. In: *Physiology, Emotion, and Psychosomatic Illness. Ciba Foundation Symposium 8,* p. 225. Associated Scientific Publishers, Amsterdam, 1972.

58. Smirk, F. H., and Hall, W. H. Inherited hypertension in rats. *Nature,* 1958, 182, 727.

59. Dahl, L. K., Heine, M., and Tassinari, L. J. Effects of chronic excess salt ingestion. Evidence that genetic factors play an important role in susceptibility to experimental hypertension. *J. Exp. Med.,* 1962, 115, 1173.

60. Okamoto, K., and Aoki, K. Development of a strain of spontaneously hypertensive rats. *Jpn. Circ. J.,* 1963, 27, 282.

61. Ben-Ishay, D., Saliternick, R., and Welner, A. Separation of two strains of rats with inbred dissimilar sensitivity to DOCA-salt hypertension. *Experimentia,* 1972, 28, 1321.

62. Schlager, G. Selection for blood pressure levels in mice. *Genetics,* 1974, 76, 537.

63. Corley, K. C., Shiel, F. O., Path, M. R. C., Mauck, H. P., and Greenhoot, J. Electrocardiographic and cardiac morphological changes associated with environmental stress in squirrel monkeys. *Psychosom. Med.,* 1973, 35, 361.

64. Montgomery, J. C., and McGregor, D. D. Blood pressure responses to stimulation of spinal sympathetic outflow in genetically hypertensive rats. *Proc. Univ. Otago Med. School,* 1974, 52, 36.

65. Clark, D. W. J., Jones, D. R., Phelan, E. L., and Devine, C. E. Blood pressure and vascular resistance in genetically hypertensive rats treated at birth with 6-hydroxydopamine. *Circ. Res.,* 1978, 43, 293.

66. Elias, M. F., Schlager, G. Discrimination learning in mice genetically selected for high and low blood pressure: Initial findings and methodological implications. *Physiol. Behav.,* 1974, 13, 261.

67. Okamoto, K. *Spontaneous Hypertension: Its Pathogenesis and Complications.* Igaku, Tokyo, 1972.

68. Department of Health, Education and Welfare, Public Health Service, National Institutes of Health, DHEW Publication No. (NIH) 77–1179. *Spontaneous Hypertension: Its Pathogenesis and Complications.* U.S. Government Printing Office, Washington, 1977.

69. Dahl, L. K., Knudsen, K. D., Iwai, J., Rapp, J. P., and Jaffe, D. Some genetically determined differences between hypertension-prone and hypertension-resistant rats. In: *Hypertension '72,* edited by J. Genest and E. Koiw, p. 337. Springer-Verlag, Berlin, 1972.

70. Dahl, L. K., and Heine, M. Primary role of renal homografts in setting chronic blood pressure levels in rats. *Circ. Res.,* 1975, 36, 692.

71. Dahl, L. K., Knudsen, K. D., and Iwai, J. Humoral transmission of hypertension: Evidence from parabiosis. *Circ. Res. [Suppl. I],* 1969, 24/25, 21.

72. Ikeda, T., Tobian, L., Iwai, J., and Goossens, P. Central nervous system pressor responses in rats susceptible and resistant to sodium chloride hypertension. *Clin. Sci. Mol. Med.,* 1978, 54, 225S.

73. Friedman, R., Tassinari, L. M., Heine, M., and Iwai, J. Differential development of salt-induced and renal hypertension in Dahl hypertension-sensitive rats after neonatal sympathectomy. *Clin. Exp. Hypertension (in press).*

74. Yamori, Y., Matsumoto, M., Yamabe, H., and Okamoto, K. Augmentation of spontaneous hypertension by chronic stress in rats. *Jpn. Circ. J.,* 1969, 33, 399.

75. Hallbäck, M., and Folkow, B. Cardiovascular response to acute mental "stress" in spontaneously hypertensive rats. *Acta. Physiol. Scand.,* 1974, 90, 684.

76. Hallbäck, M. Consequence of social isolation on blood pressure, cardiovascular reactivity and design in spontaneously hypertensive rats. *Acta. Physiol. Scand.,* 1975, 93, 455.

77. McCarty, R., Kventnansky, R., Lake, C. R., Thoa, N. B., and Kopin, I. J. Sympatho-adrenal activity of SHR and WKY rats during recovery from forced immobilization. *Physiol. Behav.,* 1978, 21, 951.

78. McCarty, R., and Kopin, I. J. Alterations in plasma catecholamines and behavior during acute stress in spontaneously hypertensive and Wistar-Kyoto normotensive rats. *Life Sci.,* 1978, 22, 997.

79. McCarty, R., Chiveh, C. C., and Kopin, I. J. Behavioral and cardiovascular responses of spontaneously hypertensive and normotensive rats to inescapable footshock. *Behav. Biol.,* 1978, 22, 405.

80. Myers, M. M., McCrorey, D., Bulman, C. A., and Hendley, E. D. Open field behavior and brain norepinephrine uptake in spontaneously hypertensive rats and Wistar-Kyoto normotensive controls. *Fed. Proc.,* 1977, 36, 1047.

81. McCarty, R., and Kopin, I. J. Patterns of behavioral development in spontaneously hypertensive rats and Wistar-Kyoto normotensive controls. *Dev. Psychobiol.,* 1979, 12, 239.

82. Myers, M. M., Whittemore, S. R., and Hendley, E. D. Forebrain catecholamine mechanisms in spontaneously hypertensive rat. In: *Second International Symposium on Catecholamines and Stress.* Elsevier, Amsterdam, 1980 *(in press).*

83. McCarty, R., Chiveh, C. C., and Kopin, I. J. Spontaneously hypertensive rats: Adrenergic hyper-responsivity to anticipation of electric shock. *Behav. Biol.,* 1978, 23, 180.

84. Lawler, J. E., Barker, G. F., and Hubbard, J. W. The borderline hypertensive rat (BHR): A genetic model for the study of stress-induced hypertension. *Psychophysiology,* 1980, 17, 314.

85. Dahl, L. K., Knudsen, K. D., Heine, M., and Leitl, G. Hypertension and stress. *Nature,* 1968, 219, 735.

86. Dahl, L. K. Psychological aspects of hypertension. *Cir. Res., [Suppl. I],* 1970, 18, 32.

87. Friedman, R., and Dahl, L. K. The effect of chronic conflict on the blood pressure of rats with a genetic susceptibility to experimental hypertension. *Psychosom. Med.,* 1975, 37, 402.

88. Friedman, R., and Iwai, J. Dietary sodium, psychic stress and genetic predisposition to experimental hypertension. *Proc. Soc. Exp. Biol. Med.,* 1977, 155, 449.

89. Friedman, R., and Iwai, J. Genetic predisposition and stress-induced hypertension. *Science,* 1976, 193, 161.

90. Friedman, R., and Dahl, L. K. Psychic and genetic factors in the etiology of hypertension. In: *Stress and the Heart,* edited by D. Wheatley, 1st edition, p. 137. Raven Press, New York, 1977.

Stress and the Heart, edited by D. Wheatley,
Raven Press, New York © 1981.

Stress-Induced Hypertension in Rats*

John F. Marwood and Mary F. Lockett

Interest in the interactions between sensory input to the central nervous system (CNS) (i.e., hearing, vision, balance, etc.) and blood pressure was stimulated by a review on the psychosomatic aspects of hypertension by Weiss in 1942 (1). Weiss pointed out that many apparent symptoms of hypertension are really manifestations of psychoneurotic conflict. In particular, he asserted, emotional tension due to chronic repressed hostility seems to bear a specific relationship to hypertension. He considered that this repressed hostility could be turned outward by psychotherapy, with resultant diminution in anxiety, often accompanied by lowering of the blood pressure. This theme will be considered in more detail in Chapter 11.

The most recent work in this field was described in the previous chapter, but it may be opportune here to consider the original work of Medoff and Bongiovanni (2) and Farris et al. (3), as these earlier studies demonstrated an association between the emotional and hypertensive effects of audiogenic stimuli. Medoff and Bongiovanni subjected rats to a constant air blast for 5 to 10 min every day from the time of weaning (at 21 days old). Identical controls were used who were not subjected to the air blast. Nearly all of the experimental animals developed dilated pupils and increased frequency of micturition and defecation, together with "running attacks." In these attacks, the mice leaped about in their pens, and the attack was usually terminated by tonic convulsions leading to tonic rigidity but rarely to death.

These authors considered that any systolic blood pressure of 160 mm Hg or over indicated hypertension, and in the younger rats (130–205 days old) there were no differences in the blood pressures of the experimental and control animals. However, in the older rats (340–890 days old), no less than 11 of 19 of the experimental rats (61%) developed hypertension based on this criterion, whereas the incidence amongst controls was only 4 out of 21 (19%). This difference was highly significant ($p < 0.01$). Furthermore, there was a good correlation between the degree of audiogenic seizures ("running attacks" and convulsions) and the development of hypertension.

Farris et al. undertook similar experiments using 23 rats, 12 of which were subjected to the air blast for 5 min per day, for 5 days per week, while the remaining 11 acted as controls. They, too, found a high incidence of hyper-

---

* Reprinted with permission from *Stress and the Heart,* edited by D. Wheatley, Raven Press, 1977, first edition.

tension (10 out of 12) among the experimental rats, compared to the controls (1 out of 11).

As a result of observational behavioral techniques, the rats were divided into those which were "emotional" and those which were "nonemotional." However, a majority of animals in both the experimental and control groups had high "emotionality" scores, although the only 2 experimental rats in which hypertension did not develop had low emotional scores. Farris et al. concluded, "Emotional make-up, therefore, seems to occupy the role of predisposing cause, and environmental stress that of the exciting factor, in the development of neurogenic hypertension in rats." Behavioral changes were also noted by Hudak and Buckley (4) in rats made hypertensive by the usual audio-visual-motion stressors. They stated, "It was also evidenced that the rats had undergone marked behavioral changes and that these animals could be utilized in the investigation of psychotropic compounds." Indeed, stress-induced hypertension of this type was first developed by Hudak and Buckley for the purpose of studying antihypertensive drugs.

It is thus clear that chronic stress in rats has a great influence on blood pressure. Our work on the effects of chronic sound withdrawal in rats, as described in this chapter, is an extension of the concept of chronic environmental stress.

EXPERIMENTAL METHODOLOGY

Wistar rats (160–190 g) were housed in pairs in a soundproof room (SPR), 3.8 × 3.0 × 2.15 meters, which was air-conditioned (eight changes per hour), maintained at 240°F, and illuminated from 6 A.M. to 6 P.M. daily. No external sounds were detectable on a Precision Sound Level meter (type 2203, Bruel and Kjoer, Sweden) within the SPR. Through breathing, eating, moving, etc., the rats themselves made noises which were never louder than 45 db. Comparable groups of rats were kept in the normal rat room (NRR) under similar conditions of temperature, air-conditioning, and lighting.

Blood pressure was measured directly via a common carotid artery catheter in rats under pentobarbital anesthesia (30 mg/kg, i.p.). The arterial catheter was attached to an E & M pressure transducer and the blood pressure was recorded on a Nesco pen recorder (model JY 110-2). Pentolinium was routinely administered (1 mg, i.v.) to block autonomic ganglia before the following pressor agents were administered, in the order and the doses shown, through a jugular venous catheter: norepinephrine, 0.25 μg; tyramine, 25 μg; angiotensin, 1.0 ng; vasopressin, 0.2 mU.

All surgery was carried out under sodium-methohexital anesthesia (45 mg/kg, i.p.). Adrenalectomy was carried out according to the method of Zarrow et al. (5) and the animals were subsequently maintained on 0.9% NaCl in the drinking water. Hypophysectomy was carried out using the method described by Burn et al. (6). Lesions were placed in the brains of rats held in a stereotactic machine (Krieg model 51200, C. H. Stoelting & Co., U. S. A.) according to Krieg's (7) method, using the stereotactic atlas of de Groot (8). Tissues for histological examination were placed in Bouin's fixative prior to processing by standard histological procedures. The areas of transverse sections of the widest part of the adrenal gland, as well as the areas of the medulla and the zones of the cortex, were measured by planimetry after the histologically prepared section was visualized on the screen of a microscope and the outlines traced onto paper.

Corticosteroids were extracted from the whole blood using ethyl acetate and then defatted by the method of Singer et al. (9), before thin-layer chromatography. The extracted steroids were estimated by the sulfuric acid-ethanol fluorescence method of Peterson (10). For corticosterone, the emission peak at 525 nm was measured using an excitation wavelength of 468 nm. For deoxycorticosterone, the emission peak at 535 nm was measured, again using an excitation wavelength of 468 nm. The epinephrine and norepinephrine content of rat urine was estimated according to the fluorometric method described by Anton and Sayre (11).

DEVELOPMENT OF HYPERTENSION

The mean systemic arterial pressure of rats maintained in the SPR rose progressively during a 4-week period to a maximum of 192.1 mm Hg (SEM± 4.9), which was significantly greater than that observed in the controls, namely 142.6 mm Hg (SEM ± 4.9). By the sixth week of sound withdrawal, blood pressure had stabilized at a slightly lower level (176.2 ± 9.2 mm Hg), although this was still significantly higher than the controls (Fig. 9-1, upper). After ganglionic blockade, the blood pressures of these rats were also significantly higher by approximately 20 mm Hg (except for week 3) than the corresponding blood pressures of the control rats (Fig. 13-1, lower).

It was established that the withdrawal of sound was the only stimulus for hypertension development; when sounds from the NRR were relayed at the same measured intensity through speakers installed in the SPR, the rats in the latter did not develop hypertension. In addition, transference of rats that had been in the SPR for 5 weeks to the NRR for a further 7 weeks did not result in a fall of blood pressure to normal.

Rats housed in the SPR showed variations in their pressor responses to norepinephrine, tyramine, and angiotensin, but not to vasopressin, over the 12 weeks following their placement in the SPR. (Fig. 13-2).

Responses to norepinephrine and tyramine were significantly different (greater) from controls only during weeks 3–5, and the responses to angiotensin were significantly different (greater) only at weeks 8 and 12.

BEFORE GANGLION BLOCK

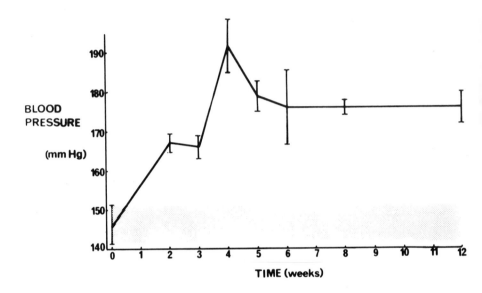

AFTER GANGLION BLOCK

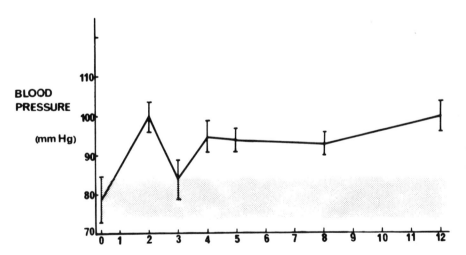

FIG. 13-1. Time course of development of hypertension in rats placed into a soundproof room (SPR). Each point is a mean supplied by 8 rats. The vertical bars represent the standard errors of the means. The shaded areas represent the blood pressure range of control rats.

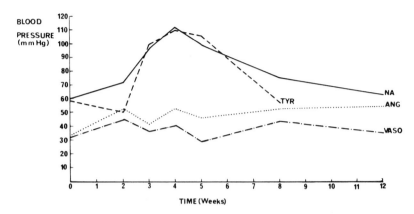

FIG. 13-2. Time courses of changes in cardiovascular reactivity of rats housed in the SPR. Pressor responses (mm Hg) to fixed i.v. doses of norepinephrine [1-noradrenaline (NA)], tyramine (TYR), angiotensin (ANG), and vasopressin (VASO).

PATHOLOGICAL CHANGES

Only after 12 weeks of sound withdrawal were histological changes in arteriolar structure demonstrable, and these are shown in Fig. 13-3.

Arterioles from the gastrocnemius muscle of rats in the SPR had thicker walls, and hence reduced lumen diameters, than arterioles of the same outside diameter from control rats in the NRR. Specific staining for elastic tissue showed there to be some thickening of the internal elastic lamina.

The organ:body weight ratios for adrenal glands, heart, thymus, and spleen were measured in rats housed in the SPR for periods of up to 12 weeks. After 2 weeks of sound withdrawal, lymphatic tissues (thymus and spleen) had increased organ:body weight ratios, whereas those of heart and adrenal tissues had decreased from control levels. These changes are shown in Table 13-1.

Between weeks 3 and 5 the organ:body weight ratios generally increased, only to fall to within normal levels (thymus, spleen) or subnormal levels (heart, adrenal) between weeks 8 and 12.

During the development of sound-withdrawal hypertension (SWH), the total area of sections of the adrenal gland did not vary greatly. However, the area of the zones of the adrenal, expressed as percentages of the total area, varied markedly, as shown in Fig. 13-4.

During the first 6 weeks of sound withdrawal there was a large increase in the size of the zona reticularis, with a slight decrease in the size of the zona glomerulosa, zona fasciculata, and medulla. During the second 6-week period of sound withdrawal, there were increases in the size of the medulla and zona glomerulosa, while the area of the zona reticularis returned to normal.

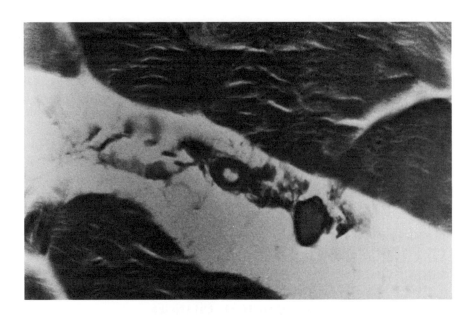

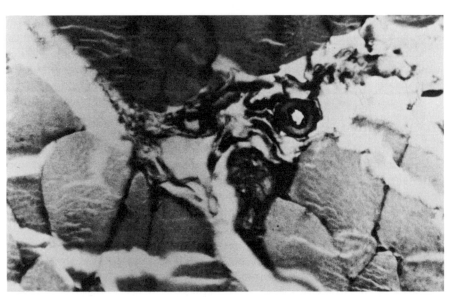

FIG. 13-3. Photomicrographs, ×520, of a small arteriole in the gastrocnemius muscle of a rat (upper) and a rat of comparable age and weight housed in the SPR for 12 weeks (lower).

TABLE 13-1. *Changes in organ: body weight ratios (mg/100 g, mean ± SE) of rats during the development of SWH*

Weeks	Tissue			
	Heart	Adrenal	Thymus	Spleen
0 (control)	3.34 ± 0.09	0.16 ± 0.07	1.09 ± 0.09	3.18 ± 0.21
2	2.98 ± 0.10[a]	0.15 ± 0.06	1.16 ± 0.08	3.56 ± 0.15
3	3.43 ± 0.09	0.18 ± 0.08[a]	1.35 ± 0.13[a]	4.20 ± 0.20[a]
4	3.17 ± 0.05[a]	0.16 ± 0.04	1.48 ± 0.05[a]	3.86 ± 0.07[a]
5	3.19 ± 0.08[a]	0.16 ± 0.07	1.47 ± 0.10[a]	3.67 ± 0.13[a]
6	3.20 ± 0.06	0.15 ± 0.02	1.28 ± 0.04[a]	2.98 ± 0.06
8	2.94 ± 0.03[a]	0.14 ± 0.05[a]	1.13 ± 0.08	3.76 ± 0.21[a]
12	2.95 ± 0.05[a]	0.13 ± 0.05[a]	1.08 ± 0.06	3.53 ± 0.36

[a] Indicates that the value is significantly different ($p < 0.05$) from control values.

NEUROHORMONAL INFLUENCES

Urine was collected once a week from rats housed in the soundproof room for a period of 8 weeks, and the catecholamine contents were measured. The rats had previously been trained to accept the procedure, and the urinary catecholamine outputs on three separate occasions served as control values. During the first 4 weeks of sound withdrawal, urinary catecholamine excretion did not change from control levels. However, urinary catecholamine during the subsequent 4-week period was markedly reduced, as shown in Fig. 13-5.

The effects of adrenalectomy and of hypophysectomy on SWH development are shown in Fig. 13-6.

After 4 weeks of sound withdrawal, when the blood pressure of intact rats would be at its highest, neither adrenalectomized nor hypophysectomized rats developed SWH. However, adrenalectomized rats maintained with glucocorticoid did develop SWH, whereas hypophysectomized rats did not, even after treatment with both glucocorticoid and growth hormone (GH).

In further experiments, rats were lesioned in specific areas of the CNS prior to being placed in the SPR for 4 weeks. As shown in Table 13-2, rats lesioned either in the hippocampal commissure (A) or in the medial septal nucleus extending into the area parolfactoria medialis (C) developed hypertension regardless of whether they were housed in the NRR or in the SPR.

Rats with lesions in the anteromedial areas of the lateral septal nucleus (B) had blood pressures which were only slightly (although significantly) above those of intact rats in the NRR. Thus, these lesions caused changes in arterial pressure which appeared to circumvent the effects of sound withdrawal.

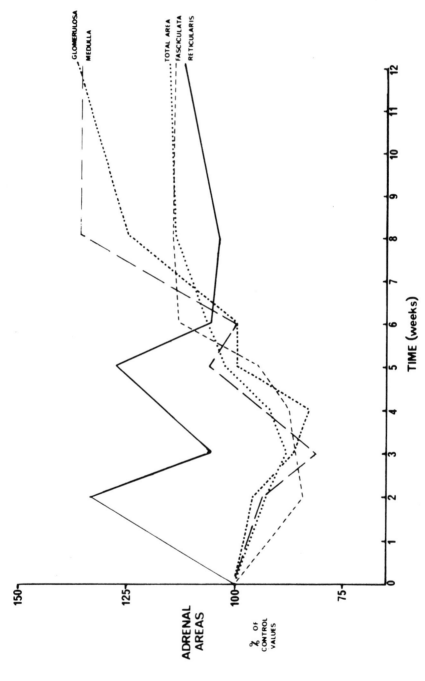

FIG. 13–4. Time courses of changes in areas of adrenal zones of rats housed in the SPR. The graphs show mean areas of adrenal zones, expressed as percentages of control values, plotted against weeks spent in the SPR.

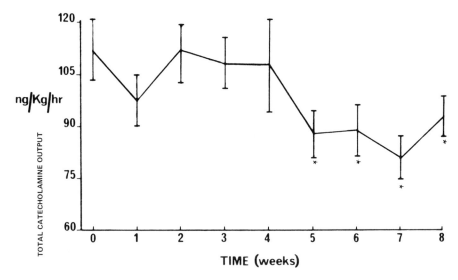

FIG. 13-5. Total urinary catecholamine outputs in ng/kg body weight of rats in the SPR. The solid line passes through mean values; the vertical bars show the standard errors of the mean. A significant difference ($p < 0.05$) from control (0 weeks) values is indicated by *.

ETIOLOGY OF SOUND-WITHDRAWAL HYPERTENSION

We have presented evidence demonstrating that the reduction of auditory input to rats resulted in the development of hypertension, which we have termed sound-withdrawal hypertension (SWH). After as brief a time as 5 weeks of sound withdrawal, the developed hypertension was not abated by replacement of normal noise levels. Furthermore, prolonged sound withdrawal resulted in histological changes in arterioles, similar to those described by Wolinsky (12), which are characteristic of all forms of chronic hypertension.

We believe that SWH is an entirely new model of experimental hypertension. This belief is based on the differences between SWH and other known models of experimental hypertension in regard to organ:body weight ratios, the cardiovascular reactivity to pressor agents, and the involvement of the pituitary-adrenal axis. Overall, organ:body weight ratios of rats housed in the SPR rose in parallel with the rising blood pressure, up to approximately the fifth week, after which they returned to the original values, whereas blood pressure remained elevated. This contrasts with organ:body weight ratios of renal hypertensive rats as described by Fregly (13), where the ratios rose sigmoidally along with the increasing blood pressure, and both remained elevated.

In rats with SWH, the early phase (weeks 3–5), was characterized by increased pressor responses to norepinephrine and tyramine, whereas the

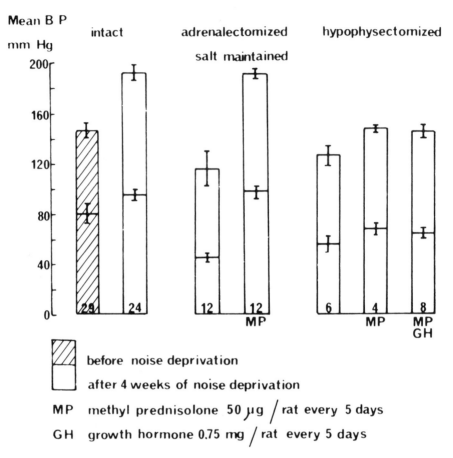

FIG. 13-6. The effect of replacement therapy on the development of hypertension of adrenalectomized and hypophysectomized rats housed in the SPR.

late phase (weeks 8–12) exhibited increased pressor responses to angiotensin only. The picture regarding cardiovascular reactivity to pressor drugs in other forms of experimental hypertension is not clear-cut. The literature is often contradictory because the distinction between acute and chronic hypertension is not always made. However, in general it appears that the chronic states of DOCA-salt hypertension (14,15), renal hypertension (16,17), and genetic hypertension (18,19) all exhibit increased pressor responses to norepinephrine and tyramine and probably to angiotensin. It is possible that the increased cardiovascular reactivity merely reflects structural changes in the arterioles, as have been described by various investigators (20-24). This appears not to be the case for SWH since the changes in

TABLE 13-2. *The effect of brain lesions on the blood pressures of rats housed either in the SPR or in the NRR*

| | Blood pressure (mm Hg) | | |
	Lesion A	Lesion B	Lesion C
NRR	187.3 ± 3.7	164.3 ± 1.5	181.9 ± 2.2
SPR	189.6 ± 3.4	159.2 ± 4.3	186.5 ± 2.4

Code for lesion sites: A = hippocampal commissure; B = lateral septal nucleus; C = medial septal nucleus extending into the area parolfactoria medialis.

cardiovascular reactivity to norepinephrine and tyramine were over before structural changes in arterioles were evident.

The urinary catecholamine output of rats transferred from the normal rat room to the soundproof room only changed after week 4 of sound withdrawal, when their output fell. Thus, the sudden withdrawal of extraneous noises did not cause the adrenomedullary adaptation known to occur following immobilization stress (25), and it is therefore unlikely that catecholamines are involved in either the genesis or the maintenance of SWH. It is generally considered that catecholamines are not of prime importance in the development of genetic hypertension (26), or in renal hypertension (27), although there is ample evidence of altered catecholamine dynamics, as described, for example, by Louis et al. (28). Catecholamines may be involved in the genesis of DOCA-salt hypertension since, in this condition, de Champlain et al. have demonstrated a defective catecholamine storage mechanism (29).

The involvement of the pituitary-adrenal axis is of paramount importance in SWH as adrenalectomized rats only became hypertensive when supplemented with glucocorticoid; hypophysectomized rats did not develop SWH even when treated with both glucocorticoid and GH. It is probable, therefore, that the pituitary plays an essential role, whereas the role of the glucocorticoid is permissive, in the sense described by Ingle (30). It would appear that pituitary substance(s) other than ACTH and GH are essential to the development of SWH. It is considered that this substance very possibly is thyrotropic stimulating hormone (TSH), for there is evidence that the thyroid is involved in the development of renal hypertension (31), DOCA-salt hypertension (32), and genetic hypertension (33). In addition, the fall in blood pressure resulting from hypophysectomy can only be reversed by the combined administration of ACTH and thyroid hormone (34).

The adrenal gland is essential for the development of genetic hypertension (35) but not for DOCA-salt hypertension (36,37) or renal hypertension (13,38), provided the animals are adequately salt maintained (39). However, there is some evidence for the involvement of the adrenal glands in renal hypertension, both in rats (40) and in man (41). Thus, the adrenal cortex is strongly implicated in the hypertensive process and adrenal steroids can also affect cardiovascular reactivity to pressor agents (42,43). Since the pituitary-adrenal axis is essential to SWH development, it is likely that the reduction of auditory input is a stressful event, in the sense described by Selye (44,45) and elaborated by Levi (46). This is in spite of the fact that plasma steroid levels after 6 weeks of sound withdrawal were lower, but not significantly, than controls (corticosterone, $\mu g/100$ ml blood; NRR, 29.8 ± 6.5; SPR, 21.5 ± 2.0; deoxycorticosterone, $\mu g/100$ ml blood; NRR, 15.9 ± 4.2; SPR, 13.6 ± 2.0). These results, together with those showing reduced adrenal medullary output after 4 weeks of sound withdrawal, may suggest that the adrenals were only required for the establishment and not the maintenance of SWH. This further suggests that the rat adrenal gland adapts during the stimulus of sound withdrawal, and this is perhaps not unexpected. Certainly there is evidence that the response of the rat adrenal can alter during continuous sound stimulation (47). Bassett et al. have shown differences between novel stress and predictable stress on rat corticosterone output (48), and so perhaps in SWH the "novelty" of sound withdrawal became a "predictable" stress. In any case, Grant et al. claim that rats require 4 weeks to adapt to a soundproof room (49); this claim is based on fluid intake data, although unfortunately blood pressure was not measured.

It is well known that the limbic system is involved, to a large degree, in behavioral patterns and also that there are two well-defined neuronal connections between the limbic system and the hypothalamus (50). These pass from the hippocampus either through the ventral portion of the fimbria to the arcuate nucleus, or through the pre- and postcommissural fornix to the septal nuclei. The limbic system is also known to influence ACTH secretion and hence adrenocortical secretion (51,52). It was intended that the brain lesions would interrupt the latter hippocampal-hypothalamic pathway mentioned above. In this way we hoped to influence adrenal cortical function and ultimately test our hypothesis that sound-withdrawal hypertension is stress-induced. However, the results did not unequivocally support the hypothesis and are open to alternative interpretations. Thus, the lesions may have caused a hypertension which was indistinguishable from SWH, or a different type of hypertension may have been induced. Clearly, more research is required to elucidate this point.

Other models of experimental hypertension, apart from those mentioned earlier using chronic environmental stress, can be considered to be stress induced. Harris et al. (53) used shock avoidance techniques in conscious baboons to raise blood pressure. A small electric shock was given and food was withheld whenever blood pressure fell below specified levels. Recently, an experimental model of hypertension has been described in which psychosocial stress was used (54). Formerly isolated mice were transferred to seven intercommunicating cages and the change in 'environment' was sufficient to raise blood pressure. Psychosocial stress has previously been shown to affect various parameters, e.g., vasopressin release, salivation, and heart rate in dogs (55). However, we believe that withdrawal of sound from rats is a stress which produces changes in CNS activity, perhaps neuronal adaptation similar to that described by Thompson (56), and these result in the development of hypertension.

CONCLUSIONS

1. Blood pressure of rats maintained in a soundproof room rises progressively to a maximum at 4 weeks, this level differing significantly from that of control rats. Furthermore, withdrawal of sound was the only stimulus for the development of hypertension since, when sounds from the normal rat room were relayed into the SPR, the rats in the latter did not develop hypertension.

2. After 5 weeks in the SPR, the rats still showed elevated blood pressure. After 12 weeks of sound withdrawal, pathological changes occurred in the arterioles, the walls of which became thicker with reduced lumen diameters.

3. After 4 weeks of sound withdrawal, neither adrenalectomized nor hypophysectomized rats developed hypertension, although adrenalectomized rats maintained with glucocorticoid did develop hypertension. On the other hand, hypophysectomized rats did not develop hypertension even after treatment with both glucocorticoid and growth hormone. Lesions in the lateral septal nucleus of the brain caused changes in blood pressure which appeared to circumvent the effects of sound withdrawal.

4. It is probable that the pituitary plays an essential role in the development of sound-withdrawal hypertension. As the pituitary-adrenal axis is essential to the development of SWH, it is likely that the reduction of auditory input is a stressful event. Therefore, we believe that withdrawal of sound from rats is a stress which produces changes in CNS activity, resulting in the development of hypertension.

REFERENCES

1. Weiss, E. Psychosomatic aspects of hypertension. *J.A.M.A.*, 1942, 120, 1081.
2. Medoff, H. S., and Bongiovanni, A. M. Blood pressure in rats subjected to audiogenic stimulation. *Am. J. Physiol.*, 1945, 143, 300.
3. Farris, E. J., Yeakel, E. H., and Medoff, H. S. Development of hypertension in emotional gray Norway rats after air blasting. *Am. J. Physiol.*, 1945, 144, 331.
4. Hudak, W. J., and Buckley, J. P. Production of hypertensive rats by experimental stress. *J. Pharm. Sci.*, 1961, 50, 263.
5. Zarrow, M. X., Yokim, J. M., McCarthy, J. M., and Sanborn, R. C. In: *Experimental Endocrinology*. Academic Press, New York, 1964, p. 194.
6. Burn, J. H., Finney, D. J., and Goodwin, L. G. In: *Biological Standardization*, 2nd edition. Oxford Medical Publications, London, 1950, p. 40.
7. Krieg, W. J. S. Accurate placement of minute lesions in the brain of the albino rat. *Q. Bull. Northwestern Med. Sch.*, Chicago, 1946, 20, 199.

8. de Groot, J. The rat forebrain in stereotaxic coordinates. *Transcr. R. Neth. Acad.*, 1969, 52, 1.
9. Singer, B., Losito, C., and Salmon, S. Effects of progesterone and adrenocortical hormone secretion in normal and hypophysectomized rats. *J. Endocrinol.*, 1963, 28, 65.
10. Peterson, R. E. The identification of corticosterone in human plasma and its assay by isotope dilution. *J. Biol. Chem.*, 1957, 255, 25.
11. Anton, A. H., and Sayre, D. F. A study of the factors affecting the aluminium oxide-trihydroxyindole procedure for the analysis of catecholamines. *J. Pharmacol. Exp. Ther.*, 1962, 138, 360.
12. Wolinsky, H. Effects of hypertension and its reversal on the thoracic aorta of male and female rats. *Circ. Res.*, 1971, 28, 622.
13. Fregly, M. J. Adrenal glands in the development of renal hypertension in rats. *Am. J. Physiol.*, 1957, 191, 542.
14. Hinke, J. A. M. *In vitro* demonstration of vascular hyperresponsiveness in experimental hypertension. *Circ. Res.*, 1965, 17, 359.
15. Beilin, L. J., and Ziakas, G. Vascular reactivity in postdeoxycorticosterone hypertension in rats and its relation to 'irreversible' hypertension in man. *Clin. Sci.*, 1972, 42, 579.
16. Finch, L. Cardiovascular reactivity in the experimental renal hypertensive rat. *Br. J. Pharmacol.*, 1971, 42, 56.
17. Page, I. H., Kaneko, Y., and McCubbin, J. W. Cardiovascular reactivity in acute and chronic renal hypertensive dogs. *Circ. Res.*, 1966, 18, 379.
18. Laverty, R. Increased vascular reactivity in rats with genetic hypertension. *Proc. Univ. Otago Med. Sch.*, 1961, 39, 23.
19. Shibayama, F., Mizogami, S., and Sokabe, H. Cardiovascular reactivity in hypertensive rats. *Jap. Heart J.*, 1971, 12, 68.
20. Conway, J. The nature of the increased peripheral resistance in hypertension. *Am. J. Cardiol.*, 1960, 5, 649.
21. Folkow, B. The haemodynamic consequences of adoptive structural changes of the resistance vessels in hypertension. *Clin. Sci.*, 1971, 41, 1.
22. Massingham, R., and Shevde, S. Aortic reactivity and electrophysiology in normotensive rats, spontaneously hypertensive rats, and rats made hypertensive with deoxycorticosterone plus salt. *Br. J. Pharmacol.*, 1971, 43, 868.
23. Folkow, B., Hallback, M., Lundgren, Y., and Weiss, L. Structurally based increase of flow resistance in spontaneously hypertensive rats. *Acta Physiol. Scand.*, 1970, 79, 373.
24. Folkow, B., Hallback, M., Lundgren, Y., Sivertsson, R., and Weiss, L. Importance of adaptive changes in vascular design for establishment of primary hypertension, studied in man and spontaneously hypertensive rats. *Circ. Res.*, 1973, 32 and 33, Suppl. 1, 2.
25. Kvetnansky, R., and Mikulaj, L. Adrenal and urinary catecholamines in rats during adaptation to repeated immobilization stress. *Endocrinology*, 1970, 87, 738.
26. Nakamura, K., Gerold, M., and Thoenen, H. Genetically hypertensive rats: Relationship between the development of hypertension and the changes in norepinephrine turnover of peripheral and central adrenergic neurons. *Naunyn-Schmiedebergs Arch. Pharmacol.*, 1971, 271, 157.
27. Lefer, L. G., and Ayres, C. R. Norepinephrine metabolism in dogs with chronic renovascular hypertension. *Proc. Soc. Exp. Biol. Med.*, 1969, 132, 278.
28. Louis, W. J., Krauss, K. R., Kopin, I. J., and Sjoerosma, A. Catecholamine metabolism in hypertensive rats. *Circ. Res.*, 1970, 27, 589.
29. de Champlain, U., Krakoff, L. P., and Axelrod, J. Catecholamine metabolism in experimental hypertension in the rat. *Circ. Res.*, 1967, 20, 136.
30. Ingle, D. J. Permissive actions of hormones. *J. Clin. Endocrinol. Metab.*, 1954, 14, 1272.
31. Fregly, M. J., and Gonzalez, J. V. Activity of thyroid gland during development of renal hypertension in rats. *Am. J. Cardiol.*, 1961, 8, 694.
32. Girerd, R. J., Salgado, E., and Green, D. M. Mechanisms of deoxycorticosterone action: XI. Influence of the pituitary. *Am. J. Physiol.*, 1957, 188, 12.
33. Field, F. P., Janis, R. A., and Triggle, D. J. Aortic reactivity of rats with genetic and experimental renal hypertension. *Can. J. Physiol. Pharmacol.*, 1972, 50, 1072.
34. Bauman, J. W., and Phillips, E. S. Failure of blood pressure restoration to repair glomerular filtration rate in hypophysectomized rats. *Am. J. Physiol.*, 1970, 218, 1605.
35. Iwai, J., Knudson, K. D., Dahl, L. K., and Tassinari, L. Effect of adrenalectomy on blood

pressure in salt-fed, hypertension prone rats. Failure of hypertension to develop in absence of evidence of adrenal cortical tissue. *J. Exp. Med.,* 1969, 129, 663.

36. Swingle, W. W., Parkins, W. M., and Remington, J. W. The effect of deoxycorticosterone acetate and of blood serum transfusions upon the circulation of the adrenolectomized dog. *Am. J. Physiol.,* 1941, 134, 503.
37. Friedman, S. M., Friedman, C. L., and Campbell, C. G. Effects of adrenalectomy and adrenal cortical extract on DCA hypertension in the rat. *Am. J. Physiol.,* 1949, 157, 241.
38. de Jong, W., Frankhuzen, A. L., and Witter, A. Renal hypertension and renin hypertension in intact and adrenalectomized animals. *Proc. Soc. Exp. Biol. Med.,* 1969, 132, 71.
39. Floyer, M. A. The effect of nephrectomy and adrenalectomy upon the blood pressure in hypertensive and normotensive rats. *Clin. Sci.,* 1951, 10:406–421.
40. Freed, S. C., and St. George, S. Adrenal cortex in the maintenance of hypertension. *Endocrinology,* 1962, 71, 422.
41. Mills, L. C., and Pontidas, E. The relationship of the adrenal cortex to hypertension. *Am. J. Cardiol.,* 1959, 40, 719.
42. Imms, F. J., and Jones, M. T. Vascular sensitivity following adrenalectomy in the rat. *Br. J. Pharmacol.,* 1968, 33, 212.
43. Drew, G. M., and Leach, G. D. H. Corticosteroids and their effects on cardiovascular sensitivity in the pithed adrenalectomized rat. *Arch. Int. Pharmacodyn.,* 1971, 191, 255.
44. Selye, H. A syndrome produced by diverse nocuous agents. *Nature (Lond.),* 1936, 138, 32.
45. Selye, H. The evolution of the stress concept. Stress and cardiovascular disease. *Am. J. Cardiol.,* 1970, 26, 289.
46. Levi, L. In: *Stress and Distress in Response to Social Stimuli.* Pergamon Press, Oxford, 1972.
47. Henkin, R. I., and Knigge, K. M. Effect of sound on the hypothalamic-pituitary-adrenal axis. *Am. J. Physiol.,* 1963, 204, 710.
48. Bassett, J. R., Cairncross, K. D., and King, M. G. Parameters of novelty, shock predictability and response contingency in corticosterone release in the rat. *Physiol. Behav.,* 1973, 10, 901.
49. Grant, L., Hopkinson, P., Jennings, G., and Jenner, F. A. Period of adjustment of rats used in experimental studies. *Nature (Lond.),* 1971, 232, 135.
50. Raisman, G. An evaluation of the basic pattern of connection between the limbic system and the hypothalamus. *Am. J. Anat.,* 1970, 129, 197.
51. Mason, J. W. Plasma 17-hydroxycorticosteroid response to hypothalamic stimulation in the conscious rhesus monkey. *Endocrinology,* 1957, 63, 403.
52. Mason, J. W. Plasma 17-hydroxycorticosteroid levels during electrical stimulation of the amygdaloid complex in conscious monkeys. *Am. J. Physiol.,* 1959, 196, 44.
53. Harris, A. J., Gilliam, W. J., Findley, J. D., and Brady, J. V. Instrumental conditioning of large magnitude, daily, 12-hour blood pressure elevations in the baboon. *Science,* 1973, 182, 175.
54. Henry, J. P., Stephens, P. M., and Santisteban, G. A. A model of psychosocial hypertension showing reversibility and progression of cardiovascular complications. *Circ. Res.,* 1975, 36, 156.
55. Corson, S. A., and Corson, E. O'L. Animal models of psychosocial stress reactions. *Psychopharmacol. Bull.,* 1973, 9, 42.
56. Thompson, R. F. Possible neuronal mechanisms of adaptation to stress. *Psychopharmacol. Bull.,* 1973, 9, 40.

Stress and the Heart, edited by D. Wheatley,
Raven Press, New York © 1981.

Yoga and Biofeedback in the Management of Hypertension

Chandra H. Patel

Hypertension is a common condition, the cause of which is unknown in 90 to 95% of cases when the condition is termed benign essential hypertension. We now know that it is neither benign nor essential. In fact, hypertension is a potent contributor to cardiovascular morbidity and mortality. In a cohort of 5,209 persons in an epidemiologic study in Framingham over a period of 18 years, it was shown that morbidity and mortality were proportional to the level of blood pressure (1). Compared with normotensives, hypertensives developed at least four times as much coronary heart disease, seven times as many strokes, and at least double the incidence of peripheral vascular disease. Examination of the data showed that 37% of men and 51% of women who died of cardiovascular disease had antecedent hypertension. If borderline hypertensives were included (BP 140/90), 73% of men and 81% of women had hypertension before cardiovascular mortality. Insurance companies' statistics also support the above observations (2). With the introduction of a number of antihypertensive drugs in the 1950s and 1960s, morbidity and mortality from hypertension were considerably reduced (3,4).

Despite these facts, a number of regional and national surveys, in both Britain and the United States (5–8), have shown that approximately half of the hypertensives are not detected; of those detected, only half are treated; and of those treated, only half as many are properly controlled. Asking hypertensives to submit to lifelong medication, especially when many antihypertensive drugs produce unpleasant side effects, is not easy. Another problem has been the failure of antihypertensive drugs to prevent myocardial infarction (9). A recent study showed that trying to lower blood pressure with drugs to a low normotensive level may, in fact, be actually harmful in this respect (10).

Hypertensive disease itself costs the British National Health Service several million pounds. When the cost of complications, such as strokes and ischemic heart disease, is added, as well as the indirect cost of sickness benefit, widows' pensions, and loss of able workers due to premature deaths, the bill becomes enormous. In view of these indirect costs and the proven benefits of drug treatment, at least in moderately severe and severe hypertension, widespread screening programs have been advocated (11,12). However, valid points have been made against this approach (13). In view of the unproven benefits in mild hypertension (14), the high cost of screening in relation to the expected yield, apparent failure of the present antihypertensive drug regimens, and problems with side effects, the first priority should be to improve the status of drug therapy and its general acceptability before attempting to apply it to a large number of people.

LEARNING BLOOD PRESSURE CONTROL

In recent years, there has been a considerable interest in learning voluntary control over autonomic functions through techniques based on biofeedback methods.

Biofeedback

Biofeedback instruments are electronic devices which, when connected to patients, measure and display some physiologic functions in the form of light or sound signals. The function measured can be one of many, e.g., blood pressure, heart rate, muscle tension (electromyogram, EMG), electrical resistance of the skin (galvanic skin resistance, GSR), or brain wave pattern (electroencephalogram, EEG). The person connected to the device then tries to change the function in a desired direction by cognitive or subjective states. Any change in the function immediately becomes known, which helps the individual to change his cognitive strategies until, by trial and error, he learns to control that function. The rationale of the procedure is that knowledge of success reinforces the learning. A large part of this biofeedback work has focused on the control of cardiovascular activity, such as the levels of arterial blood pressure.

It has been shown that human subjects can learn to increase or decrease systolic or diastolic blood pressure by operant conditioning methods (15–18). Shapiro and his colleagues (15), at Harvard Medical School, have been pioneers in this field. In this study, their blood pressure feedback instrument consisted of an arm cuff with a crystal microphone placed over the brachial artery. The cuff was inflated to a median systolic pressure, and each time the pressure was either increased or decreased, feedback signals were produced in the form of light and sound to indicate the direction in which the pressure was deviating from the median systolic pressure at each heartbeat. In addition to this sensory feedback, the subjects were otherwise reinforced after 20 correct responses (by presentation of slides of a nude female or landscapes and by money). Typically, subjects were given 25 trials per session, each trial lasting for 50 heartbeats, with an interval of 30 to 45 sec between trials. In the final block of five trials, the average increases were 1 to 2 mmHg, while the average decreases were 4 to 6 mmHg. Subsequent interviews of the best learners failed to identify any consistent cognitive or somatic strategies (19). It may also be noted that, as these investigators themselves have indicated, the pressure changes observed in the foregoing experiments were not of sufficient magnitude for therapeutic application.

In a related experiment, Benson et al. (20) studied seven patients with essential hypertension who received daily feedback sessions for decreasing systolic blood pressure until no further reduction occurred over five consecutive sessions. The change in systolic pressure ranged from +1 to −34 mmHg, with an average reduction of 16 mmHg. After the training stopped, however, pressures gradually returned to their previous levels. These results were encouraging but raised two questions: (a) Can patients learn to control their blood pressure outside the laboratory without the feedback equipment when confronted with the noisy and stressful situations of modern life? (b) What were the somatic or cognitive strategies used by the successful patients?

In the biofeedback control of blood pressure, the biofeedback instrument gives an objective measure of blood pressure to the patient, who tries to control it by an act of volition. This knowledge of objective measure guides him to control his pressure, but with every change in the objective measure, there is an associated subjective or cognitive state responsible for that change. It is this subjective state by which the patient must learn to control his blood pressure, both inside and outside the laboratory. Unfortunately, in most biofeedback experiments, the patient has either been unable to describe this state in a known language, or such widely variable accounts have been given that no definite pattern has emerged.

An alternative approach is to identify a behavior that will reduce blood pressure and then teach that behavior using biofeedback instruments as teaching aids. Formulation of therapeutic behavior requires a knowledge of pathogenesis.

PATHOGENESIS OF ESSENTIAL HYPERTENSION

It is generally agreed that hypertension results from the interaction between hereditary predisposition and environmental factors (21). Since genetic factors cannot be removed, therapeutic efforts must be concentrated on counteracting environmental factors with the hope of mitigating genetic influence. Pickering (21) stated: "environmental factors acting through the mind are important." Evidence for this belief is based on clinical observations, epidemiologic studies, and experimental work.

The environment can affect us in two different ways: (a) the noxious effects of the environment itself, and (b) the physiologic response of the individual to his environment.

Environment

Only a few studies are mentioned here as they have been discussed in other chapters of the book.

In their review of the literature, Scotch and Geiger (22) concluded that hypertension results from a failure of the individual to adapt to changing environment. Cruz-Coke et al. (23,24) introduced the concept of the "ecologic niche" to explain the consistently low pressures found in groups living in isolated regions and enjoying an unchanging and unchallenged tradition. When people from the same group migrate to areas of Western urban civilization, their blood pressures begin to rise.

Henry and Cassel (25) arranged data from 18 epidemiologic studies from various parts of the world into three groups according to the social and psychologic environment of the groups. They showed that where the population did not show a rise in blood pressure with age, the culture had remained stable; traditional forms were honored, and group members were secure in their roles, having adapted to them from an early age. With the onset of industrialization, urbanization, and migration, social, cultural, and economic values change, and the individual is required to make continuous behavioral adjustments. As people age, this process of adaptation becomes more stressful and is reflected in rising blood pressure.

Nearly 25 centuries ago, Hippocrates (26) told his contemporaries that ". . .those things which one has been accustomed to for a long time, although worse than the things which one is not accustomed to, usually give less disturbance." Those who advocate environmental stress as one of the important contributory factors in the pathogenesis of essential hypertension are constantly criticized by those who cannot conceive that there can be more stress today, with so much available material comfort. Strange as it may seem, the more an individual gets, the more he strives, the more responsibility he is prepared to accept, and the longer he works. The rich feel just as insecure and worried about the future as do the poor. It has been said that "hypertension is a new disease and a stress disease, the price a millionaire pays for his directorship and a clerk for his failure"(27).

On the basis of these observations, it is reasonable to suggest that a susceptible man in competitive, industrialized, urban society, living at an ever-increasing pace and exposed to psychosocial and environmental stimuli, may also develop chronic hypertension. However, it is difficult to prove a clear-cut relationship between hypertension and specific environmental stress. Emotion is a highly subjective experience determined by its appeal to each individual. Stress, whether emotional, occupational, or social, is also difficult to measure. A constant search to identify specific environments may not be productive because of the rapidity with which our environments are changing. Even if the specific environmental factors were to be found, it is doubtful if people would want to give up the fruits of civilization. Better preventive or therapeutic methods may be achieved by altering his physiologic response to the environment.

Physiologic Mechanisms

A suggested pathogenesis of essential hypertension is shown schematically in Fig. 14.1. It is generally accepted that the defense reaction or the "fight-or-flight" response is a basic stress response activated by a wide range of stimuli. An important component of this reaction is cardiovascular in nature and

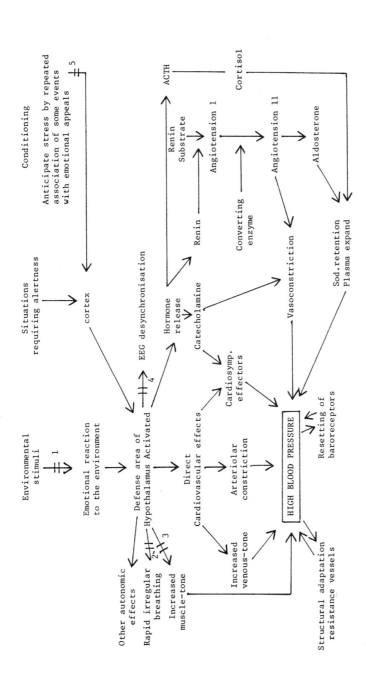

FIG. 14.1. Suggested pathogenesis of essential hypertension and behavior modification: 1, educational program; 2, breathing exercise; 3, muscle relaxation; 4, meditation; and 5, deconditioning.

consists of a rise in blood pressure, increase in heart rate, vasoconstriction in skin, splanchnic, and renal vessels, and vasodilation in skeletal muscles (28–30). The other changes in this physiologic response are an increase in muscle tone in anticipation of fight-or-flight behavior, irregular breathing pattern, and other autonomic changes, such as increased sweating and blood clotting tendency. Desynchronization of the EEG also occurs, and the fast low-amplitude waves, characteristic of the alert brain, are present. In brief, the picture is that of increased sympathetic nervous system activity (31).

As indicated in Fig. 14.1, a rise in blood pressure may result directly from increased stimulation of the sympathetic effectors or indirectly through hormonal release of catecholamines and mobilization of the renin-angiotensin-aldosterone system or the hypothalamic-pituitary-adrenal axis. Both central and peripheral nervous systems, as well as the endocrine system, participate in bringing about the final result. The noxious stimuli from the environment are received by the brain through sensory organs and then integrated in the cortex, which interprets events and consciously or subconsciously relates them to attitudes, conditioning, experience in early life, and other characteristics peculiar to that individual. If the cortical interpretation is one of threat, the physiologic reaction is mediated through the intimately connected pathways of the cerebral cortex, hypothalamus, and reticular activating system. By stimulating these areas directly through electrical or mechanical means or indirectly through environmental stress, the defense reaction, with its cardiovascular and hormonal components, can be mobilized (30).

The Autonomic Nervous System

The autonomic nervous system is thought to play a role in the pathogenesis of essential hypertension. Several observations are pertinent. The fall in blood pressure during sleep is probably due to a fall in sympathetic vasoconstrictive tone; it has been shown that marked reduction occurs in the flow of impulses in sympathetic nerves during desynchronized sleep (32), and that such fall in blood pressure during sleep can be reduced by bilateral thoracolumbar sympathectomy (33). Increased sympathetic activity in this disorder is also indicated by the fact that most hypotensive drugs interfere in some way with the functioning of the sympathetic nervous system, and that they produce a greater fall in blood pressure in hypertensive than in normotensive subjects (34,35).

Although most investigators would agree that emotional stress can transiently raise blood pressure, its relationship to the development of permanent hypertension is disputed. There is, however, a considerable amount of evidence to suggest that frequent neurohormonal pressure rises would lead to "resetting" of the baroreceptors at a higher level, as well as to structural hypertrophy of the resistance vessels. These factors could maintain high blood pressure, even in the absence of the initiating factors.

The Baroreceptors

The baroreceptors are stretch receptors, situated beneath the adventia of the expanded origin of the internal carotid artery and of the arch of the aorta. A rise in blood pressure increases the frequency of impulses from these baroreceptors to the reticular formation of the brain, reflexively slowing the heart and dilating the peripheral vessels, thus reducing the blood pressure to its original level. On the other hand, a fall in blood pressure reflexively quickens the heart and constricts the peripheral vessels. In hypertension, this regulatory mechanism is disturbed (36–39). For example, McCubbin et al. (40) showed that the baroreceptors were reset at a new and higher level in chronic experimental hypertension in the dog.

Resistance Vessels

It has been frequently observed that when arterial pressure has been elevated for some time, it is neither immediately nor fully reversible when the original cause, such as coarctation of the aorta, is removed (41). Furthermore, resistance vessels have been shown to hypertrophy in response to an increased pressure load (42,43), and these structural changes maintain high blood pressure even in the absence of initiating factors. This may be one of the reasons it is sometimes difficult to find emotional factors, or biochemical evidence of them, in established hypertensives. In contrast to the foregoing observations, Folkow et al. (44) have provided some evidence that if the arterial pressure is reduced and effectively maintained at the lower level, these structural changes in the resistance vessels reverse.

Autonomic Response Stereotypy

According to this concept, the individual responds to stress by a generalized increase in sympathetic activity but consistently shows maximal response in only one or two physiologic functions (45,46). For example, Wolf and Wolff (47) compared 103 hypertensive subjects with 203 normotensive controls. During stressful interviews, the hypertensives showed a greater rise in blood pressure than the controls, despite an affable exterior. Schachter (48) subjected both normotensive and hypertensive subjects to three types of stimuli—pain (immersion of hand in ice-cold water), fear (the threat of an electric shock), and anger (frustration caused by an irritating technician)—and found a greater rise in the blood pressure of hypertensives. Similar findings have been reported by others (49,50).

That such an idiosyncratic specific individual pattern seems to persist has been experimentally verified over a period of 4 years (46). The suggestion is that there are "blood pressure reactors" just as there are "pulse reactors, stomach reactors, or nose reactors." The high reactivity of a given response system, whether it is gastrointestinal, respiratory, or cardiovascular, frequently leads to malfunction of the system when it is repeatedly stimulated. This constitutional pattern is probably what is inherited. Theoretically, the concept could be stretched even further and put to experimental test to explain individual differences in hemodynamic and humoral factors. Why do some patients have an increase in cardiac output while others have a predominant increase in peripheral vascular resistance? Why are there high, normal, and low renin hypertensives? Why are catecholamine or corticoids not uniformly increased in all hypertensives? Since the body's compensatory processes are continuously trying to adjust to the internal environment, the net effect may be different in different individuals and also in the same individual at different times (51).

A PROPOSED BEHAVIORAL APPROACH

The factors involved in the pathogenesis of essential hypertension are suggested in Fig. 14.1. The hypothesis advanced was that by modifying some of the peripheral manifestations of the response, it may be possible to alter the sensitivity of the central hypothalamic response (52) (points 1 to 5 in Fig. 14.1). A number of studies, conducted to test the hypothesis, are discussed.

The suggested approach, essentially an "unlearning" of maladaptive responding under psychosocial stress, has both behavioral and relaxation components. In its behavioral aspects, this approach includes learning to discriminate between realistic and unrealistic fear and aggression, and between appropriate and inappropriate physiologic responses to situations in daily life. The aim is to learn a coping response to reduce fear and hence an inappropriate response to it. It is accomplished by an education program aimed at cognitive restructuring to alter the response pattern (point 1 in Fig. 14.1).

Relaxation and Meditation

The major component in my approach is the mastery of a thorough relaxation technique based on a Yoga principle. It is known that breathing is erratic when a person is excited, yet slow and regular when he is calm and composed. The patient, therefore, is taught a simple breathing exercise. By a slow, rhythmic, diaphragmatic breathing exercise, a certain amount of physical calmness is induced (point 2 in Fig. 14.1), the additional advantage being that the exercise can be performed anywhere and in any position without other people even noticing it.

This is followed by a systematic deep relaxation. The patient is advised to perform this exercise on an empty stomach and bladder. He is asked to lie down, close his eyes, and systematically relax each part of his body (point 3 in Fig. 14.1). After a few sessions of breathing exercises and deep muscle relaxation, a type of mental relaxation is introduced in the form of passive concentration and eventually meditation (point 4 in Fig. 14.1). It is uncertain whether any of the patients reach a meditative state; nevertheless, the process itself leads to mental calm. Another advantage is that the slight mental activity involved in meditation prevents sleep. Relaxation is conducive to sleep because of the mechanisms of sleep, but if the patient is allowed to sleep, the concept of voluntary control is nullified. Meditative practices are also known to change the EEG pattern into a more synchronized one with high amplitude, slow wave pattern of the relaxed brain, not passing into sleep (53). They also increase the coherence between the cerebral hemispheres, as well as between the anterior and posterior parts of each hemisphere (54).

The assumption that deep muscle relaxation reduces the intensity of the hypothalamic response is implicit in the results of animal experiments. It has been shown that increased flow of proprioceptive and exteroceptive impulses leads to increased intensity of the hypothalamic responsiveness, producing not only a highly emotional state with appropriate somatic expression but also cortical desynchronization and a rise in blood pressure. The changes produced can be as great as those produced by direct electrical and mechanical stimulation of the hypothalamus (30,55–57). On the other hand, a reduction in proprioception with curare-like drugs has been shown to induce behavioral sleep and, in general, reduce intensity of the hypothalamic responsiveness (58,59). Yogic relaxation also has been shown to reduce blood pressure in hypertensive patients (60).

In this context, it is interesting to note that an increase in isometric contraction, such as a tight hand grip or weight lifting, causes a considerable rise in blood pressure (61,62). It is assumed that a dramatic decrease in proprioception, exteroception, and visceroception, implied in the relaxation technique, should reduce the sympathetic responsiveness of the hypothalamus and eventually lower blood pressure; it may even partially reverse the perpetuating factors.

Reducing Arousal Level

The points discussed are aimed at reducing the level of arousal. The resulting condition may be regarded as opposite in nature to the fight-or-flight response and has been variously described as a "wakeful hypometabolic state" (53), a relaxation response (63), and an "antistress response" (64). The biofeedback principle is used to train patients more efficiently to move into a low arousal state. One of two instruments is mainly used. The one measuring GSR informs the patient about his level of sympathetic arousal; the EMG displays his level of muscle tension. As used by myself, both types of machine give continuous sound signals. As the patient relaxes, the sound becomes fainter and the clicks fewer, until they stop. The sensitivity is then turned up to give further signals, and the patient must relax further to stop the signals. His task is made more difficult as he becomes more expert at relaxing.

In addition to this relaxation feedback, the patient is given an overall feedback of his blood pressure level at the end of each session. Every success the patient has is taken as an opportunity to raise his self esteem and his motivation to continue the program on a long-term basis. He is asked to practice this relaxation technique for 15 to 20 min twice a day and, later, to integrate relaxation into everyday life.

A specific method of overcoming unrealistic fear or inappropriate aggression is through a procedure of counterconditioning. The fear of an aggression-inducing stimulus is paired with some stimulus or condition, such as relaxation, that acts to inhibit the fear or aggression response (65). Patients are encouraged to practice regular breathing and muscle relaxation prior to, or during, stressful activities, such as driving, public speaking, flying, or interviews (point 5 in Fig. 14.1). The idea behind this procedure is to desensitize the susceptible patient to the stressful stimuli of everyday life.

YOGA AND BIOFEEDBACK IN HYPERTENSION

A behavioral program proposed on therapeutic grounds was tested in a series of studies involving hypertensive patients.

Pilot Study

In a pilot study (66), 20 patients (nine males and 11 females; average age, 57.3 years) were trained in the techniques proposed. They attended three times each week over a period of 3 months (for details, see ref. 67), having been stablised on antihypertensive medications before the study began. In addition to relaxation feedback, the patients were also given an overall feedback of blood pressure readings at the end of each session, and a success was verbally praised. The dosage of drugs were adjusted according to the response, allowing each patient to participate in the decision to reduce any drug, thus allocating to the patient some responsibility for his own health.

The control group patients were matched for age and sex from the hypertensive age-sex register kept in our medical practice and were added to the study retrospectively (68). The demographic data of the patients are given in Table 14.1.

History taking, investigations, number of attendances, time spent at each session, and procedure for blood pressure measurement were the same for both the control and treatment groups, but instead of being trained in relaxation and behavior modification, the patient in the control group was asked to rest on a couch. The results at the end of the 3-month trial are shown in Table 14.2.

In the treatment group, mean systolic and diastolic pressures were reduced by 20.4 and 14.2 mmHg, respectively ($p = < 0.001$). In addition to these significant reductions, five patients were able to stop their antihypertensive drugs altogether; seven were able to reduce their drug requirements from between 33 and 60%, four had their blood pressure controlled better without any drug reduction; and in the remaining four patients, there was no significant change.

TABLE 14.1. *Pilot study: details of patients*

Group	Treatment	Control
Total number	20	20
Males	9	9
Females	11	11
Average age (years)	57.35	57.2
Duration of hyper- tension (years)	6.8	7.05
Number of patients on hypotensive drugs	19	18
Original BP[a]		
Systolic[b]	201.5 ± 24.2	197 ± 31.8
Diastolic[b]	121.8 ± 12.4	115 ± 17.3

[a] Original BP = blood pressure at the time of diagnosis.
[b] Average plus or minus standard deviation.

In the control group, the reductions in systolic and diastolic pressure were 0.5 and 2.1 mmHg, respectively, which were not significant.

Spontaneous fluctuations and regression to the mean are so common in high blood pressure, that the value of any claimed therapy can only be assessed by its long-term effectiveness. The patients in the above trial were followed up

TABLE 14.2. *Pilot study: results*

Blood pressure	Treatment group	Control group
Pretrial BP[a]		
Systolic[b]	159.1 ± 15.9	163.1 ± 20.9
Diastolic[b]	100.1 ± 6.4	99.1 ± 12.8
End of trial BP[c]		
Systolic[b]	138.7 ± 16.0	162.6 ± 24.4
Diastolic[b]	85.9 ± 8.7	97.0 ± 12.0
Difference		
Systolic[b]	20.4 ± 11.8	0.5 ± 14.5
Diastolic[b]	14.2 ± 7.5	2.1 ± 6.2
Paired *t* test		
Systolic[b]	7.75	0.15
Diastolic[b]	8.50	1.52
p =	<.001	NS[d]
Additional benefit		
Total drug reduction	41.7%	Nil

[a] Pretrial BP = baseline blood pressure (average of 18 measurements).
[b] Average plus or minus standard deviation.
[c] End-of-trial BP = blood pressure at the end of treatment (average of 24 measurements).
[d] NS = not significant.

TABLE 14.3. *Pilot study: follow-up results*

Blood pressure	Treatment group	Control group
End-of-trial arrival BP		
Systolic	144.6 ± 11.0	167.1 ± 9.73
Diastolic	86.0 ± 5.74	97.1 ± 6.54
3-month follow-up:		
Systolic	143.9 ± 13.38	167.6 ± 8.08
Diastolic	84.0 ± 3.84	97.4 ± 7.74
6-month follow-up:		
Systolic	146.7 ± 10.72	164.1 ± 15.0
Diastolic	88.3 ± 6.84	97.3 ± 8.0
9-[a] and 12-month[b] follow-up		
Systolic	144.4 ± 9.83	163.6 ± 9.42
Diastolic	86.7 ± 3.33	98.1 ± 7.83
$p =$	NS[c]	NS[c]

[a] Control group.
[b] Treatment group.
[c] NS = not significant.

monthly for 12 months in the treatment group and 9 months in the control group, after the initial 3-month trial period. Mean blood pressure for the groups are given in Table 14.3.

Because there was a change in the procedure of blood pressure measurements, pretrial pressures were adjusted for comparison with follow-up blood pressures. Despite some individual variations, the reduction in mean blood pressure in the treated group was maintained, and only slight and insignificant variations in the antihypertensive drugs were made on clinical grounds during this follow-up period. Motivating these patients to continue this regular, time-consuming practice of relaxation and meditation was the most difficult task. Better methods of integrating relaxation in everyday life may partly offset this requirement.

Randomized Controlled Study

The previous study shows that behavioral techniques designed to produce low levels of arousal were effective in significantly reducing blood pressure; while mere rest, increased medical attention, or repeated blood pressure measurements were not effective in producing lasting reductions in patients who were already familiar with the physician and with the procedure of blood pressure measurements. The next study (69) was designed to establish the effectiveness of the treatment more scientifically by randomly allocating patients to the treatment and control groups. The period of training was reduced to 6 weeks, two sessions per week, and the training technique was improved as a result of previous experience.

Thirty-four patients, known to be hypertensive for 6 months to 20 years and controlled on antihypertensive medications, took part in the study. Blood pressures were recorded on 3 separate days to provide baseline blood pressure. A trained nurse, using a random zero sphygmomanometer (70), made all the measurements. Pressures were recorded in the standing, sitting, and supine positions and repeated similarly after a 30-min rest in the supine position. The patients were then randomly allocated to treatment or control groups.

In the first phase of the trial, blood pressure was recorded before and after each of 12 30-min sessions, twice a week, for 6 weeks. The patients in the treatment group were motivated to follow the program as closely as possible by means of meetings during which they were shown films and slides about high blood pressure, the different ways in which emotions affect bodily processes, the physiology of relaxation, the concept of biofeedback, self-control, and so forth. Queries and problems were discussed freely. The rapport created between doctor and patients, as well as among the patients themselves, helped to strengthen the program and ensure maximum cooperation. The patients were asked to keep their medications constant. The patients in the control group attended the same number of sessions for the same length of time. They were asked to relax on the couch or reclining chair but were not given specific instructions and were not connected to biofeedback instruments. At the end of the study, patients in both groups were followed every 2 weeks for 3 months.

An extension of this study, phase 2, was undertaken as a precaution against the possibility that the original random allocation of patients may have resulted in groups that were not strictly comparable. Phase 2 began 2 months after the end of the follow-up for phase 1. The previous control group now became the treated group, with 12 treatment sessions, as in phase 1. (One patient dropped out because he could not attend sessions regularly.) Patients in the previously treated group were used as controls but were seen only at the beginning and end of this phase to provide blood pressure readings for comparison purposes. There was only one initial and one follow-up session in each group in phase 2.

Seventeen patients in each group completed phase 1. Every blood pressure reading used in the analysis was the mean of three readings taken with the patient standing, sitting, and lying down. Although measurements were made at the beginning and end of each session, only those made at the beginning of sessions have been used here (blood pressures at the end of sessions were invariably lower). In addition, figures for "initial" pressures in phase 1 are the means of readings at the three preliminary sessions, and those for "final" pressures the means of the six follow-up sessions. During the first phase, systolic blood pressure fell by an average of 26.2 mmHg in the treated group and by 8.9 mmHg in the control group ($p = < 0.005$). The corresponding figures for diastolic pressure were 15.2 and 4.2 mmHg ($p = < 0.001$). Although there was a significant fall in both systolic and diastolic pressure in the control group, this was not true for all patients. Two patients in the control group showed a rise in both systolic and diastolic pressure and another six a rise in one of the two. No patients in the treated group showed a rise in pressure. The means of each group, week by week, in phase 1 are shown in Fig. 14.2.

At the beginning of the second phase, blood pressure was higher in the new treatment group (formerly control) than at the beginning of the first phase (possibly because only one reading was taken). The blood pressure in the former treated group, however, was close to the level at the end of phase 1. This group was not seen again until the end of phase 2. The results for the treated group were similar to those in phase 1, while the control group changed very little. No significance tests were performed for this phase, as their validity seemed doubtful; but it is clear that the difference was of comparable magnitude to that previously obtained. Again, no member of the treated group showed a rise in blood pressure.

In phase 1, the treated group showed a much larger reduction in blood pressure than did the control group. Evidence that this was due primarily to the relaxation technique they had learned is provided by the fact that at the start of phase 2, their blood pressure remained at lower levels, while those of the control group had risen to at least the initial level. Admittedly, placebo responding can reduce blood pressure (71–73) (see also the following chapter). Grenfell et al. (74), in a double-blind study of patients whose initial blood pressures were more than 200/120 mmHg, found that both guanethidine (average dose, 60 mg/day) and an oral placebo produced comparable and statistically significant reductions in blood pressure over a 12-week period. The average decreases in the placebo group were 25 and 12 mmHg for systolic and diastolic pressures, respectively. These results show that blood pressure can be reduced without

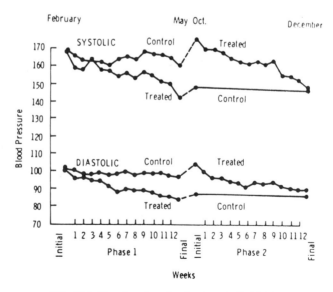

FIG. 14.2. Results of randomized controlled trial.

the help of active drugs, and that the higher the initial blood pressure the greater the reduction. Although the term placebo often implies that the beneficial effects are only transient and are possibly attributable to a favorable doctor/patient relationship and other psychologic mechanisms (75), it should be noted that in this study, the beneficial effect in the treatment group has lasted for as long as 1 year and is still continuing. The doctor/patient relationship was the same for both groups; hence, the mechanisms of the therapeutic effect must have been different.

MODIFICATION OF PRESSOR RESPONSE TO "STRESS"

It is well known that physical and emotional stimuli are effective in modifying blood pressure. Pressor responses to various stimuli have been shown to be exaggerated and protracted in hypertensive patients (44–50,76–82), as well as hypertensive rats, as described in the previous chapter. The true pressure load on the left ventricle and vessel walls can neither be the resting pressure nor the occasional peak of pressure in response to a mental or emotional stress but the integrated average pressure over longer periods. As Smirk (83) pointed out, if the psychologically induced peaks of increased pressure are added to a high baseline blood pressure, the two carry the final height of the pressure to degrees that contribute to hypertensive cardiovascular disease. As the individual grows older, various organs begin to deteriorate under the onslaught of transient blood pressure elevations. The advantages of any therapy that could reduce the magnitude or duration of these pressure rises are obvious.

A study was undertaken to determine, in a controlled experiment, whether the pressor response to laboratory stressor stimuli would change as a result of training in behavioral modification (84). Thirty-two patients, 21 females and 11 males between the ages of 34 and 75 years (average age, 58.5 years), with essential hypertension of known duration of from 6 months to 13 years (average, 5.7 years), were randomly allocated to a treatment and control group. Fourteen patients in the treatment group and 15 in the control group were receiving antihypertensive drugs. The patients were given two stress tests—an exercise test and a cold pressor test—at the beginning of the study and again after 6 weeks. Baseline blood pressure was first obtained after a 20-min rest in the supine position; and the exercise test consisted of climbing a 9-inch step 25 times. In the cold pressor test, the patient was alerted 60 sec in advance about the test to be performed; the left hand was then immersed in water at 4°C for 80 sec. Blood pressure was taken during the alert phase, at the end of each test, and every 5 min thereafter until it returned to the original value (or up to a maximum of 40 min). The maximum rise in systolic and diastolic pressures and the time taken for recovery (to reach baseline blood pressure) were calculated in each case. Differences in the above measurements and those obtained during the repetition of the tests were compared within the groups by Student's *t*-test and between the groups by an unpaired *t*-test (two-tailed).

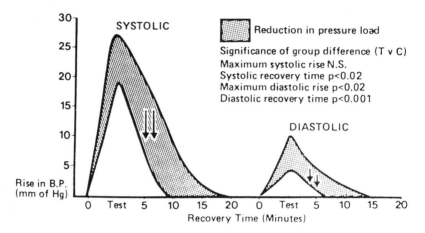

FIG. 14.3 Results of exercise test for the treatment group ($n = 16$).

In the 6 weeks between test periods, all patients attended the clinic twice weekly. The patients in the treatment group were given 30 min of training in behavior modification, as previously described.

The results are shown in Figs. 14.3–14.6, the peaks representing the maximum rise in systolic and diastolic blood pressures following the stress test. Recovery times are plotted along the axes. The shaded area represents change in the pressure load, and the arrows indicate direction in which the pressure load changed between pre- and posttrial tests.

Merely telling the patient about the test to be performed (alert phase) caused blood pressure to rise in most patients, although the average changes were small. In the treatment group, there was a significant reduction in pressure rises as well as in recovery time ($p = < 0.05$). That mere repetition of the

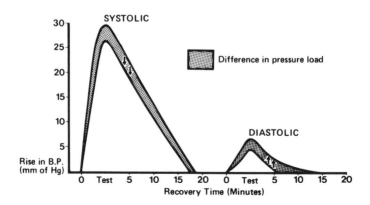

FIG. 14.4. Results of exercise test for the control group ($n = 16$).

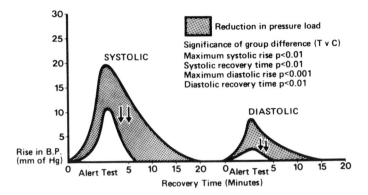

FIG. 14.5. Results of cold pressor test for the treatment group (*n* = 16).

tests, or an habituation effect, did not account for these alterations in stress responding is shown by the results in the control group. When the differences between the groups were compared by unpaired *t*-tests, all measurements except the systolic pressure rise after exercise showed significant improvement in the treated group ($p = < 0.02$).

Although the pathologic consequences of such stresses have been difficult to document precisely, there is some pertinent information. For example, Taylor (85), taking 100 to 120 heartbeats per minute as a criterion of sympathetic drive, observed that the majority of healthy young males engaged in business activity reached this range more than 50 times per day, many executives 100 times each day, and a few more than 250 times per day. Business and professional activities, as well as bus driving, showed high levels of heart rate (85). If the

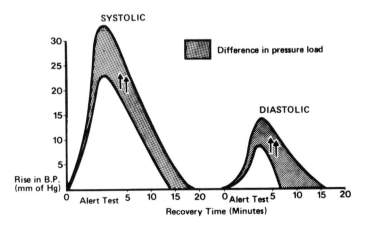

FIG. 14.6. Results of cold pressor test for the control group (*n* = 16).

same sort of reactivity holds for blood pressure, the savings in pressure load afforded by a reduction in the magnitude and duration of pressure rise (see Figs. 14.3–14.6), multiplied by the frequency of such daily activities over a number of years, could be considerable. At present, these are purely speculative presumptions; until proven in a strictly controlled study in unmedicated subjects with bias-free data collection, caution must be maintained in making any claims.

BEHAVIORAL METHODS IN REDUCING CORONARY HEART DISEASE RISK

As already outlined in the first section of this book, numerous risk factors for coronary heart disease (CHD) have been identified, such as hypertension, elevated blood lipids, cigarette smoking, diabetes mellitus or hypoglycemia, obesity, sedentary living, and a positive family history (86). The data from the pooling project (86), which reports on the prospective studies of heart disease in the United States, show a large number of false positives and false negatives. Only 14% of the people in the high risk group develop CHD in the next 10 years. Thus 83% of the total cases of CHD occurring in the population do not come from the high risk group, and 86% of those classified in the high risk group do not develop CHD in 10 years (87). It is reasonable to conclude that, although the ability to predict CHD from the presence of risk factors is impressive, a substantial proportion of CHD must occur for reasons other than conventional risk factors.

Psychosocial Stress

It is well recognized that emotional stress may lead to overeating, excessive drinking and smoking, aggressive behavior and possibly physical inactivity by promoting early fatigue (88). Its contribution to hypertension has already been discussed, and its link with serum cholesterol level is gradually being revealed (see Chapter 3).

Many astute physicians in the past have recognized this association, e.g., Heberden in 1768 (89) and Hunter in 1794 (90). The classic studies of Friedman and Rosenman (91) and Russek and Zohman (92) have already been described. Of particular relevance is the study by the former, concerned with occupational deadlines and increased pressure of work in a group of accountants before tax deadlines. These were associated with a small (8%) but significant increase in serum cholesterol (93). Other investigators (94–98) have also shown elevations in various lipids associated with psychosocial and other stressors.

Epidemiologic Studies

The association between dietary cholesterol and CHD remains controversial in the face of numerous conflicting transcultural studies (86,99–107).

For example, Gordon et al. (108) compared the incidence rates of CHD from studies that had used uniform methods in Framingham, Honolulu, and Puerto Rico. The incidence of CHD in Framingham was 2 to 3 times higher than that in Puerto Rico and Honolulu, but this could not be accounted for by the conventional risk factors. Smoking, for example, had no effect on the incidence rate of CHD in Puerto Rico. Similarly, in a longitudinal study of 17,530 civil servants in London over a period of 7.5 years, men in the lowest grade (messengers) were shown to have 3.6 times the CHD mortality of men in the highest grade (administrators) (109). Again, a large part of this mortality difference could not be accounted for by the conventional risk factors.

Transcultural Factors

There is some evidence that social and cultural factors may interact with biologic risk factors in an important manner which influences the incidence rate of CHD. Japan has the lowest rate of CHD of any industrialized nation, while the United States has one of the highest rates. There is an increasing gradient in mortality from CHD in Japanese living in Japan, Hawaii, and California, respectively (110,111), which is explained by serum cholesterol, blood pressure, and smoking levels.

Marmot and Syme (112) suggested that, among the Californian Japanese, the traditional Japanese would have lower rates of CHD than those Japanese-Americans who had changed their culture to the American way of living. In an elegant study, they showed that prevalence of definite CHD and, indeed, each characteristic (angina pectoris, pain of myocardial infarction, and major EKG abnormality for each age group) were greater in the American Japanese than in the traditional Japanese. These differences could not be accounted for by the differences in the conventional risk factors, e.g., age, levels of blood pressure, serum cholesterol and triglycerides, cigarette smoking, and body weight.

RELAXATION AND BLOOD LIPIDS

If relaxation-based behavior modification can reduce high blood pressure as well as emotional and occupational stresses, it is possible that it may also reduce blood cholesterol and other lipids. In a pilot study (113) in 14 hypertensive patients, I found that, over a 6-week period, there was a reduction in mean systolic pressure from 170.6 to 147.9 mmHg, while reduction in mean diastolic pressure was from 102.5 to 89 mmHg ($p = 0.001$). The mean cholesterol level in this group of patients was reduced from 214.6 to 217 mg/100 ml ($p < 0.001$), and 13 of 14 patients showed some decrease in serum cholesterol. However, this was an uncontrolled study.

In another pilot study in collaboration with Carruthers (114), four groups of subjects were studied. A group of 18 normotensive subjects acted as controls; another group of 18 normotensive subjects was treated by the biofeedback-relaxation-meditation-behavioral modification program. A group of 22 hypertensives and a group of 18 current smokers were similarly treated. There was a significant reduction in blood pressure in all the treated groups, with no significant change in the control group, while plasma cholesterol, triglycerides, and free fatty acids were reduced significantly in some but not all the treated groups, with no change in the control group. In smokers, the number of cigarettes smoked was reduced by 48% at the end of the first week, dropping gradually week by week until an approximate 80% reduction was achieved by the end of a 6-week training period. Not all the reduction was maintained, however, although at 6 months follow-up, the total number of cigarettes smoked was still 60% less than the original (see Fig. 14.7). Most of these smokers wanted to give up smoking and had themselves approached the local antismoking clinic for help.

The coronary risk factor reduction study (115) was planned to replicate the results in a properly controlled trial involving people with risk factors who were also unselected, previously unknown to the therapist, unmedicated, relatively young, and engaged in full-time occupational work. Of 1,132 industrial employees, 230 had two or more risk factors. The risk factors were defined as: (a) an average of four blood pressure measurements to be 140/90 or more (116), (b) serum cholesterol level of 6.3 mmoles/liter or more (nonfasting), and (c) current cigarette smoking of 10 or more cigarettes per day. Eventually, 204 of these individuals consented to take part in the study and were randomly allocated to biofeedback and control groups, which were similar for age, sex, number of subjects with raised blood pressure, raised cholesterol, and mean levels of each blood pressure, plasma cholesterol, and number of cigarettes smoked per day by smokers, but the proportion of current smokers was slightly higher in the treatment groups.

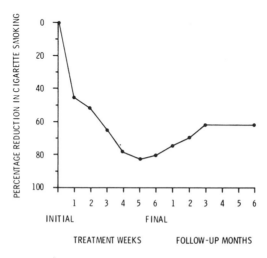

FIG. 14.7. Reduction in cigarette smoking in smokers group, achieved by behavioral methods.

The management protocol for both groups consisted of (a) 10 min of individual counseling, and (b) allocation of health education literature, including "Why should I stop smoking?," "How to stop smoking," "Cholesterol and heart disease," "Eating for a healthy heart," and "Information about high blood pressure." The treatment group included eight 1-hour training sessions (weekly) and 3 hr of stress education program.

Reduction in Risk Factors

Table 14.4 shows reduction in each risk factor after 8 weeks. The reductions in both systolic and diastolic pressures were significantly greater in the biofeedback group than the control group, not only for all patients but also for those with initial high blood pressures. Although there was no significant difference between serum cholesterol reductions for all patients in the two groups, for patients with initial cholesterol of 6.3 mmoles/liter or more, there was a reduction of 0.9 mmoles/liter in the biofeedback group compared with 0.5 mmoles/liter in the control group ($p < 0.025$). Finally, for people in the two groups who initially were smokers, 68% of the biofeedback group reduced the number of cigarettes smoked per day, compared with 39% in the control group. Of these, 11% of the biofeedback and 7.8% of the control group completely stopped

TABLE 14.4. *Reduction in risk factors after eight weeks*

	Biofeedback group Mean ± S.E.	Control group Mean ± S.E.	Between group diff. t value
Reduction in system B.P.	***	***	***
Whole group	13.8 ± 1.34	4.0 ± 1.30	5.30
	***	***	***
Initial BP high 140 mm Hg or more	18.0 ± 1.72	8.8 ± 1.42	4.07
Reduction in diastolic B.P.	***		***
Whole group	7.2 ± 0.91	1.4 ± 0.81	4.75
	***	***	***
Initial BP high 90 mm Hg or more	10.6 ± 1.37	3.8 ± 1.04	3.90
Reduction in cholesterol	***		
Whole group	0.71 ± 0.12	0.53 ± .11	1.15
	***	***	*
Initial cholesterol high 6.3 mmol/l or more	0.90 ± 0.12	0.52 ± .12	2.3
Reduction cigarette smoking	***		***
% reduced smoking	67.9 ± 5.19	39.1 ± 6.10	3.58(SND)
	***	***	**
Average no. of cigarettes/day less	5.8 ± .73	2.6 ± .75	3.01

* $.01 < p < .05$
** $.001 < p < .01$
*** $p < .001$

TABLE 14.5. *Changes in log plasma renin activity*

	Difference between initial and 8 weeks
Biofeedback n = 25	0.56 ± .10 log pg/ml/hr.
Control n = 27	0.10 ± .12 log pg/ml/hr.

smoking. The mean number of cigarettes consumed per day fell by 5.8 in the biofeedback group and 2.6 in the control group ($p < 0.01$).

We also measured plasma renin and aldosterone levels in some subsamples. The results are shown in Tables 14.5 and 14.6. The reduction in log plasma renin activity in the biofeedback group was significantly greater at 0.56, compared with 0.10 in the control group. However, there was no correlation between changes in blood pressure and changes in plasma renin activity, suggesting that these effects may be independent of each other. There was a mean decrease of 78 pmoles/liter in plasma aldosterone in the treatment group, compared with a rise of 33 pmoles/liter in the control group ($p < 0.05$). Examining the data in a different manner, we identified 15 of 25 subjects in the treatment group, compared with only six of 29 in the control group, who showed a fall of 50 pmoles/liter or more ($p = < 0.01$). There was also a greater fall in plasma norepinephrine in the treatment group, but the changes were less clear.

Results at 6 Months

The greater reduction in both systolic and diastolic BP in the biofeedback group was maintained at 6 months. The differences between the groups were still highly significant. Confining our analysis of serum cholesterol to the subjects with high initial levels, the reduction was less pronounced in the biofeedback group, being 0.77 mmoles/liter in comparison to 0.56 mmoles/liter in the control group, thus narrowing the gap between the groups. As mentioned earlier, both the groups were given literature on modified fat diets. Did they change their

TABLE 14.6. *Changes in plasma aldosterone after eight weeks*

	Biofeedback group n = 25	Control group n = 29	2 Tail probability
Mean change pmol/l	−78	+33	<.05
Proportion showing a fall of 50 pmol/l	60%	20%	<.01

diets? If so, were the changes identical in both the groups? Our analysis of their 24-hr recall dietary diaries is still proceeding.

The proportion of smokers who reduced smoking was 67.5% in the biofeedback group compared with 37.5% in the control group; of these, 10% in the treatment group compared with 5% in the control group stopped smoking. The mean number of cigarettes consumed per day was five in the biofeedback group and two in the control group, a statistically significant difference.

Thus psychosocial stress may be an important risk factor. Assuming that these reductions in risk factors would reduce the mortality from CHD, we can calculate the potential reduction in mortality using the multiple logistic function from the Whitehall study. The figure at 8 weeks is a 21% reduction in the predicted risk of CHD death; at 6 months, the figure is 18%.

This may not be very impressive, but if one considers that the subjects in this study had elevations of risk factors sufficient to increase their risk of serious complications but too mild to warrant the hazards of pharmacologic intervention, this reduction in risk would be no mean achievement. It is possible that reduction in CHD risk may occur through paths other than the conventional risk factors. Estimation of this, however, is beyond the scope of this study.

CONCLUSIONS

A behavior modification program, which includes training and regular practice of breathing exercises, deep muscle relaxation, meditation, proper discrimination between appropriate and inappropriate responses, and adequate coping with situations in everyday life, can result in highly significant reductions in both systolic and diastolic blood pressures in essential hypertension. The results also suggest that psychosocial-occupational stress may play an important etiologic role in hypertension.

My personal experience suggests that motivating symptomless hypertensive patients to comply with the time-consuming practice of relaxation is probably as difficult as persuading them to take long-term antihypertensive medications, which often produce unpleasant side effects. Most patients, however, show a preference for nondrug or minimal drug approaches, if possible. The motivation to follow a behavioral program can be strengthened by an adequate health education program and by instilling a sense of participation in the patient. The magnitude of blood pressure reduction, its long-term maintenance, and the reduction of pressor response to experimental stressors reported are such that it would be worthwhile to improve the program as well as to produce better evidence of its efficacy.

The results of international epidemiologic studies show that the difference in CHD incidence, prevalence, and mortality in different parts of the world cannot be completely accounted for by the differences in conventional risk factors. Clinical observations, as well as animal and human studies, show that psychosocial-occupational stress and certain personality characteristics might be causative or contributory factors.

A hypothesis is formulated suggesting that psychosocial stress may be an important causative factor leading to sudden death or myocardial infarction, either directly or indirectly through the conventional risk factors. Although not yet proved, the results suggest that the behavioral modification program mentioned can at least reduce measurable risk factors. The reductions in serum cholesterol and cigarette smoking are not impressive, but when added to the reduction in blood pressure, a worthwhile reduction in coronary risk can be calculated.

ACKNOWLEDGMENT

Studies reviewed in this chapter were supported by the South West Thames Regional Health Authority and the British Heart Foundation.

REFERENCES

1. Kannel, W. B., and Dawber, T. R. Hypertension as an ingredient of cardiovascular risk profile. *Br. J. Hosp. Med.*, 1974, 11, 508–523.
2. Metropolitan Life Insurance Company. Blood pressure: Insurance experience and its implications. 1961.
3. Veterans Administration Cooperative Study Group on Antihypertensive Agents. Effects of treatment on morbidity in hypertension: Results in patients with diastolic blood pressures averaging 115 through 129 mm.Hg. *JAMA,* 1967, 202, 1028–1034.
4. Veterans Administration Cooperative Study Group on Antihypertensive Agents. Effects of treatment on morbidity in hypertension II. Results in patients with diastolic blood pressure averaging 90 through 114 mm.Hg. *JAMA,* 1970, 213, 1143–1152.
5. Reid, D., Hamilton, P. J. S., Keen, H., Brett, G. Z., Jarrett, R. J., and Rose, G. Cardiorespiratory diseases and diabetes among middle-aged male civil servants. *Lancet,* 1974, i, 469–473.
6. Miall, W. E., and Chinn, S. Screening for hypertension: Some epidemiological observations. *Br. Med. J.,* 1974, 3, 595–600.
7. Hawthorne, V. M., Greaves, D. A., and Beevers, D. G. Blood pressure in a Scottish town. *Br. Med. J.,* 1974, 3, 600–603.
8. National Heart and Lung Institute. The public and high blood pressure. DHEW publication no. (NIH) 74–356, 1973.
9. Breckenridge, A., Dollery, C. T., and Parry, E. H. O. Prognosis of treated hypertension. *Q. J. Med.,* 1970, 39, 411–429.
10. Stewart, I. McD. G. Relation of reduction in pressure to first myocardial infarction in patients receiving treatment for severe hypertension. *Lancet,* 1979, i, 861–865.
11. Wilber, J. A., and Barrow, J. G. Hypertension: A community problem. *Am. J. Med.,* 1972, 52, 653–663.
12. Schoenberger, J. A., Stamler, J., Shekelle, R. B., and Shekelle, S. Current status of hypertension control in an industrial population. *JAMA,* 1972, 222, 5, 559–562.
13. Sackett, D. L., and Holland, W. W. Controversy in the detection of disease. *Lancet,* 1975, ii, 357–359.
14. Peart, W. S., and Miall, W. E. M.R.C. treatment for mild hypertension. *Lancet,* 1979, 2, 41–42.
15. Shapiro, D., Tursky, B., Gershon, W., and Stern, M. Effects of feedback and reinforcement on the control of human systolic blood pressure. *Science,* 1969, 163, 588–589.
16. Shapiro, D., Tursky, B., and Schwartz, G. E. Control of blood pressure in man by operant conditioning. *Circ. Res. [Suppl. I]*, 1970, 26 and 27, I-27–32.

17. Shapiro, D., Schwartz, G. E., and Tursky, B. Control of diastolic blood pressure in man by feedback and reinforcement. In: *Biofeedback and Self Control 1972*, edited by D. Shapiro, T. X. Barber, L. V. Dicara, J. Kamiya, N. E. Miller, and J. Stoyva, pp. 217–226. Aldine, Chicago, 1973.

18. Brener, J., and Kleinman, R. A. Learned control of decreases in systolic blood pressure. *Nature*, 1970, 226, 1063–1064.

19. Schwartz, G. E., and Shapiro, D. Biofeedback and essential hypertension: Current findings and theoretical concerns. In: *Seminars in Psychiatry. Biofeedback Behavioral Medicine*, edited by L. Birk, pp. 493–503. Grune & Stratton, 1973.

20. Benson, H., Shapiro, D., Tursky, B., and Schwartz, G. Decreased systolic blood pressure through operant conditioning techniques in patients with essential hypertension. *Science*, 1971, 173, 740–742.

21. Pickering, G. W. *High Blood Pressure*, second edition, Churchill, London, 1968.

22. Scotch, N. A., and Geiger, H. J. The epidemiology of essential hypertension. A review with special attention to psychologic and socio-cultural factors. II. Psychologic and socioculture factors in etiology. *J. Chronic Dis.*, 1963, 16, 1183–1213.

23. Cruz-Coke, R. Environmental influences and arterial blood pressure. *Lancet*, 1960, ii, 885–886.

24. Cruz-Coke, R., Etcheverry, R., and Nagel, R. Influence of migration on blood pressure of Eastern Islanders. *Lancet*, 1964, i, 697–699.

25. Henry, J. P., and Cassel, J. C. Psycho-social factors in essential hypertension. Recent epidemiological and animal experimental evidence. *Am. J. Epidemiol.*, 1969, 90, 3, 171–200.

26. Hippocrates, cited by Wolf, S. In: *Society, Stress and Disease*, Oxford University Press, London, 1971.

27. Ogilvie, H. In praise of idleness. *Br. Med. J.*, 1949, 1, 645–651.

28. Brod, J., Fencl, V., Hejl, Z., and Zirka, J. Circulatory changes underlying blood pressure elevation during acute emotional stress (mental arithmetic) in normotensive and hypertensive subjects. *Clin. Sci.*, 1959, 18, 269–279.

29. Abrahams, V. C., Hilton, S. M., and Zbrozyna, A. Active muscle vasodilation produced by stimulation of the brain stem: Its significance in the defence reaction. *J. Physiol.*, 1960, 154, 491–513.

30. Folkow, B., and Rubinstein, E. H. Cardiovascular effects of acute and chronic stimulations of the hypothalamic defence area in the rat. *Acta Physiol. Scand.*, 1966, 68, 48–57.

31. Gellhorn, E. The emotions and the ergotropic and trophotropic systems. *Psychol. Forsch.*, 1970, 34, 48–94.

32. Iwamura, Y., Uchino, Y., Ozawa, S., and Torii, S. Spontaneous and reflex discharge of a sympathetic nerve during "para-sleep" in decerebrate cat. *Brain Res.*, 1969, 16, 359–367.

33. Zanchetti, A., Bacelli, G., Guazzi, M., and Mancia, G. The effect of sleep on experimental hypertension. In: *Hypertension: Mechanisms and Management*, edited by G. Onesti, K. E. Kim, and J. H. Moyer. Grune & Stratton. New York, 1972.

34. Doyle, A. E., and Smirk, F. H. The neurogenic component in hypertension. *Circulation*, 1955, 12, 543–552.

35. Smirk, F. H. The neurologenically maintained component in hypertension. *Circ. Res.*, [*Suppl. 2*], 1972, 26–27, II-55–63.

36. Kezdi, P. Sinoaortic regulatory system role in pathogenesis of essential and malignant hypertension. *AMA Arch. Int. Med.*, 1953, 91, 26–34.

37. Kubicek, W. G., Kottke, F. J., Laker, D. J., and Visscher, M. B. Adaptation in pressor receptor reflex mechanisms in experimental neurogenic hypertension. *Am. J. Physiol.*, 1953, 175, 380–382.

38. Pickering, T. G., Gribbin, B., and Oliver, D. O. Baroreflex sensitivity in patients on long term haemodialysis. *Clin. Sci.*, 1972, 43, 645–657.

39. Sleight, P. Baroceptor function in hypertension. In: *Pathophysiology and Management of Arterial Hypertension*, edited by C. Berglund, L. Hansson, and L. Werko, pp. 45–43. Lindgren & Soner, Sweden, 1975.

40. McCubbin, J. W., Green, J. H., and Page, I. H. Baroreceptor function in chronic renal hypertension. *Circ. Res.*, 1956, 4, 205–210.

41. Benson, W. R., and Sealy, W. C. Arterial necrosis following resection of coarctation of the aorta. *Lab. Invest.*, 1956, 5, 359–376.
42. Folklow, B., Grimby, G., and Thulesius, O. Adaptive structural changes of the vascular walls in hypertension and their relation to the control of the peripheral resistance. *Acta Physiol. Scand.*, 1958, 44, 255–272.
43. Sivertsson, R. The haemodynamic importance of structural vascular changes in essential hypertension. *Acta Physiol. Scand.* [*Suppl.*], 1970, 343, 6–56.
44. Folklow, B., Hallbäck, M., Lundgren, Y., Sivertsson, R., and Weiss, L. Importance of adaptive changes in vascular design for establishment of primary hypertension studied in man and in spontaneously hypertensive rats. *Circ. Res.*, [*Suppl. I*], 1973, 32–33, 2–16.
45. Malmo, R. B., Shagass, C., and Davis, F. H. Symptom specificity and bodily reactions during psychiatric interview. *Psychosom. Med.*, 1950, 12, 362–366.
46. Lacey, J. I., and Lacey, B. C. The law of initial value in longitudinal study of autonomic constitution. Reproducibility of autonomic responses and response patterns over a four year interval. *Ann. NY Acad. Sci.*, 1962, 98, part 4, 1257–1290.
47. Wolf, S., and Wolff, H. G. A summary of experimental evidence relating life stress to the pathogenesis of essential hypertension in man. In: *Hypertension*, edited by E. T. Bell. University of Minnesota Press, Minneapolis, 1951.
48. Schachter, J. Pain, fear and anger in hypertensives and normotensives. *Psychosom. Med.*, 1957, 19, 17.
49. Innes, G., Miller, W. M., and Valentine, M. Emotion and blood pressure. *J. Med. Sci.*, 1959, 105, 840–851.
50. Shapiro, A. P. An experimental study of comparative responses of blood pressure to different noxious stimuli. *J. Chronic Dis.*, 1961, 13, 293–311.
51. Page, I. Arterial hypertension in retrospect. *Circ. Res.*, 1974, 34, 133–142.
52. Patel, C. *Biofeedback-Aided Behavioural Modification in the Management of Hypertension.* Doctoral dissertation, University of London, 1976.
53. Wallace, R. K., and Benson, H. The physiology of meditation. *Sci. Am.*, 1972, 226(2), 84–90.
54. Banquet, J. P. Spectral analysis of the EEG in meditation. *Electroencephalogr. Clin. Neurophysiol.*, 1973, 35, 143–151.
55. Hess, W. R. In: *Functional Organisation of Diencephalon*, edited by J. R. Hughes. Grune & Stratton, 1957.
56. Gellhorn, E. Motion and emotion: The role of proprioception in the physiology and pathology of the emotions. *Psychol. Rev.*, 1964, 71, 6, 457–472.
57. Bernhaut, M., Gellhorn, E., and Rasmussen, A. T. Experimental contributions to problem of consciousness. *J. Neurophysiol.*, 1953, 16, 21–35.
58. Hodes, R. Electrocostical synchronisation resulting from reduced proprioceptive drive caused by neuromuscular blocking agents. *Electroencephalogr. Clin. Neurophysiol.*, 1962, 14, 220–232.
59. Gellhorn, E., and Kiely, W. E. Mystical states of consciousness: Neurological and clinical aspects. *J. Nerv. Ment. Dis.*, 1972, 154, 399–405.
60. Datey, K. K., Deshmukh, S. N., Dalvi, C. P., and Vineker, S. L. "Shavasan." A yogic exercise in the management of hypertension. *Angiology*, 1969, 20, 325–333.
61. Lind, A. R., Taylor, S. H., Humphreys, P. W., Kennelly, B. M., and Donald, K. W. The circulatory effects of sustained voluntary muscle contraction. *Clin. Sci.*, 1964, 27, 229–244.
62. Kivowitz, C., Parmley, W. W., Donoso, R., Marcus, H., Ganz, W., and Swan, H. J. C. Effects of isometric exercise on cardiac performance. The grip test. *Circulation*, 1971, 44, 994–1002.
63. Benson, H., Beary, J. F., and Carol, M. P. The relaxation response. *Psychiatry*, 1974, 37, 37–46.
64. Stoyva, J., and Budzynski, T. Cultivated low arousal. An antistress response? In: *Biofeedback and Self Control 1974*, edited by L. V. Dicaria, T. X. Barber, J. Kamiya, N. E. Miller, D. Shapiro, and J. Stoyva. Aldine, Chicago, 1975.
65. Wolpe, J. *Psychotherapy by Reciprocal Inhibition.* Stanford University Press, Stanford, 1958.
66. Patel, C. H. Yoga and biofeedback in the management of hypertension. *Lancet*, 1973, ii, 1053–1055.

67. Patel, C. Biofeedback-aided relaxation and meditation in the management of hypertension. In: *Biofeedback and Self Regulation,* Plenum Press, New York, 1977.

68. Patel, C. A 12 month follow up of yoga and biofeedback in the management of hypertension. *Lancet,* 1975, i, 62–65.

69. Patel, C. H., and North, W. R. S. Randomised controlled trial of yoga and biofeedback in management of hypertension. *Lancet,* 1975, ii, 93–95.

70. Wright, B. M., and Dore, C. F. A random zero sphygmomanometer. *Lancet,* 1970, i, 337–338.

71. Althausen, T. L., and Keer W. J. Water-melon seed extract in the treatment of hypertension. *Am. J. Med. Sci.,* 1929, 178, 470–489.

72. Ayman, D. Evaluation of therapeutic results in essential hypertension: Interpretation of blood pressure reduction. *JAMA,* 1930, 95, 246.

73. Ayman, D., and Godshine, A. D. Blood pressure determinations by patients with essential hypertension: Differences between clinic and home readings before treatment. *Am. J. Med. Sci.,* 1940, 200, 465–474.

74. Grenfell, R. F., Briggs, A. H., and Holland, W. C. Antihypertensive drugs evaluated in a controlled double-blind study. *South. Med. J.,* 1963, 56, 1410–1415.

75. Crisp, A. Therapeutic aspects of the doctor/patient relationship. *Psychother. Psychosom.,* 1970, 18, 12–33.

76. Barath, E. Arterial hypertension and physical work. *Arch. Intern. Med.,* 1928, 42, 297–300.

77. Brod, J. Essential hypertension: Haemodynamic observations with a bearing on its pathogenesis. *Lancet,* 1960, ii, 773–778.

78. Engel, B. T., and Bickford, A. F. Response specificity stimulus: Response and individual response specificity in essential hypertensives. *Arch. Gen. Psychiatry,* 1961, 5, 478–489.

79. Sannerstedt, R. Haemodynamic response to exercise in patients with arterial hypertension. *Acta Med. Scand., [Suppl.],* 1966, 458, 5–83.

80. Amery, A., Julius, S., Whitlock, L. S., and Conway, J. Influence of hypertension on the haemodynamic response to exercise. *Circulation,* 1967, 36, 231.

81. Sokolow, M., Werdegar, D., Perloff, D. B., Cowan, R. M., and Porenenstuhl, H. Preliminary studies relating portably recorded blood pressures to daily life events in patients with essential hypertension. In: *Psychosomatics in Essential Hypertension,* edited by W. Koster, H. Musaph, and P. Visser. Karger, Basel, 1970.

82. Lorimer, A. R., Macfarlane, P. W., Provan, G., Duffy, D. T., and Lawrie, T. D. V. Blood pressure and catecholamine responses to stress in normotensive and hypertensive subjects. *Cardiovasc. Res.,* 1971, 5, 169–173.

83. Smirk, H. F. Pathogenesis of hypertension. In: *Anti-Hypertensive Agents,* edited by E. Schlitter. Academic Press, London, 1967.

84. Patel, C. Yoga and biofeedback in the management of stress in hypertensive patients. *Clin. Sci. Mol. Med. [Suppl.],* 1975, 48, 171–174.

85. Taylor, S. H. The circulation in hypertension. In: *Hypertension—Its Nature and Treatment.* Horsham, England, 1975.

86. Intersociety Commission for Heart Disease Resources. Primary prevention of the atherosclerotic diseases. *Circulation,* 1970, 42, A55–A95.

87. Marmot, M., and Winkelstein, W. Epidemiologic observation on intervention trials for prevention of coronary heart disease. *Am. J. Epidemiol.,* 1975, 101, 177–181.

88. Nixon, P. Human function curve with special reference to cardiovascular disorders. Part I. *Practitioner,* 1976, 217, 765–770.

89. Heberden, W. Some account of a disorder of the breast. In: *Cardiac Classics,* edited by F. A. Willins and T. E. Keys. C. V. Mosby, St. Louis, 1941.

90. Hunter, J. A treatise on the blood, inflammation and gunshot wounds. 1794. In: *Cardiac Classics,* edited by F. A. Willins and T. E. Keys. C. V. Mosby, St. Louis, 1941.

91. Friedman, M., and Rosenman, R. H. Association of specific overt behaviour pattern with blood and cardiovascular findings. Blood cholesterol level, blood clotting time, incidence of archus senilis and clinical coronary artery disease. *JAMA,* 1959, 169, 1286–1296.

92. Russek, H. I., and Zohman, B. L. Relative significance of heredity, diet and occupational stress in coronary heart disease of young adults. *Am. J. Med. Sci.,* 1958, 235, 266–277.

93. Friedman, M., Rosenman, R. H., and Carroll, V. Changes in the serum cholesterol and blood

clotting time in man subjected to cyclic variation of occupational stress. *Circulation,* 1958, 17, 852–861.

94. Thomas, C. B., and Murphy, E. A. Further studies on cholesterol levels in the Johns Hopkins Medical students, the effect of stress at examinations. *J. Chronic Dis.,* 1958, 8, 661.

95. Grundy, S. M., and Griffin, A. C. Effects of periodic mental stress on serum cholesterol levels. *Circulation,* 1959, 19, 496–498.

96. Dreyfuss, F., and Czaczkes, J. W. Blood cholesterol and uric acid of healthy medical students under the stress of an examination. *AMA Arch. Int. Med.,* 1959, 103, 708–711.

97. Taggart, P., and Carruthers, M. Endogenous hyperlipidaemia induced by emotional stress of racing driving. *Lancet,* 1971, i, 363–366.

98. Wolf, S., McCabe, W. R., Yamamoto, J. Changes in serum lipids in relation to emotional stress during rigid control of diet and exercise. *Circulation,* 1962, 26, 379–387.

99. Kennel, W. B. The role of cholesterol in coronary atherosclerosis. *Med. Clin. North Am.,* 1974, 58, 363–379.

100. Keys, A. Coronary heart disease in seven countries. *Circulation [Suppl. I],* 1970, 41–42, 1–199.

101. Groen, J. J., Tijong, B. K., Willebrandt, A. F., and Kamminga, C. J. Influence of nutrition, individuality and different forms of stress on blood cholesterol. Results experiment of a 9 months duration in 60 normal volunteers. *Proc. First Int. Congress Dietetics,* Voeding, 1959.

102. Medalie, J. H., Kahn, H. A., Neufeld, H. N. et al. Myocardial infarction over a five year period. I. Prevalence, incidence and mortality experience. *J. Chronic Dis.,* 1973, 26, 63–83.

103. Medalie, J. H., Kahn, H. A., Neufeld, H. N. et al. Five year myocardial infarction incidence II. Association of single variables to age and birthplace. *J. Chron. Dis.,* 1973b, 26, 329–349.

104. Prior, I. M., Harvey, H. P. B., Neave, M. I., and Davidson, F. *The Health of Two Groups of Cook Island Maoris.* Medical Research Council of New Zealand, Dept. of Health, 1966.

105. Labarthe, D., Reed, D., Brody, J., and Stallones, R. A. Health effects of modernisation in Palau. *Am. J. Epidemiol.,* 1973, 98, 161–174.

106. Keys, A., Aravanis, C., Blackburn, H. et al. Probability of middle aged men developing coronary heart disease in five years. *Circulation,* 1972, 45, 815–828.

107. Morris, J. N., and Gardener, M. J. Epidemiology of ischaemic heart disease. *Am. J. Med.,* 1969, 46, 674–683.

108. Gordon, T., Garcia-Palmieri, M. R., Kagan, A., Kannel, W. B., and Schiffman, J. Differences in coronary heart disease in Framingham, Honolulu and Puerto Rico. *J. Chron. Dis.,* 1974, 27, 329–344.

109. Marmot, M. G., Rose, G., Shipley, M., and Hamilton, P. J. S. Employment grade and coronary heart disease in British civil servants. *J. Epidemiol. Community Health,* 1978, 32, 244–249.

110. Gordon, T. Mortality experience among the Japanese in the United States, Hawaii and Japan. *Public Health Rep.,* 1957, 72, 543–553.

111. Marmot, M. G., Syme, S. L., Kagan, A., Kato, H., Cohen, J. B., and Belsky, J. Epidemiologic studies of coronary heart disease and stroke in Japanese men living in Japan, Hawaii and California: Prevalence of coronary and hypertensive *Am. J. Epidemiol.,* 1975, 102, 514–525.

112. Marmot, M. G., and Syme, S. L. Acculturation and coronary heart disease in Japanese-Americans. *Am. J. Epidemiol.,* 1976, 104, 225–246.

113. Patel, C. Reduction of serum cholesterol and blood pressure in hypertensive patients by behaviour modification. *J. R. Coll. Gen. Pract.,* 1976, 26, 211–215.

114. Patel, C., and Carruthers, M. Coronary risk factor reduction through biofeedback aided relaxation and meditation. *J. R. Coll. Gen. Pract.,* 1977, 27, 401–405.

115. Patel, C. H., Marmot, M., Terry, D. J., Carruthers, M., and Sever, P. Coronary risk factor reduction through biofeedback aided relaxation and meditation. Paper presented at the 52nd Annual Scientific Meeting, Anaheim, California. Oct., 1979, American Heart Association Abstracts, Circulation 60, No. 4, Abstract 882, II-226.

116. Rose, G. Standardisation of observers in blood pressure measurement. *Lancet,* 1965, i, 673–674.

117. Rose, G. Calculation of coronary risk using multiple logistic function from the London Whitehall study based on seven and a half years' mortality experience. *(Personal communication.)*

Stress and the Heart, edited by D. Wheatley,
Raven Press, New York © 1981.

Anxiety and Hypertension

David Wheatley

In the human, as in the animal experiments described, the physiologic response
to stress falls mainly on the cardiovascular system, adrenergic stimulation resulting in peripheral vasoconstriction and an increase in systemic blood pressure
(1). The analogous effects that occur in anxiety-provoking situations immediately
suggest an association, whether causal or effectual, between raised blood pressure
and anxiety.

The relationship between catecholamines and blood pressure has been investigated in two studies in age-matched hypertensives and normotensive controls.
In the first of these, Philipp et al. (2), in Germany, measured the plasma norepinephrine (NE) concentrations in 29 patients with essential hypertension aged
between 20 and 49 years and in 29 normotensive subjects aged between 20
and 48 years. These measurements were made both at rest and after a standardized exercise workload. The plasma NE concentration in the hypertensive patients was slightly elevated during recumbency, differing significantly from that
in the controls. This difference became even more significant during physical
exercise. The pressor response to exogenous NE was also measured. In the
normotensive subjects, it showed an inverse correlation with the plasma NE
concentration during physical exercise. In the hypertensive patients, this relationship was invariably disturbed, since the pressor response to NE was not diminished appropriately in the hypertensive patients with high plasma NE levels.
In those hypertensive patients with normal NE levels, the reactivity to exogenous
NE was inappropriately increased, the degree of disturbance increasing with
the severity of hypertension. The authors commented: "The findings suggest
that sympathetic nervous activity and pressor response to noradrenaline together
form an important determinant of the arterial blood-pressure levels."

In the second study, from the Netherlands, Hofman et al. (3) measured plasma
NE concentrations in 38 young people (aged 13 to 23 years) with potential
hypertension (initial BP, 140/90 mm Hg or more) compared to 39 aged-matched
controls from the same open population who were not potentially hypertensive.
The potentially hypertensive subjects had a significantly higher plasma NE concentration (mean, 351 pg/ml) compared with their controls (mean, 248 pg/
ml). These subjects were followed up for periods of 2 to 4 years. The findings
suggested that in teenagers and young adults, a persistently raised blood pressure
is associated with increased plasma NE concentrations. Furthermore, systolic
rather than diastolic pressures seem to be related to the excessive sympathetic

activity, since the plasma NE concentrations and systolic blood pressure levels were positively correlated.

CLINICAL BACKGROUND

Anxiety may be temporary or sustained, physiologic or pathologic. Acute anxiety, as a normal physiologic and emotional response to conflict situations occurring during life, can undoubtedly elevate blood pressure, in particular the systolic level. This is a normal defense mechanism, designed to enable an individual to respond to whatever emotional or stressful influence may have evoked the response. Nevertheless, such elevations of blood presssure are temporary and confined to the duration of the stress situation.

Anxiety symptoms that are inappropriate to the patient's emotional situation constitute a form of psychiatric illness that bears no relation to physiologic responses to stress. To what extent such individuals may be more susceptible to the development of hypertension is relatively unknown. Research studies undertaken by Heine and his colleagues (4) have produced some evidence to suggest that affective disorders may, in fact, lead to the development of hypertension. They investigated blood pressure in patients who had undergone prolonged periods of emotional disturbance (a long history of depressive illness with agitation). Their results supported the hypothesis that prolonged emotional disturbance leads to an irreversible increase in blood pressure, although contrary to their expectations, they found that ratings of anxiety and agitation (but not those of depression) were correlated with blood pressure levels when ill. Furthermore, patients who showed a fall in diastolic pressure on recovery were significantly more anxious and agitated when referred than those who did not. Robinson (5) investigated the relationship between symptoms (fatigue, palpitations, insomnia, breathlessness, anxiety, headache, dizziness, and depression) and the discovery of high blood pressure, and concluded: "Either people with high blood pressure have relatively severely a high number of the symptoms measured, or a certain pattern of symptoms is typical of them."

The Influence of Stress

There are a number of reports associating the stress of danger-involving situations with elevation in blood pressure. As long ago as 1945, Graham (6) reported an incidence of symptomless hypertension of 27% in 695 men after they had been involved in desert warfare for 1 year. For days on end even when there was no immediate danger, these men showed rapid pulse, pale face, and enlarged pupils. He speculated that this was the probable cause of the blood pressure elevation, particularly since this dropped after rest and relief of anxiety.

Cobb and Rose (7) investigated the incidence of hypertension, peptic ulcer, and diabetes in air traffic controllers and found that the incidence of hypertension was four times greater than in second class airmen (subjected to considerably less stress). Furthermore, air traffic controllers working with high traffic densities showed more cases of hypertension than those working with low traffic densities. Hypertension was diagnosed at an earlier age among high stress controllers as compared to their low stress colleagues. Finally, investigating the relationship between arterial pressure and automobile driving, Littler et al. (8) found: "There were short periods of raised arterial pressure during driving, related to such episodes as overtaking."

Mental stress of an intellectual nature has been studied by Bridges (9), who obtained data from 42 students, as measured by various physiologic responses to the strain of an academic oral examination. Anxiety was measured at the same time, using various psychologic tests. Highly significant rises were seen in both systolic and diastolic blood pressure after the stressful situation, as compared to the control period; this was associated with "high prevailing anxiety."

An example of extreme, life-endangering stress producing elevation in blood pressure was the 1947 Texas City disaster (10). On that occasion, a ship loaded with explosive chemicals blew up, setting off an even more disastrous explosion from a nearby chemical works. Reporting the incident, Ruskin et al. (10) commented that the force of the explosion "approached that of the Bikini atom bomb." These authors studied 408 casualties who were admitted to a local hospital, 180 of whom had previously attended the hospital, so that accurate records of their blood pressure prior to the explosion were available. They found a systolic blood pressure of 150 mm Hg or more in 90 of these 180 victims (50%) and a diastolic pressure of 95 mm Hg or more in 103 (i.e., over 50%). They then compared these records to 100 hospital patients who were not blast victims and, using the same criteria, found that the systolic pressure was only elevated in 25% and the diastolic in 34% of these patients. They found that in the blast victims blood pressure had risen during the 2- to 28-hr period after the explosion, and in most cases the rise took place 7 to 8 hr after. Blood pressure had returned to normal by 10 to 14 days later in most of these cases. Indeed, this would seem to be an example of nature providing the confirmation in man of the animal experiments described by Buckley.

An example of a more day-to-day stress causing elevation in blood pressure has been provided by Morrison and Morris (11) in their survey of 302 London busmen and conductors. They based their study on the assumption that the driver's job of negotiating busy London traffic is considerably more stressful than that of the conductor, who only collects fares from the passengers. They found that in the drivers, the average systolic blood pressure increased with age, the mean pressure being 147 mm Hg at ages 45 to 54 and 158 mm Hg at 55 to 60. However, the blood pressure elevations were confined to a small group of drivers whose parents had died in middle life. In those bus drivers whose parents lived to old age, systolic blood pressure in the 55- to 60-year-old group was distributed in a manner almost identical to that in the 45- to 54-year-old group; the average pressure of these men did not, in fact, rise with age. Furthermore, there were substantially more drivers with high blood pressure than conductors. Morrison and Morris commented that this evidence strongly suggests a hereditary cause for hypertension, but that this may be modifiable by environment, since use of the same classification (parents dying in middle age) for conductors revealed considerably fewer conductors with hypertension.

An association between stress of a different kind and hypertension was provided by Cruz-Coke (12) who studied 50 Peruvian policemen raised in the primitive environment of Cuzco in the eastern Andean highland and later trained in Lima. Twenty-one migrated to the capital some years before entering the police school, while 29 remained in Cuzco living in a non-Western society of the past until just before their police training began. Cruz-Coke compared blood pressure between these two groups and found that for those who left their native environment later, the mean diastolic was 65.1 mm Hg, whereas for the other group who settled in Lima earlier, it was 76.8 mm Hg. In other words, blood pressure tended to rise in those who moved to the capital where they were subjected to far greater stress and a more hectic way of life.

As long ago as 1939, Alexander (13) suggested that hypertension might be a manifestation of "repressed hostility." He suggested that one neurotic way of handling a conflict between aggressive impulses and social control is to repress those impulses, whereupon they provide a constant source of irritation, which produces a chronic elevation of blood pressure. He concluded that hypertensives should differ from normal individuals in two ways: they should exhibit a higher level of repressed hostility and be more neurotic.

ENVIRONMENTAL AND PERSONALITY INFLUENCES

A number of studies have been undertaken over the past two decades to investigate the effects of induced emotional stress on both normal subjects and those with elevated blood pressure. Wolf and Wolff (14), for example, administered stressful interviews to 16 normotensive and 21 hypertensive persons and found that both systolic and diastolic pressures were elevated in both groups of subjects as a result of the interviews. Several investigations of psychosocial factors in relation to raised blood pressure have been undertaken. Wolf et al. (15) studied 58 hypertensive patients and compared them to 42 normal individuals and 150 patients suffering from vasomotor rhinitis and asthma. This was a prospective study undertaken over 1 to 3 years, and personalities, attitudes, habits, and general behavior were studied in these cases. The authors found that the hypertensives were more offensive than the normal individuals, and that the asthmatics, on the other hand, were more defensive. In their comments on the study, they drew a comparison between reactions of the car driver who is faced with an emergency situation and the development of hypertension. The driver becomes tense and sits on the edge of the seat, this being the primitive "readiness to spring" reaction to a stressful situation. In the context of a car crash, it is, in fact, the most inappropriate attitude, and the driver would do better to relax and curl up on the floor! Similarly, hypertensives may meet threats arising out of problems in their day-to-day living with an attitude of restrained aggression inappropriate to their illness. Thus hypertension may be an illness that occurs when this essentially emergency pattern is adopted as a way of life.

An even more fundamental approach to the problem has been made by Kalis et al. (16), who assessed a group of young female college students exposed to an emotion-provoking, interpersonally stressful situation. They divided their subjects into two groups designated, respectively, as "prehypertensives" and "normals." The criteria for this division were: a systolic blood pressure of at least 140 mm Hg and/or a diastolic blood pressure of at least 90 mm Hg for the prehypertensives, and a systolic pressure of less than 120 mm Hg and/or less than 80 mm Hg diastolic for the normals. They found that the prehypertensive women were less well controlled, more egocentric, and generally less adaptable than the control subjects. In other words, they would be more vlunerable in life situations involving emotional stress, and it is just such situations that may initiate the processes leading to hypertension. They reexamined their subjects 4 years later and found that these characteristics were even more apparent in the prehypertensive women now that they had assumed their postcollege roles.

Returning to the clinical field of established hypertension, Gressel et al. (17) studied 50 hypertensives, comparing these to 50 matched patients with psychosomatic complaints and 50 with chronic medical or surgical illnesses (i.e., with low psychologic factors). These investigators used a six-item rating scale, each item being assessed on a defined five-point severity scale. The assessed items were: impulsiveness, subnormal assertiveness, obsessive-compulsive behavior, depressive behavior, anxiety, and hysteria. They then calculated correlations between the three groups of patients on the one hand and the psychologic ratings on the other. They found that the ratings of obsessive-compulsive behavior and subnormal assertiveness significantly differentiated the hypertensive patients from those with personality disorders who were nonhypertensive, but this was not so with any of the other ratings. All the rated items, with the exception of impulsiveness, significantly differentiated the hypertensive patients from those with chronic somatic disorders. On the other hand, all items except obsessive-compulsive behavior and subnormal assertiveness differentiated the two control groups from each other. The authors concluded that obsessive-compulsive behavior and subnormal assertiveness were characteristics peculiar to the hypertensives, although they were careful to point out that these were concomitant associations and not necessarily etiologic relationships.

Finally, Harburg et al. (18) examined 800 male college students and selected 74 who were classified as having either high or low systolic blood pressures. These two groups were then subclassified according to three blood pressure parameters as follows: paired casual blood pressure, usual blood pressure, and sustained blood pressure levels. The "casual blood pressure" was defined as being the average of two casual readings taken on separate occasions 1 month apart: the "paired casual" was defined as a systolic pressure that remained either high or low for both of these readings. The "usual" blood pressure was the median of six self-determined measurements together with the average of three measurements taken by the physician after 20 min bed rest (there was, in fact, a high correlation between these two methods). Finally, "sustained" blood pressure was determined in those cases where the blood pressure was either high or low as measured by both the average casual reading and the usual reading. The definitions used to signify high and low were over 140 mm Hg and under 110 mm Hg, respectively. All diastolic pressures in these patients were below 90 mm Hg.

These investigators then assessed psychiatric morbidity on the Cattell 16 PF Test and the Mandler-Sarason Test Anxiety Questionnaire and found some significant correlations. On nine items from the Cattell scale, with the average casual blood pressure, there were significant correlations with: submissiveness, sensitivity, warm-sociable, dependent, suspecting, neurotic, and introversion. For the usual blood pressure, there were significant correlations with: sensitivity, neuroticism, anxiety, and test-anxiety; for the paired casual blood pressure, there were significant correlations with: submissiveness, sensitivity, warm-sociable, and anxiety. Finally, there was one significant correlation with sustained blood pressure, namely, sensitivity. These correlations were all significant at the 5% level. These findings raised the possibility that anxiety and neuroticism are more closely associated with a tendency to greater blood pressure lability than with sustained hypertension.

Thus there is considerable clinical evidence for some association between psychiatric symptoms and hypertension. In particular, stressful and anxiety-provoking situations have been implicated, as have depressive illness and individual aggressiveness. Therefore, we decided to initiate a survey, the overall object of which was to determine whether there is more psychiatric morbidity associated with hypertension, and, if so, to understand its nature (19) and determine whether or not concomitant treatment with an appropriate psychotropic drug might be indicated.

PSYCHIATRIC SYMPTOMATOLOGY IN HYPERTENSION

The survey was undertaken by 90 members of the General Practitioner Research Group in England, each investigator recording data on four cases as follows:

Group 1. The first new (undiagnosed) case of hypertension.

Group 2. The next patient seen, for whatever cause, matched for age and sex (i.e., new hypertensive control).

Group 3. The first old case of hypertension (i.e., already diagnosed and probably under treatment).

Group 4. The next patient seen, for whatever cause, matched to the old hypertensive case for age and sex.

For each of these cases, four forms were completed as follows:

1. Demographic data (personal and social history over the past 18 months).
2. Symptom self-rating scale (58 psychiatric symptoms experienced over the past 12 months) (20,21).
3. Life situation form (good and bad events over the past 18 months) completed by patient (22).
4. Physician's report. This included the relevant data concerning hypertension, together with details of other medical conditions and complaints, with records of blood pressure readings in the recumbent position after 3 min at rest, pulse rate, weight, and height. In addition, records were made of all medications the patient was taking, both for hypertension and for other conditions, including psychotropic drugs. Finally, the physician assessed the following psychiatric symptoms on a five-point severity scale (not present, mild, moderate, severe, and extremely severe): (a) anxiety (fearful, nervous, tense, etc.); (b) depression (sad, blue, hopeless about the future, etc.); and (c) anger-hostility (sullen, short-tempered, irritable, etc.).

Analysis of variance was used to test for significant differences.

The objects of the survey were as follows. In new cases, hypertension is discovered from routine examination or because symptoms (i.e., headache) lead the doctor to take the blood pressure. In most cases, because the patient is unaware that he has raised blood pressure, any associated psychiatric symptomatology, if greater than the controls, suggests cause rather than effect. (It can be argued that the establishment of the diagnosis of hypertension by taking the blood pressure will almost certainly induce anxiety symptoms in most cases, but the self-rating scale was recorded as it applied to the past 1 year, i.e., symptoms that were present before the current consultation.)

In the old cases, there may be more or less psychiatric morbidity, for the patient now knows he has high blood pressure and may worry over this, or, alternatively, as a result of treatment he may feel more reassured. If, therefore, psychiatric morbidity is higher than in the controls and higher than in new cases, this would suggest an effect. In the new cases, there will not as yet have been any medication; these can be compared to old cases under treatment, and this should determine whether lowering the blood pressure relieves psychiatric symptoms and whether the concomitant use of psychotropic drugs is indicated.

The systolic blood pressure is markedly affected by emotional factors, whereas the diastolic is not. Comparison of psychiatric symptoms to these separate measures may give further insights into the role of psychiatric abnormality in the condition. Thus an association between high psychiatric symptomatology and high systolic blood pressure would suggest a functional relationship, whereas a similar association with high diastolic blood pressure would suggest an organic relationship.

Demographic Data

A total of 348 case reports were suitable for analysis, 87 in each of the four groups. The following data were recorded: sex, age, marital status, number of children, number of children living at home, proportion living with spouse, proportion with up to 11 years + education (less than 7 years of school), and proportion with other medical conditions.

With the exception of mean age and percentage of patients with other medical conditions, the four groups matched one another very well in the various items of demographic data recorded. The mean age was higher in the older hypertensive and control groups (3 and 4), as would have been expected, and the percentage of patients with other medical conditions was higher in the two control groups, also as expected.

Results of the Survey

On the physicians' ratings, there were no patients with extremely severe symptoms. Figure 15.1 shows the proportions of patients in the four groups, with the other degrees of psychiatric symptoms.

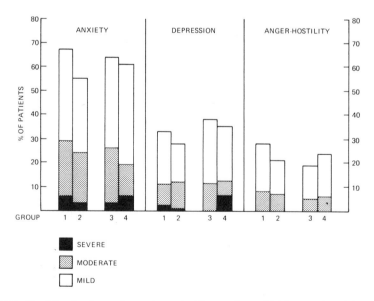

FIG. 15.1. Physicians' ratings of symptoms. Incidence of psychiatric symptomatology in new cases of hypertension (Group 1) and old cases (Group 3), as compared to their respective controls (Groups 2 and 4). (Reproduced by kind permission of the editor of the British Journal of Psychiatry.

It is apparent that, in all four groups, anxiety symptoms were more frequent than those of either depression or anger-hostility. Thus no fewer than 58 (67%) of the new hypertensive patients and 56 (64%) of the old hypertensive patients exhibited symptoms of anxiety, although in the majority these were only mild or moderate. Although the incidence of anxiety symptoms was less in the control groups, the differences were not statistically significant. There were no significant differences between the hypertensive groups and their respective controls for symptoms of either depression or anger-hostility.

On the self-rating assessments, there were no significant differences in any of the four groups with respect to the various factor and cluster scores of the scale or in relation to the total scores.

Both new and old hypertensive cases had raised systolic and diastolic blood pressures in relation to their control groups, indicating that despite hypotensive drug treatment, blood pressure was not fully controlled in group 4. The incidence of complications directly attributable to hypertension was comparatively high also in the old hypertensive cases.

ANTIANXIETY DRUGS IN HYPERTENSION

The survey on psychiatric factors in hypertension failed to show significant differences in psychiatric symptomatology between patients with hypertension and their matched controls. This is in keeping with an investigation undertaken by Meyer et al. (23), who evaluated manifest psychologic symptom levels associated with hypertension among primarily black patients of lower socioeconomic status. The authors also used the HSCL self-rating scale and a semistructured interview which involved a total of 698 patients, aged between 16 and 65 years for men and 16 and 62 years for women. On a number of their test measures, there was a significantly lower incidence of emotional disturbance in the hypertensive as compared to the normotensive subjects. There was good agreement between the scores recorded on the symptom dimensions in this study and those recorded in our own survey. The majority of hypertensive patients in this study, however, were presumably receiving specific treatment for their hypertension; this may act as an anxiety-relieving factor, although it did not appear to be the case in the old hypertensive patients in our survey. Another negative report of an association between affective disorder and hypertension is provided by Seidel (24), who found such a relationship for paranoid states (205 patients) but not for affective disorders (nonparanoid) (320 patients), schizophrenias (100 patients), or personality disorder (79 patients).

Nevertheless, in our survey of the three main symptom groups investigated, anxiety symptoms occurred considerably more frequently than symptoms of either depression or anger-hostility. Although these symptoms were only of mild or moderate severity in the majority of cases, and although other patients without hypertension may exhibit a similar degree of mild and moderate anxiety symptoms, it is important to assess whether such symptoms play a part in the control of hypertension by drug therapy.

That both systolic and diastolic blood pressures in hypertensive patients are susceptible to psychologic control is amply demonstrated in the previous chapter by Patel. Similar results in less hypertensive individuals have been obtained by Benson et al. in Boston (25), with relaxation induced by transcendental meditation. Conversely, central sympathetic stimulation may increase blood pressure, and psychologic stresses are important factors in producing this effect (26–28). Kristt and Engel (29) have demonstrated that blood pressure can be brought under voluntary control through "operant conditioning," using colored-light instructions and audible recordings of the patient's own blood pressure. Thus their five patients learned to raise or lower their blood pressure at will, and this ability was still retained 3 months after the instruction period. Changes of systolic blood pressure of 40 to 50 mm Hg in either direction were achieved by this method.

It is apparent that control of blood pressure, and particularly the systolic levels, may be influenced by a number of stress factors, of which anxiety may be a significant one. It is important to determine whether or not the use of anxiety-relieving drugs may be beneficial in the treatment of hypertension.

Trial of a Benzodiazepine

The following advantages might be achieved by adding an antianxiety drug to standard treatment with hypotensive drugs: (a) better control of systolic and/or diastolic blood pressure, (b) better control of anxiety symptoms, (c) less postural hypotension (systolic more susceptible to psychic influences), (d) a lower dose of hypotensive drugs to achieve the same effect, and (e) a reduced incidence of complications (which may be related to systolic "swings").

Accordingly, a double-blind comparative trial was undertaken by the General Practitioner Research Group (30) to compare treatment of hypertension with methyldopa + placebo and methyldopa + the antianxiety drug medazepam (Nobrium®) (31). Methyldopa (Aldomet®) was chosen as the standard antihypertensive drug, because at the time of the trial (1974) this was the drug most frequently used to treat hypertension in Great Britain (32). The use of this drug has since declined owing to its side effects; it has been replaced mainly by the beta-blocking drugs (33). Medazepam is a benzodiazepine that has been available in Great Britain for some time and has been shown to be equally effective to, if not slightly better than, established drugs of this series, such as chlordiazepoxide (Librium®) and diazepam (Valium®) (34).

The trial was conducted over a 2-month period with subsequent follow-up assessments at 6-month intervals. The dose of medazepam was 10 to 20 mg t.d.s. and that of methyldopa 250 to 500 mg q.d.s. or whatever might be appropriate to control blood pressure. The trial involved a total of 71 patients. On breaking the code, it was found that 38 patients had received medazepam together with methyldopa, whereas the remaining 33 had received placebo together with methyldopa.

Blood pressure was measured in the upright position and again after 3 min in the recumbent position. Anxiety was measured in three ways: (a) GPRG physicians' rating (maximum score, 36) (30), (b) HSCL 58-item self-rating checklist (maximum score, 174) (20,21,30), and (c) defined global ratings (maximum score, 3) (30).

Results on the three anxiety rating scales were similar. Figure 15.2 shows the mean changes in the physicians' anxiety ratings and systolic and diastolic pressure in the resting position for the 2-month period of the trial and the first 6-month follow up.

Between-period mean values were tested for statistical significance using analysis of covariance, but no significant differences were present in relation to either relief of anxiety or reduction in blood pressure in either the supine or upright position.

Further analyses were undertaken in relation to cases where normotension was achieved (systolic, 150 mm Hg or less; diastolic, 95 mm Hg or less) by the end of the trial period and, conversely, in relation to those patients experiencing a satisfactory relief of anxiety symptoms (final score of 3 or less on the GPRG rating). These results are shown in Tables 15.1 and 15.2.

It should be noted that the initial mean anxiety rating was relatively low compared to trials in anxiety states, where the usual level is between 16 to 20 on this scale. Nevertheless, all but two patients in the medazepam-treated group and all but three patients in the placebo group exhibited some symptoms of anxiety initially. Furthermore, taking a score of 10 as indicating an appreciable degree of anxiety, in the medazepam group there were nine such cases (27%)

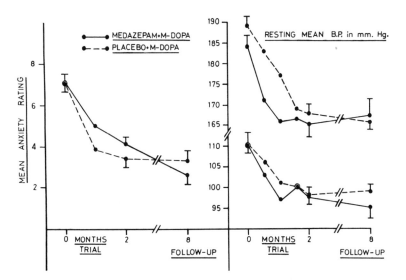

FIG. 15.2. Relief of anxiety and reduction in blood pressure in patients treated with either medazepam + methyldopa or placebo + methyldopa.

TABLE 15-1. *Hypotensive effect and relief of anxiety: medazepam and placebo*

	Systolic normal			Systolic still raised		
	Mean anxiety score			Mean anxiety score		
	Initial	8 Weeks	Improvement (%)	Initial	8 Weeks	Improvement (%)
Medazepam	8.0	2.7	66[a]	7.0	4.8	31
Placebo	7.7	3.9	49	6.6	3.2	52[b]
Totals	7.8	3.3	58[b]	6.8	4.0	41[b]
	Diastolic normal			Diastolic still raised		
Medazepam	9.8	5.1	48[a]	4.9	3.2	35
Placebo	6.3	2.6	59[a]	7.3	3.9	47[a]
Totals	8.5	4.1	52[a]	6.2	3.6	42[b]

[a] $p < 0.05$; [b] $p < 0.01$.

initially and in the placebo group, eight cases (24%). The figures for the incidence and severity of anxiety symptoms in hypertension, as recorded in this clinical trial, confirm those recorded in the survey described earlier. In fact, the incidence of anxiety symptoms in the patients treated in this study was even higher than that recorded in the survey. It is apparent, however, that neither relief of anxiety nor control of blood pressure was any better when the antianxiety drug was added to the hypotensive drug treatment than when the placebo was added.

When the systolic pressure became normal by the end of the trial, there was a greater relief of anxiety symptoms with medazepam (66%) than with placebo (49%) When it remained raised at the end of the trial, however, the improvement in anxiety symptoms was considerably less with medazepam (31%) than with placebo (52%) Analysis of covariance did not show any significant differences between the two types of patients. In the patients treated with meda-

TABLE 15-2. *Relief of anxiety and blood pressure changes in mm Hg: medazepam and placebo*

Relief of anxiety	Medazepam					Placebo				
	Initial		Final	Fall		Initial		Final	Fall
Good	179	→	156	24		187	→	166	21
	—		—	—		—		—	—
	110	→	95	15		108	→	96	12
Poor	189	→	180	9		201	→	182	19
	—		—	—		—		—	—
	110	→	102	8		117	→	107	10

zepam in whom there was good relief of anxiety symptoms, there were greater falls in the mean levels of both systolic and diastolic pressures than in the placebo-treated patients. None of the differences was statistically significant. The most marked difference was a negative one; when relief of anxiety was poor with medazepam, mean blood pressure falls were considerably less than in any of the other three groups of patients.

The results of this study do not provide any evidence that the addition of the antianxiety drug medazepam to standard hypotensive drug therapy resulted in either better relief of anxiety symptoms or better control of either systolic or diastolic blood pressures; nor was there any "sparing" effect on the methyldopa dosage required to control blood pressure. As postural hypotension was negligible in both groups of patients, there was no advantage in this respect either.

Propranolol

It is well established in the treatment of hypertension that the beta-adrenergic blocking drugs are also effective antianxiety agents (see Chapter 6) A further study was undertaken to assess relief of anxiety symptoms and control of blood pressure, along similar lines, in a comparison between propranolol alone and methyldopa alone (31,35).

This trial was slightly different from the previous one; there was an initial "run-in" dose-adjustment period of 2 to 4 weeks, followed by a trial period of 12 instead of 8 weeks. This was to allow for the relatively slow build-up of the antihypertensive effect that occurs with propranolol.

Results were obtained on 78 patients, 36 treated with propranolol and 42 with methyldopa. Figure 15.3 shows the changes in the anxiety ratings and the supine systolic and diastolic blood pressures.

As in the case of the previous trial, the initial anxiety levels were relatively low; as before, the proportion of patients with anxiety symptoms of whatever degree was relatively high. There were only three patients who did not complain of any anxiety symptoms initially in the group treated with propranolol (9%) and only four such patients in the group treated with methyldopa (10%). Using the same criterion of a score of 10 or more as indicating an appreciable level of anxiety symptoms, in the propranolol group there were seven such cases (20%) and in the methyldopa group 11 (26%).

The differences between pre- and postscores were tested for significance, using Student's *t*-test. In the patients treated with propranolol, the mean anxiety score fell from 5.6 (SE $\pm$ 0.8) initially to 3.5 (SE $\pm$ 0.8) by the end of the trial, a difference which is not statistically significant. In the case of the patients treated with methyldopa, the equivalent mean anxiety score fell from 6.8 (SE $\pm$ 0.8) initially to 2.9 (SE $\pm$ 0.6) by the end of the trial, a difference which is highly significant ($p < 0.001$). The patient self-rating scales were analyzed in like manner; it was found that in the patients treated with propranolol, there was again a nonsignificant reduction in anxiety symptoms but a significant reduction in

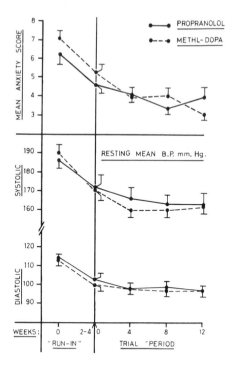

FIG. 15-3. Relief of anxiety and reduction in blood pressure in patients treated with either propranolol or methyldopa.

the patients treated with methyldopa at 4, 8, and 12 weeks ($p < 0.05$ at each period, respectively).

These results are strongly against any specific antianxiety effect being exerted by the beta-blocking drug. The reductions in both systolic and diastolic blood pressures were virtually identical with the two drugs, raising the possibility that methyldopa may have exerted specific antianxiety effects in these patients. Alternatively, of course, the improvement may have been entirely nonspecific and associated with the reduction in blood pressure achieved as a result of drug therapy.

To elucidate this point, the cases were stratified as in the previous study, with selection of those in whom normal systolic and diastolic pressures were achieved by the end of the trial, and also those where significant relief of anxiety was achieved. It was found that when either systolic or diastolic pressure became normal by the end of the trial, there was a highly significant relief of anxiety symptoms for all cases taken together, this relief being statistically significant for the methyldopa-treated cases but not for those treated with propranolol. In the patients where normotension was not achieved (either systolic or diastolic), relief of anxiety was statistically significant with methyldopa but not with propranolol.

With propranolol, there were greater reductions in mean systolic and diastolic pressures (both statistically significant) in those patients in whom relief of anxiety was good, as compared to those in whom relief of anxiety was poor (no significant differences). In the case of methyldopa, the falls in mean systolic and diastolic pressures were similar in these two groups of patients, and statistically significant in both groups. Moreover, the level of statistical significance was much greater in those patients in whom there was good relief of anxiety ($p < 0.001$) than in those in whom there was poor relief ($p < 0.05$). This finding applied to the changes in both systolic and diastolic pressures.

These results confirm the conclusions made from the previous trial, namely, that there was an association between relief of anxiety and the degree of reduction of both systolic and diastolic pressures, whether this association might be cause or effect.

Depression and Somatic Symptoms

As discussed in Chapter 6, it has been claimed that propranolol specifically relieves the somatic manifestations of anxiety but not the psychic component (36), and that the drug may induce rather than relieve depressive symptoms (37). On the other hand, Snaith and McCoubrie (38) were unable to find any evidence of a relationship between the administration of methyldopa and other antihypertensive drugs and depressive illness.

It was of interest to analyze separately the two items from the rating scale concerned, respectively, with "anxiety" and "hysterical symptoms and somatization." In the scale used, these are single items, both of which can score a maximum severity of four. Many of the patients did not complain of either depression or somatic symptoms at any stage of the trial; such patients were excluded from this analysis. Regarding depression, the analysis concerns 15 patients treated with propranolol and 24 with methyldopa; regarding somatization, it concerns 15 treated with propranolol and 22 with methlydopa. Table 15.3 shows the mean prepost scores for depression and somatization in these patients.

Although the mean depression score fell somewhat with propranolol by the end of the trial, this change was not statistically significant, whereas with methyldopa there was a considerable fall, which was significant at the 1% level. For

TABLE 15-3. *Changes in mean scores for depression and somatization*

Item	Propranolol (± SEM)		Methyldopa (± SEM)	
Depression	1.1 (± 0.2)	→ 0.7 (± 0.2)	1.2 (± 0.2)	→ 0.4[b] (± 0.1)
Somatization	1.5 (± 0.2)	→ 0.7[a] (± 0.2)	1.1 (± 0.2)	→ 0.4[b] (± 0.1)

[a] $p < 0.05$; [b] $p < 0.01$.

somatic symptoms, there were significant falls in severity with both drugs, although the fall was greater with methyldopa ($p < 0.01$) than for propranolol ($p < 0.05$). It is clear that there was no specific effect of propranolol in the relief of somatic symptoms, as compared to methyldopa, but neither was there any increase in severity of depressive symptoms with the beta-blocking drug.

INITIAL SEVERITIES OF ANXIETY AND HYPERTENSION

Further analyses were made of the data from these two trials to answer the following questions. (a) Is a high initial blood pressure associated with a high level of anxiety? (b) Does the previous response to treatment influence the relief of anxiety symptoms?

Initial Blood Pressure and Anxiety

Cases from both trials were stratified into two groups according to the initial scores on the GPRG ratings as follows: score 10 or more = high anxiety; score 5 or less = low anxiety.

Cases coming between these two categories were discarded, and these two groups of patients were analyzed in relation to the initial level of supine blood pressure. Table 15.4 shows the mean initial blood pressures in these two groups of patients. When the initial level of anxiety was high, the mean systolic blood pressure was higher (191.7 mm Hg) than when the initial level of anxiety was low (182.8 mm Hg). This difference does not even approach statistical significance.

Whether the initial level of anxiety was high or low made little difference in the initial mean diastolic pressure. It does not appear that anxiety symptoms as recorded in this trial were related to the initial levels of either systolic or diastolic pressure.

Effects of Previous Treatment

In both studies, patients were included who had had no previous treatment for their blood pressure, as well as patients to whom previous treatment had been given with varying degrees of effectiveness in reducing blood pressure. Patients from both studies were divided into three groups: those where no previ-

TABLE 15-4. *Initial anxiety in relation to initial blood pressure*

Initial anxiety	No.	Mean blood pressure	
		Systolic	Diastolic
High	33	191.7 ± 5.4	112.4 ± 2.2
Low	61	182.8 ± 3.5	111.0 ± 1.7

ous treatment had been given, those where previous treatment had been successful, and those where previous treatment had failed. For the purpose of allocating patients to the results-of-treatment categories, the initial supine blood pressure levels were used according to the following definitions:

Success: systolic 160 mm Hg or less, *or*
           diastolic 95 mm Hg or less
Failure: systolic 200 mm Hg or more, *or*
         diastolic 115 mm Hg or more.

Cases in the intermediate categories were discarded, leaving a total of 41 cases in whom there had been no previous treatment, 14 in whom previous treatment had been successful, and 42 in whom previous treatment had failed. The initial and final mean anxiety ratings for these three groups of patients are shown in Table 15.5.

The initial mean anxiety scores were similar in all three groups. It might have been expected that patients for whom previous treatment had failed might have exhibited more anxiety symptoms than either those in whom previous treatment had been successful or those in whom there had been no previous treatment. It is apparent from the analysis of the initial mean anxiety ratings that this was not the case, and that the degree of anxiety was not associated with previous treatment.

Considering the degrees of improvement in the three treatment groups, the greatest improvement (63%) was exhibited by the patients who had not received previous treatment, whereas the improvement shown in the remaining two groups was exactly the same, namely, 42%. The improvements in anxiety ratings shown by the two groups where there had either been no previous treatment or where previous treatment had failed were both highly significant, although the improvement shown in the remaining group, where previous treatment had been successful, was not significant (however, this is probably because there was only a relatively small number of cases in this group). A further analysis, using Student's *t*-test, was undertaken to compare the final mean ratings between the group where there had either been no previous treatment and the group where previous treatment had failed, but the difference was not statistically significant.

TABLE 15-5. *Relief of anxiety in relation to previous treatment*

Previous treatment	Mean anxiety scores ±SEM		
	Initial	Final	Improvement (%)
None	6.7 ± 0.8	2.5 ± 0.6	63[b]
Successful	6.9 ± 1.6	4.0 ± 1.3	42
Failure	6.9 ± 0.7	4.0 ± 0.6	42[a]

[a] $p < 0.01$; [b] $p < 0.001$.

It does not appear that improvement in anxiety symptoms during these two trials was related to previous treatment either.

LORAZEPAM AND BENDROFLUAZIDE

The tranquilizing effects of reserpine were well known (39) for only a brief period before it was superceded by the phenothiazines and its effects in lowering blood pressure were discovered. Methyldopa, in addition to having antihypertensive actions, exerts effects on the central nervous system analogous to those of reserpine (40,41). Indeed, as with reserpine, drowsiness and depression may occur in clinical use.

Our choice of methyldopa as the standard antihypertensive drug to combine with antianxiety drugs in the treatment of hypertension was an unfortunate one. In the two trials described, antianxiety effects were produced by methyldopa, and these may have obscured any beneficial effects from the other drugs used. To continue our studies, it was necessary to choose an antihypertensive drug without any potential antianxiety effects per se. The thiazide diuretics are a standard form of antihypertensive drug therapy, either alone in the milder cases of hypertension or, more commonly, combined with other antihypertensive drugs. Indeed, Wilcox (42), following a comparative study between six beta-blocking drugs and bendrofluazide in essential hypertension, came to the conclusion that: "Bendrofluazide was equal or superior to all the beta-blockers except atenolol in reducing resting blood pressure, and its cheapness still makes it an agent of first choice in mild or moderate essential hypertension." We had in fact been deterred from using this drug previously, owing to its relatively mild antihypertensive effect; but clearly, since neither sedation nor tranquilization has ever been recorded with this type of compound, it became the most suitable agent for our further studies.

The trial was a double-blind comparison between the antianxiety drug lorazepam (Ativan®) and placebo added to bendrofluazide (or placebo) as the antihypertensive drug (43). After an initial control period of 2 weeks, during which no treatment was given, treatment with the trial preparations was for 6 weeks with one of the following medication combinations: (a) lorazepam (20 to 30 mg nocte) + bendrofluazide (5 to 10 mg mane) (group LB); (b) lorazepam (20 to 30 mg nocte) + placebo (1 to 2 mane) (group L); (c) bendrofluazide (5 to 10 mg mane) + placebo (2 to 3 nocte) (group B); (d) placebo lorazepam (2 to 3 nocte) + placebo bendrofluazide (1 to 2 mane) (group P).

Allocation to treatment groups was determined by random selection.

Patient Characteristics

A number of items of patient data were recorded which might have an influence on either blood pressure or anxiety. Table 15.6 summarizes some of the more important of these. Forty-four patients were included in the trial, females exceed-

TABLE 15.6. *Various items of data concerned with the characteristics of the patients in the four treatment groups*

	L	LB	B	P	Totals
Male:female	5:4	4:6	5:6	2:12	16:28
Mean age	52.9	54	50.8	57.6	54 (±1.7)
Married	6	7	9	13	35 (80%)
Hypertension					
No family history	4	6	8	9	27 (69%)
Mild:moderate	5:4	7:3	5:6	8:5	25:18
Under 3 years	7	8	9	12	36 (88%)
No previous drugs	7	8	9	8	32 (73%)
Anxiety					
Previous symp-					
toms	6	8	10	8	32 (73%)
No previous drugs	6	6	7	10	29 (66%)
Nonsmokers	4	8	5	8	25 (57%)
Nondrinkers	4	6	5	9	24 (55%)

ing males, with a mean age of 54 years (SEM ± 1.7) and the majority (80%) married. In most cases, there was no family history of hypertension (69%). Since we were not using a particularly potent antihypertensive drug in this trial, only mild (diastolic 90 to 104 mm Hg) and moderate (diastolic 105 to 114 mm Hg) cases were included, and there was a small preponderance of the former. The majority of patients had had hypertension for less than 3 years (88%) and had not received any previous antihypertensive drugs (73%). On the other hand, the majority of patients had had previous anxiety symptoms (73%), although the majority had not received any previous antianxiety drug treatment (66%). Finally, patients were almost equally divided between non-smokers and smokers, and nondrinkers (alcohol) and drinkers, respectively.

Hypotensive Effects

Blood pressure was recorded after the patient had been supine for 3 min and again in the upright position. The mean systolic and diastolic levels in the supine position are shown in Fig. 15.4

Using the paired t-test to test for significant pre-post differences, during the 2-week control period, there were nonsignificant reductions of similar order in systolic and diastolic pressures in all four treatment groups. At the end of 5 weeks of treatment with the trial preparations, the reductions in mean systolic and diastolic pressures with lorazepam (as compared to the end of the control period) were not statistically significant, although the reduction in diastolic pressure was nearly significant ($p = 0.053$). On the other hand, in the group treated with lorazepam + bendrofluazide, there was a significant reduction in both systolic and diastolic blood pressures ($p < 0.01$). In the group treated

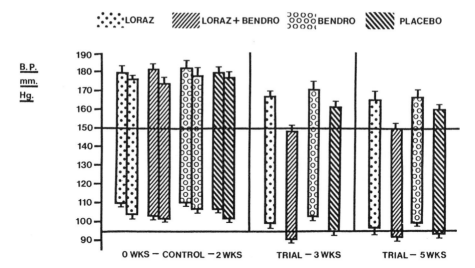

FIG. 15.4. Mean B.P. (supine) in mm Hg in the four treatment groups. Reprinted with permission of Elsevier/North Holland.

with bendrofluazide, there were also significant reductions in both mean systolic pressure ($p < 0.05$) and mean diastolic pressure ($p < 0.01$); this was also the case in the placebo group (systolic $p < 0.002$, diastolic $p < 0.02$).

The greatest reductions in mean systolic and diastolic pressures were recorded in the group of patients treated with lorazepam + bendrofluazide and the next greatest in the group treated with bendrofluazide. Analysis of covariance was used to test for between-group differences, but there were no significant differences for either systolic or diastolic pressure in any of the four groups.

Diurnal Variations

That there is a circadian variation of blood pressure has been demonstrated by Millar-Craig et al. (44). Continuous intraarterial blood pressure and electrocardiogram recordings were obtained in 20 hypertensive and five normotensive ambulant patients. The authors found that blood pressure was highest midmorning and then fell progressively throughout the day, being lowest at 3 a.m. and beginning to rise again during the early hours of the morning before waking.

During the sixth and final week of our trial, blood pressure was measured every day, morning and evening, to assess the importance of diurnal blood pressure variations. The results, shown in Fig. 15.5, are presented as the extent to which the mean systolic and diastolic pressures varied during this last week above the lowest reading recorded at any one measurement. It can be seen that this variation was comparatively slight in all four groups, not exceeding 10 mm Hg in the case of systolic pressures and little more than 5 mm Hg in the case of diastolic pressures. Diurnal variation was not an important factor

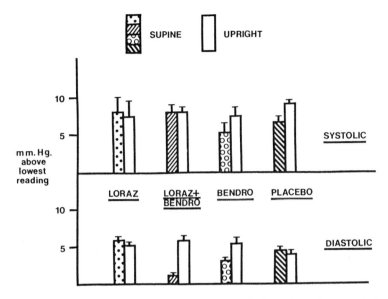

FIG. 15.5. Mean B.P. readings (supine) in mm Hg above the lowest reading recorded during last week of trial when B.P. was measured twice daily. Reprinted with permission of Elsevier/ North Holland.

in this trial. Nevertheless, in trials of this nature, it is probably important to ensure that blood pressure is taken at approximately the same time of day in individual patients at each assessment.

Relief of Anxiety

Two rating scales were used to assess psychiatric symptomatology: the Leeds Patient Self-Rating Scale (45) and the GPRG Physicians Anxiety Rating Scale (30).

Although there were reductions in the mean severity score in each of the three active treatment groups on the self-rating scale, none was statistically significant for either the total scores or the depression or anxiety subscale scores. In the placebo group, however, there were statistically significant reductions for both total and anxiety scores ($p < 0.03$ and < 0.01, respectively). There were no significant prepost differences in any of the four groups on the physicians rating scale.

As in the previous studies, the occurrence during the course of the trial of adverse or beneficial life events in the patients' lives was recorded. Few good events occurred in any of the 4 weeks, and the proportions between good and bad events were similar among the first three groups, although the proportion of bad to good events in the placebo group was higher than in the other three. Therefore, this finding would have favored the active treatment groups at the expense of the placebo group, although as we have seen, this was not the case.

Implications for Further Research

The most striking finding of the trial was the marked and statistically significant reductions in mean blood pressure which occurred in the group treated with only placebo medication. It had been anticipated that 5 weeks would have been an adequate period for any placebo effect to wear off, but it is apparent that, in future studies, a much longer trial period must be employed. Over a longer period of time, the reductions in blood pressure recorded in the placebo group probably would be replaced by subsequent rises, in contrast to the sustained reductions in blood pressure to be expected with active medications.

Despite the deficiencies of the trial in relation to the shortness of the trial period and the numbers of subjects involved in the treatment groups, the results do not suggest that lorazepam alone exerted any significant antihypertensive effects. In the three other groups, although there were significant reductions in both systolic and diastolic pressures, the mean reductions were greatest in the group treated with the combination of lorazepam and bendrofluazide. Furthermore, as seen in Fig. 15.4, at both 3 and 5 weeks, this was the only group of patients in whom the mean reductions in both systolic and diastolic blood pressures fell below the normal range for this age of patient (systolic 150 mm Hg, diastolic 95 mm Hg). However, with the relatively small numbers involved, the comparative differences were not statistically significant. This may indicate that this combination of drugs might be useful in the treatment of hypertension, although clearly larger numbers and a longer trial period will be needed to test this hypothesis. It is of interest that this particular combination of drugs was well tolerated in the trial, since this group had the lowest incidence of side effects of all four groups, including the placebo group.

The next finding of interest is that concerning the last week of the trial, when multiple blood pressure recordings were made in the morning and evening. There was considerable variation between patients during this last week, in that both systolic and diastolic blood pressures remained relatively constant in some, while in others there were appreciable swings. Averaging out the recordings for the full week's period, however, the four treatment groups were comparable in this respect. The trial did not provide any evidence that lorazepam exerted any better control of these swings of systolic and/or diastolic pressures. It is apparent that taking blood pressure every morning and evening every day for a period of even one week is difficult to achieve under the conditions of general practice. The implications for future research are that a random blood pressure recording made at the end of a week of treatment may not reflect the variations in blood pressure that have occurred during that week. In future, it might be wise to take several readings on different days during the assessment week and average these out to give a single final reading for comparative purposes. Alternatively, home recording of blood pressure by the patients might be considered (46).

We shall now endeavor to undertake a further trial, perhaps with an initial placebo period of, say, 4 weeks, to be followed by a double-blind comparison between lorazepam + bendrofluazide and bendrofluazide alone for a longer period of, say, 3 months.

CONCLUSIONS

The initial data recorded in the drug trial studies confirmed the results of the survey on the psychiatric aspects of hypertension. Also in these studies, it was found that the majority of patients suffering from hypertension exhibited anxiety symptoms, although mostly of mild or moderate severity. For all patients, including those from a study of acebutolol described in the first edition of the book (47), the initial mean GPRG anxiety score was 6.0 (SE ± 0.5). The total possible score on this scale is 36, and the usual mean severity recorded in cases of anxiety neurosis is between 15 and 20. Of the total of 236 hypertensive patients involved, 211 (89%) exhibited anxiety symptoms of varying degrees.

The results of these three studies showed that relief of anxiety symptoms accompanied reduction in blood pressure, although it is not yet possible to deduce from the results that anxiety is a factor influencing the response to hypotensive drug therapy. We were unable to find any evidence that there was a relationship between the severity of anxiety symptoms and the response to antihypertensive drug treatment.

Relief of anxiety in these hypertensive patients under treatment could have been due merely to a sedative or depressant action of the drugs being used. In view of this possibility, a further analysis was undertaken of the cases in the trial of propranolol versus methyldopa to compare the results in those patients who complained of drowsiness and in those who did not. Combining all the drowsy patients in this trial (irrespective of drug given), there were 18 who completed the full trial period. The mean anxiety score on the GPRG ratings in this group of patients was 7.4 initially; this fell progressively to 4.1 by the end of the trial. However, the only significant prepost difference was the one between the initial mean level of anxiety and the final level, and this was only significant at the 5% level. None of the other pre-post differences in this group of patients achieved statistical significance. Therefore, far from the drowsy patients achieving a better relief of anxiety, the converse was the case. The antianxiety effects of both drugs in this trial (and methyldopa in particular) were not associated with the production of drowsiness.

The reduction in the level of anxiety in the first two studies described in this chapter may have been due to the antianxiety effects of the antihypertensive drug methyldopa. Therefore, the study comparing the addition of another benzodiazepine, lorazepam, to bendrofluazide, an antihypertensive drug with no antianxiety or sedative actions, was undertaken. This study also did not provide an answer to the question, since it was a short-term trial involving a placebo group, and no significant relief of anxiety symptoms was demonstrated in any but the placebo group.

It will now be necessary to conduct a further clinical trial to compare a benzodiazepine to placebo, added to a thiazide diuretic alone, for a longer trial period of 2 to 3 months, as in the initial studies undertaken. Only when the results of such a trial have been recorded can we determine for how long the placebo effect may be maintained and to what extent the use of an antianxiety drug may assist in the control of blood pressure in patients suffering from hypertension, as an adjunct to long-term treatment of the condition.

These studies have demonstrated that a high proportion of hypertensive patients do exhibit anxiety symptoms, albeit mainly of mild or moderate severity. Furthermore, these studies have shown that relief of these anxiety symptoms parallels reduction in blood pressure, although it cannot be determined at present whether this may be cause or effect, or coincidence. It is hoped that further studies to be undertaken by our group will provide more definitive answers to these questions.

ACKNOWLEDGMENTS

Part of this work was supported by a U.S. Public Health Service research contract (HSM-42–71–65) (to D.W.) from the National Institute of Mental Health.

Figures 15.4 and 15.5 are reproduced by kind permission of the editors of *Biological Psychiatry Today* (Elsevier, 1979).

REFERENCES

1. Levi, L. *Stress and Distress to Psychosocial Stimuli.* Pergamon Press, Oxford, 1972.
2. Philipp, T., Distler, A., and Cordes, U. Sympathetic nervous system and blood pressure control in essential hypertension. *Lancet,* 1978, ii, 959.
3. Hofman, A., Boomsma, F., Schalekamp, M. A. D. H., and Valkenburg, H. A. Raised blood pressure and plasma noradrenaline concentrations in teenagers and young adults selected from an open population. *Br. Med. J.,* 1979, 1, 1536.
4. Heine, B. E., Sainsbury, P., and Chynoweth, R. C. Hypertension and emotional disturbance. *J. Psychiatr. Res.,* 1969, 7, 119.
5. Robinson, J. O. Symptoms and the discovery of high blood pressure. *J. Psychosom. Res.,* 1969, 13, 157.
6. Graham, J. D. P. High blood pressure after battle. *Lancet,* 1945, i, 239.
7. Cobb, A., and Rose, R. M. Hypertension, peptic ulcer and diabetes in air traffic controllers. *JAMA,* 1973, 224, 489.
8. Littler, W. A., Honour, A. J., and Sleight, P. Direct arterial pressure and electrocardiogram during motor car driving. *Br. Med. J.,* 1973, ii, 273.
9. Bridges, P. K. Practical aspects of the use of some psychological tests of anxiety in a situation of stress. *Br. J. Psychiatry,* 1973, 123, 587.
10. Ruskin, A., Beard, O., and Schaffer, R. L. Blast hypertension: Elevated arterial pressure in victims of the Texas City disaster. *Am. J. Med.,* 1948, 4, 228.
11. Morrison, S. L., and Morris, J. N. Epidemiological observations on high blood pressure without apparent cause. *Lancet,* 1959, ii, 864.
12. Cruz-Coke, R. Environmental illnesses and arterial blood pressure. *Lancet,* 1960, ii, 885.
13. Alexander, F. Emotional factors in essential hypertension: Presentation of a tentative hypothesis. *Psychosom. Med.,* 1939, 1, 173.

14. Wolf, A., and Wolff, H. G. In: *Hypertension,* edited by E. T. Bell, p. 288. Minnesota Press, Minneapolis, 1950.
15. Wolf, S., Pfeiller, J. B., Ripley, H. S., Winter, O. S., and Wolff, H. G. Hypertension as a reaction pattern to stress: Summary of experimental data on variations in blood pressure and renal blood flow. *Ann. Intern. Med.,* 1948, 29, 1056.
16. Kalis, B. L., Harris, R. E., Bennett, L. F., and Sokolow, M. Personality and life history factors in persons who are potentially hypertensive. *J. Nerv. Ment. Dis.,* 1961, 132, 457.
17. Gressel, G. C., Shobe, F. O., Saslow, G., Dubois, P. H., and Schroeder, H. A. Personality factors in arterial hypertension. *JAMA,* 1949, 140, 265.
18. Harburg, E., Julius, S., McGinn, N. F., McLeod, J., and Hoobler, S. W. Personality traits and behavioural patterns associated with systolic blood pressure levels in college males. *J. Chronic Dis.,* 1964, 17, 405.
19. Wheatley, D., Balter, M., Levine, J., Lipman, R., Bauer, M. L., and Bonato, R. Psychiatric aspects of hypertension. *Br. J. Psychiatry,* 1975, 127, 327.
20. Derogatis, L. R., Lipman, R. S., Rickels, K., Uhlenhuth, E. H., and Covi, L. The symptom distress checklist: A measure of primary symptom dimensions. *Behav. Sci.,* 1974, 19, 1.
21. Derogatis, L. R., Lipman, R. S., Rickels, K., Uhlenhuth, E. H., and Covi, L. Hopkins symptom checklist (HSCL). In: *Psychological Measurements in Psychopharmacology. Modern Problems of Pharmacopsychiatry, Vol. 7,* edited by P. Pichot, p. 79. Karger, Basel, 1974.
22. Paykel, E. S., Myers, J. K., Dienelt, M. N., Klerman, G. L., Lindenthal, J. J., and Peooer, M. D. Life events and depression. *Arch. Gen. Psychiatry,* 1969, 21, 753.
23. Meyer, E., Derogatis, L. R., Miller, M., and Reading, A. Hypertension and psychological distress. *Psychosom. Med.,* 1978, 19, 161.
24. Seidel, U. P. Hypertension and paranoid states. *Lancet,* 1977, i, 906 (Letter).
25. Benson, H., Rosner, B. A., Marzetta, B. R., and Klemchuk, H. M. Decreased blood pressure in pharmacologically treated hypertensive patients who regularly elicited the relaxation response. *Lancet,* 1974, i, 289.
26. Brod, J., Fencl, V., Hejl, Z., and Jirka, J. Circulatory changes underlying blood pressure elevation during acute emotional stress (mental arithmetic) in normotensive and hypertensive subjects. *Clin. Sci.,* 1959, 18, 269.
27. Nestal, P. J. Blood pressure and catecholamine excretion after mental stress in labile hypertension. *Lancet,* 1969, i, 692.
28. Gutman, M. C., and Benson, H. Interaction of environmental factors and systemic arterial blood pressure: A review. *Medicine,* 1971, 50, 543.
29. Kristt, D. A., and Engel, B. T. Learned control of blood pressure in patients with high blood pressure. *Circulation,* 1975, 51, 370.
30. Wheatley, D. *Psychopharmacology in Family Practice.* Heinemann, London, 1973.
31. Wheatley, D. Circulatory manifestations of soma and psyche. In: *Therapy in Psychosomatic Medicine,* edited by F. Antonelli. Edizioni Luigi Pozzi, S.p.A, Rome, 1976, 163.
32. Smith, A. J. Drug treatment of hypertension. *Br. J. Hosp. Med.,* 1974, 533.
33. Editorial. Beta-blockers for hypertension. *Lancet,* 1976, ii, 551.
34. General Practitioner Clinical Trials. Medazepam: A new tranquillizer. *Practitioner,* 1971, 206, 688.
35. Collaborative Study. Propranolol in hypertension. *J. Pharmacother.,* 1977, 1, 7.
36. Tyrer, P. J., and Lader, M. H. Response to propranolol and diazepam in somatic and psychic anxiety. *Br. Med. J.,* 1974, 2, 14.
37. Waal, H. Propranolol-induced depression. *Br. Med. J.,* 1967, 2, 50.
38. Snaith, R. P., and McCoubrie, M. Antihypertensive drugs and depression. *Psychol. Med.,* 1974, 4, 393.
39. Schlittler, E., and Plummer, A. J. Tranquillizing drugs from Rauwolfia. In: *Psychopharmacological Agents. Vol. I,* edited by M. Gordon. Academic Press, New York, 1964.
40. Sourkes, T. L. The action of α-methyldopa in the brain. *Br. Med. Bull.,* 1965, 21, 66.
41. Oates, J. A., Seligmann, A. W., Clark, M. A., Rousseau, P., and Lee, R. E. The relative efficacy of guanethidine, methyldopa and pargyline as antihypertensive agents. *N. Engl. J. Med.,* 1965, 273, 729.
42. Wilcox, R. G. Randomised study of six beta-blockers and a thiazide diuretic in essential hypertension. *Br. Med. J.,* 1978, ii, 383.

43. Wheatley, D. Stress and hypertension: Clinical implications. In: *Biological Psychiatry Today,* edited by J. Obiols, C. Ballus, E. González Monclús, and J. Pujol, Elsevier/North Holland, Amsterdam. p. 821. 1979.
44. Millar-Craig, M. W., Bishop, C. N., and Raftery, E. B. Circadian variation of blood-pressure. *Lancet,* 1978, i, 795.
45. Snaith, R. P., Bridge, G. W. K., and Hamilton, M. The Leeds scales for the self-assessment of anxiety and depression. *Br. J. Psychiatry,* 1976, 128, 156.
46. O'Brien, E. T., and O'Malley, K. ABC of blood pressure measurement: Future trends. *Br. Med. J.,* 1979, ii, 1124.
47. Wheatley, D. A new beta-adrenergic blocking drug in hypertension. *Practitioner,* 1976, 216, 218.

Prologue: Psychopharmacologic Aspects of the Cerebral Circulation

Hypertension is a systemic illness that may produce its most profound effects in the brain. The alterations that occur in the cerebral circulation due to age produce similar effects without the intervention of a rise of systemic blood pressure. With the present trend toward increasing longevity, psychogeriatric disturbances are becoming increasingly important, not only because of individual disability but also as a result of far-reaching effects on the community as a whole. Therefore, a better understanding of the factors underlying mental and psychiatric disorders in the elderly is as important as the study of coronary heart disease in younger patients. Furthermore, efforts to modify, with both cardiac and psychotropic drugs, the effects of cerebral disease accompanying old age are of paramount importance, although the therapeutic gains may seem small in extent.

In the first chapter of this section, Sourander and Sourander outline the problem, with a comprehensive review of the pathologic changes contributing to organic brain syndromes. They lay considerable emphasis on underlying changes in the cerebral vasculature and proceed to describe methods for investigating the effects of dysfunction in this system on various physiologic functions in man. They then describe some of the drugs that are being used to treat the manifestations of mental disorders in the elderly, in relation to cerebral circulation and the effects that it may have on bodily functions. In this context, both drugs affecting psychiatric function and drugs affecting the circulation itself are of some help, although, as the Souranders point out, it is necessary to employ precise methods for measuring the various facets of cognitive function. Without the use of such measures, small but significant gains in well being can be overlooked and valuable therapeutic drug effects denigrated.

In the second chapter of this section, the emphasis moves from the clinical investigation of the effects of cardiovascular drugs on the brain to the wider field of nootropic drugs generally and methods of measuring their cerebral effects. The electroencephalogram (EEG) provides a precise method of recording these effects in both normal individuals and elderly patients suffering from a variety of brain disorders. Saletu considers a whole range of drugs that have been advocated for the improvement of mental functioning in the elderly and shows that the majority of these produce changes in the EEG recordings that differ from those produced by placebo. As he remarks, quantitative pharmaco-EEG, along with psychometric tests, is an outstanding tool to evaluate the encephalotropic, psychotropic, and pharmacodynamic properties of drugs that may be useful in treating mental ailments of old age.

Although some of the drugs described in this chapter may be unfamiliar to American and British readers, their active investigation in European countries emphasizes the importance of this field for the application of effective drug therapy. In this context, the emphasis is on the use of drugs that may counter the effects of hypoxia on the aged brain, rather than on psychotropic drugs per se. For the comparative evaluation of future compounds for this indication, this methodology should prove invaluable as a prelude or adjunct to clinical assessment in patients. Unfortunately, the methods for clinical assessment are crude; and in the elderly, even minor gains in a few functional parameters, or even prevention of deterioration in the same parameters, may be of immense value in the management of the geriatric patient.

In the next chapter, James describes a more specialized investigation into the effects of one particular type of psychotropic drug, namely, tricyclic antidepressants, on brain function as directly measured by the effects of these drugs on cerebral metabolism. Not only is James able to correlate precisely an experimental procedure in laboratory animals with the exact counterpart of the experiments in man, he is able to establish a correlation between changes in cerebral metabolism and response by depressed patients to antidepressant drugs.

In the last chapter of this section, the large part still to be played by the use of psychotropic drugs in the elderly is comprehensively surveyed, the main contribution in this context coming from Hordern. The present state of the art in relation to the use of cerebral vasodilators and cerebral activators is also considered, but it is apparent that, from the clinical point of view, the use of cardiac and other drugs for these indications is still in its infancy.

These chapters should provide fresh stimulus to the study of both psychotropic drugs and drugs affecting the cerebral circulation for the control of the distressing manifestations of mental disease in the elderly.

Stress and the Heart, edited by D. Wheatley,
Raven Press, New York © 1981.

Organic Brain Syndromes and Circulatory Disorders in Old Age*

Leif Sourander and Patrick Sourander

Organic brain syndromes (OBS) comprise those neuropsychiatric disorders which are caused by, or associated with, organic brain tissue changes manifested as functional impairment. This impairment can have intra- or extracranial causes and be of either vascular, hemodynamic, or nonvascular and nonhemodynamic origin. OBS are common in old age and increase in the highest decades. The symptomatology is characterized by a multitude of neuropsychiatric functional impairments, and it is thus misleading to speak about a defined syndrome as a clinical entity. The clinical interpretation of OBS has often been simplified, especially in old age, the most common belief being that narrowing of the arteriosclerotic cerebral vessels is the all-embracing explanation for the syndrome. As a result of this, there is a trend either toward therapeutic nihilism or to uncritical treatment, based on misunderstanding of the basal changes leading to impaired brain tissue function in old age.

The aim of this chapter is to present some aspects of vascular involvement, circulation, and clinical findings in OBS, in order to shed some light on the possibilities for treatment of aged patients suffering from these conditions.

CEREBRAL CIRCULATION IN THE ELDERLY

It is generally assumed that cerebral blood flow (CBF) and cerebral metabolic rate (CMR) diminish with increasing age. Fazekas et al. (1) showed significantly reduced CBF and CMR in subjects over 90 years of age, as compared to findings in normal subjects less than 50 years old. However, the values for both parameters were not significantly different from those noted for normal subjects between 50 and 91.

This seems to indicate that factors responsible for the age-dependent decline of CBF and CMR proceed at an extremely low rate in healthy elderly individuals. The reduced cerebral blood flow in old age was thought to be caused by an increased cerebrovascular resistance (CVR) due to arteriosclerosis. Whether the reduced metabolic rate in the brain was second-

---

*Reprinted with permission from *Stress and the Heart,* edited by D. Wheatley, Raven Press, 1977, first edition.

ary to cerebrovascular insufficiency, as defined by Corday et al. (2), or was a consequence of decreased capacity of brain tissue to utilize oxygen (decreased neuronal metabolic demand?) could not be determined. Although the available evidence supports the opinion that advancing age is generally accompanied by a decrease in CBF and CMR and an increase in CVR, there seem to be notable exceptions. Thus, studies by Sokoloff (3,4,4a) have indicated that, in carefully selected elderly individuals who are healthy, actively at work, and well adjusted to their community, CBF and CMR remain largely intact.

A number of different changes affecting small arteries, arterioles, and capillaries, particularly in the cerebral cortex and leptomeninges, have been described as occurring in healthy elderly individuals and particularly in patients with senile dementia (5–7). A common characteristic of these vascular alterations is that they occur in subjects without morphological or clinical evidence of atherosclerosis or hypertensive disease and thus are considered to be due to primary senile degeneration. Some of the vascular deformities such as "glomerular loop formation" may possibly contribute to a reduced CBF, as indicated by physical model experiments and calculations (7). Theoretically, the most interesting change is represented by the accumulation of amyloid (possibly as the result of an unknown immunological disturbance) in the media of small arteries, particularly in the occipital cortex and sometimes in the leptomeninges of patients with presenile or senile dementia. The pathogenesis and clinical significance of all these changes has not yet been determined.

MENTAL CHANGES DUE TO INFARCTION AND ATHEROSCLEROSIS

As pointed out by Fisher (8), "There are no pathological data supporting the idea that a small stroke in a 'silent' area of the brain may produce a sudden change in intellect, personality or character." Infarctions and changes of degenerative "senile type" (senile plaques, Alzheimer's fibrillary tangles, and granulovacuolar degeneration of hippocampal neurons), either alone or in combination, may also occur in brains of old, nondemented people. An attempt to quantitate such lesions showed that cases with functional psychosis and acute confusion did not reveal greater pathological changes than those dying of purely physical disease (9). Moderate to severe atherosclerosis of the basal cerebral arteries without substantial brain damage does not appear to be of importance for the manifestation of dementia in old age (10). Obviously great caution is needed in the interpretation of the possible clinical significance of minor ischemic brain lesions, as well as atherosclerosis of the basal cerebral arteries.

Hachinski et al. (11), summarizing the results of recent clinical and pathological studies, stated that the previously held view, that a gradual narrowing of the cerebral arteries due to arteriosclerosis may lead to a state of chronic brain ischemia and mental deterioration, is fundamentally false. Supported by the previous findings of Worm-Petersen and Pakkenberg (10), Hachinski et al. introduced the concept of multi-infarct dementia, which implies that "when vascular disease is responsible for dementia it is through the occurrence of multiple small or large cerebral infarcts." Furthermore, they suggested that the majority of small cerebral infarcts are secondary to disease of the extracranial arteries and the heart and associated with thromboembolism, as previously indicated by the studies of Torvik and Jorgensen (12).

CEREBRAL VASCULAR INSUFFICIENCY

A new epoch in research on cerebral circulatory disturbances began with the advent of modern techniques for measurement of the total mean cerebral blood flow (m CBF) in patients with various kinds of encephalopathies. The original inert gas diffusion (nitrous oxide) method of Kety and Schmidt for determining m CBF has now been superseded by the 133 Xenon intracarotid injection method for measurement of regional cerebral blood flow (r CBF) [cf. Ingvar and Lassen (13)].

On the theoretical side, a definite advance was achieved with the introduction of the concept of "cerebral vascular insufficiency" (CVI) by Corday et al. (2,14). The reality of this new entity was supported by results from animal experimentation (15). CVI means the inadequacy of the cerebral circulation to provide the brain or its parts with the blood flow necessary to maintain normal metabolic activities under various physiological conditions. Such conditions may imply either an impaired CBF or an increased metabolic demand because of an additional load on the metabolic activities of the brain. CVI may be present continuously or occur intermittently, and it is precipitated by a broad spectrum of heart affections associated with diminished cardiac output and leading to a reduction of intracerebral blood pressure. The pathogenesis of diminished cardiac output may consist of a heart block (e.g., Adams-Stokes syndrome), ventricular arrhythmia, coronary artery insufficiency, myocardial infarction, acquired valvular diseases, or hypertonia resulting in cardiac decompensation, etc. Because symptoms of arrhythmia and myocardial infarction may be silent and remain undetected without laboratory tests, the pathogenesis of CVI may be hidden.

It is fortunate that the vascular system of the brain has the capacity to maintain normal volume flow through a wide range of perfusion pressures. This capacity for adaptation, called autoregulation, is affected through changes in CVR. These changes are the consequences of constriction or dilatation of small cerebral arteries and arterioles. However, autoregulation ceases if maximal vasodilatation occurs throughout the brain. In such a state, the CBF is the direct function of the cerebral diffusion pressure. It is generally assumed that suspended autoregulation is the necessary prerequisite for the subsequent oligemic brain damage.

According to Brierley (16), data from limited clinical experience and animal models indicate that the extension of the oligemic brain damage is determined by "the rate at which blood pressure falls, the lowest pressure attained and its duration and the rate of its return to normal." Furthermore, according to this author, "cardiac arrest of abrupt onset, followed by a rapid restoration of CBF, will result in generalized damage in at least the neocortex and cerebellum. A shorter period of circulatory arrest preceded and/or followed by appreciable periods of reduced CBF, will lead to ischaemic alterations that are concentrated in the anterior boundary zones of the cerebrum, cerebellum, and sometimes the basal ganglia."

The brain is composed of a great number of structures, differing in rates of flow of their blood supplies, metabolic activities, and function. The various types of danger zones supplied by the ramifications of the cerebral vascular tree can be identified, as described by Zülch and Behrend (17). One type involves cortical and subcortical areas directly in the center of a region supplied by terminal branches of a main cerebral artery. An example of such an area is the calcarine cortex, supplied by the posterior cerebral artery. The other type is represented by border zones ("watershed areas") between two or several arteries, e.g., between the anterior and middle or middle and posterior cerebral arteries. If the cerebral circulatory insufficiency is transient or intermittent, the concomitant functional disturbances may be confined to the same topographical brain territories. The theory advocated by Zülch implies that neurologic deficits localized to the danger zones may occur as a result of an overall reduction of CBF. Depending on the degree of vascular insufficiency, the symptoms and the underlying brain lesions are either reversible or permanent.

CONFUSIONAL SYNDROMES

It has been suggested that whether or not occlusive arterial disease of varying severity may be present, hemodynamic factors appear to be the important determinant of reversible as well as permanent brain damage, following from a major reduction in the overall CBF. A substantial decline of CBF associated with mental symptoms, such as confusion and aphasia in elderly people, does not necessarily imply that occlusive arterial disease of the brain is present. Thus, in such patients without angiographic signs of cerebrovascular disease, extracerebral circulatory disturbances, probably contributive to the "cerebral circulatory insufficiency," were frequently observed by Riishede (18). Lassen (19) showed that in cardiac decompensation associated with confusion, the total mean CBF was considerably reduced, whereas CVR was not significantly lowered. Furthermore, following adequate therapy, the confusional state disappeared and the cerebral blood flow was restored to normal values. On the other hand, even in some extremely severe cases of atherosclerosis of the basal cerebral arteries, e.g., in patients with occlusion of both carotid arteries and one vertebral artery, neurologic deficits and mental symptoms may be entirely absent sometimes (20).

In recent years several studies have indicated that not only acute or subacute confusional syndromes but also chronic encephalopathies in elderly people may be associated with, and in some cases probably caused by, recurrent episodes of CVI. Dalessio et al. (21) reported on neurologic and mental symptoms in aged subjects, with different forms of heart block leading to diminished cardiac output. In 1973 Abdon and Malmcrona (22) called attention to the frequent occurrence of clinically significant but hidden bradyarrhythmias in the elderly population in Sweden. Furthermore, it was revealed that undiagnosed intermittent arrhythmias were common in aged subjects considered to be suffering from senile dementia (23). Thus, a careful examination of the cardiovascular system should be performed in any patient with an unexplained chronic encephalopathy, especially if senile dementia is suspected.

The limbic structures and adjacent cortical areas at the inferomedial portion of the temporal lobes, as well as the visual cortical fields, represent terminal territories supplied by the posterior cerebral arteries. Recently, it has been suggested that transient ischemic attacks (TIA) affecting these cerebral regions, manifested as episodes of transitory global amnesia (TGA) and sometimes associated with visual field defects, may be caused by vertebrobasilar insufficiency (VBI) (24,25). Recurrent attacks of VBI are not uncommon in elderly people and are assumed to lead to progressive memory loss and dementia. Hemodynamic disturbances in the vertebrobasilar system between episodes of TGA, and stenotic as well as occlusive lesions in one or both posterior cerebral arteries, have been observed (24).

CLINICOPATHOLOGICAL INVESTIGATION

In order to illustrate the incidence of extra- and intracerebral arteriosclerosis and of cerebral lesions induced by circulatory disturbances in various gerontopsychiatric disease categories, some results of an extensive clinical and pathoanatomical investigation are now briefly presented.

The data, collected during the years 1940 to 1964, were recorded from 318 female patients treated at Clinic I, Lillhagen Hospital (for mental diseases). Since 75% of the patients included in the investigation died at an age of over 70 years, we are dealing with a predominantly gerontopsychiatric population. All the patients were repeatedly examined and followed up by the same neuropsychiatrist, Dr. Hakon Sjögren. The neuropathological investigations were initiated by the late Prof. Nils Gellerstedt and, since 1953, continued by one of the present authors (P.S.)

The data were divided into five groups according to the *clinical diagnosis*. The first group was designated the functional division (FD) and included 60 cases with neuroses and affective disorders. The next group consisted of a mixture of cases of neuropsychiatric diseases with symptoms and signs suggestive of organic encephalopathies but unrelated to Alzheimer's disease, senile dementia, and cerebrovascular disease (other organic encephalopathies, OOE). This group was comprised of 54 cases including 25 characterized by confusional syndromes and cardiac disease. Alzheimer's disease (Alz) was represented by 68 cases fulfilling the clinical criteria for this disease as defined by H. Sjögren (Sjögren, Sjögren, and Lindgren, 1952), and senile dementia (DS) by 60 cases. The principal clinical difference between Alz and DS was the occurrence of focal symptoms in the Alz group (aphasia, agnosia, apraxia, spatial disorientation, and symptoms of the Klüver-Bucy syndrome) and the absence of such symptoms in the DS group. The final group of cerebrovascular disorders (CV) consisted of 72 cases. Clinically these cases were characterized by acute onset, symptoms and signs of focal cerebral lesions, and a fluctuating course.

RESULTS

The results are presented in relation to the cerebral vascular abnormalities disclosed at autopsy. These abnormalities fall into three main groups: arteriosclerosis of basal cerebral arteries (ABCA), arteriosclerosis of intracerebral arteries (AICA), and infarction (Inf). The varying degrees of these different vascular abnormalities are now presented in relation to the five clinical groups already described.

Arteriosclerosis of Basal Cerebral Arteries (ABCA)

Figure 16-1 shows the percentages of patients in the various clinical groups who were found to have varying degrees of ABCA. Some degree of ABCA was present in the majority of all disease groups examined. In good agreement with the clinical diagnosis, ABCA was most marked in the CV group, being present in moderate or severe degree in no less than 93% of the cases. On the other hand, in the DS group, ABCA was slight or even absent in 56% of the cases, moderate in 31%, and severe in only 13%. A previous study on the same material revealed that most of the cases with severe ABCA were found in subjects over 80 years of age (26).

In contrast, in the FD, OOE, and Alz groups, ABCA was absent or slight in the majority of cases.

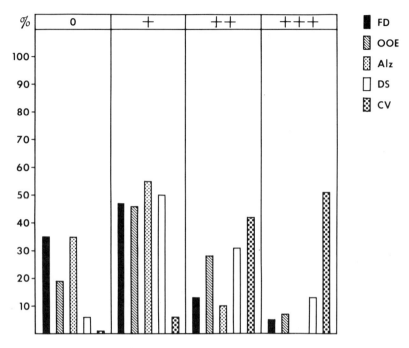

FIG. 16-1. Incidence of various degrees of ABCA in the five clinical groups. 0 = Absent. + = Mild. ++ = Moderate. +++ = Severe.

Arteriosclerosis of Intracerebral Arteries (AICA)

Figure 16-2 shows the incidence and severity of this pathological finding in the five clinical groups in similar manner to the previous figure.

In the evaluation of the incidence of intracerebral vascular changes, arteriosclerosis as well as arteriolosclerosis was considered. Signs of AICA were lacking in the great majority of cases in all disease groups except in the CV group. When present in these disease groups it was mostly to a slight degree. However, in the CV group, AICA was noticed in moderate or severe degree in 85% of the cases; it was of slight degree in the remaining 15%. In the DS group, AICA was seen in only 25% of the cases and it was usually of slight degree.

Infarction (Inf)

Results for this pathological finding are shown in Fig. 16-3.

In the FD and Alz groups, infarctions were observed in less than 20% of the cases and in the OOE and DS groups in a little more than 20%. In contrast, single or multiple infarctions of considerable size (+++) were present

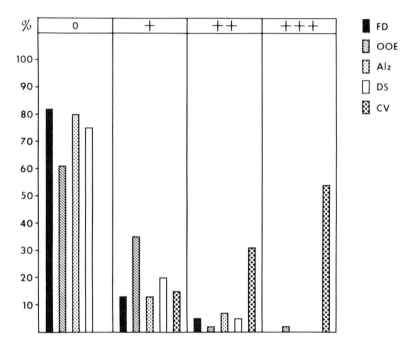

FIG. 16-2. Incidence of various degrees of AICA in the five clinical groups. 0 = Absent. + = Mild. ++ = Moderate. +++ = Severe.

in 54% of CV cases and in only 5% of DS cases. Single or a few macroscopic infarctions of small size (++) were observed in 33% of the CV cases and in less than 11% of the other disease groups. Only microscopic infarctions (+) were seen in a small minority of cases in all groups.

Thus, arteriosclerosis of basal cerebral and intracerebral arteries, as well as infarctions, occurred in all clinically diagnosed disease groups and were, as expected, most prominent in patients clinically diagnosed as suffering from cerebrovascular disease. Arteriosclerosis of basal cerebral arteries, varying from slight to severe, was a much more common phenomenon in all disease groups than intracerebral arteriosclerosis. Severe degrees of intracerebral arteriosclerosis occurred almost exclusively in patients clinically diagnosed as having cerebrovascular disorders. Severe degrees of infarction were seen in the majority of cases with cerebrovascular disorders, but in only 16% of the cases with senile dementia.

As for the cases of confusional syndromes associated with cardiac disease and belonging to the OOE group, some remarks should be made. Psychiatrically the 25 cases included in this category were characterized by acute confusion, sometimes progressing to delirious states, and by hallucinations and delusions. Progressive dementia was not a typical feature,

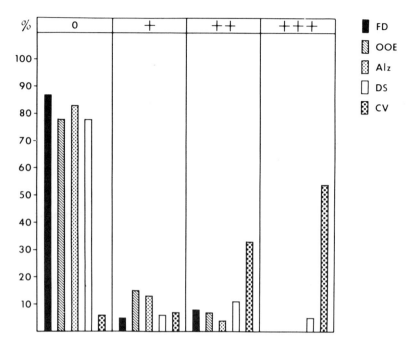

FIG. 16-3. Incidence of various degrees of infarction in the five clinical groups. 0 = Absent. + = Mild. ++ = Moderate. +++ = Severe.

but in some advanced cases symptoms reminiscent of those in Alzheimer's disease were noted. The mental illness lasted from a few months to 3 years and was preceded by periods of progressive and recurrent heart failure. During the course of the illness, cardiac arrhythmias were observed in 10 patients and Adams-Stokes syndrome in an additional 3 of the 25 patients. Autopsy revealed chronic valvular disease in 12, severe coronary sclerosis in 11, and myocardial infarctions in 6 of the 25 cases. The age at death was above 75 years in 80% of the cases. The principal cerebral changes consisted of loss of neurons, "ischemic neuronal disease" of Spielmeyer, and astrocytic proliferation in the cortex. These changes were considered to be caused mainly by severe cardiac disease (Fig. 16-4).

From the study presented, the following conclusions may be drawn:

1. Provided that the clinical observations are carried out by an experienced clinician and over a length of time, it seems possible to single out, with considerable accuracy, cases of mainly cerebrovascular disorders from the bulk of gerontopsychiatric diseases.

2. A significant number of elderly patients who died in a mental hospital revealed confusional syndromes associated with cardiac diseases. For adequate treatment the early identification of such cases appears important.

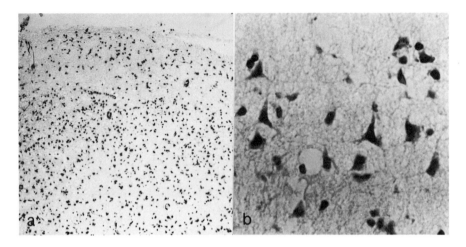

FIG. 16-4. Frontal cortex. Cresyl violet. **a.** Low power view showing loss of neurons, particularly in third cortical layer. Note the considerable increase in the number of glial nuclei. **b.** Higher magnification revealing nerve cells with pale, shrunken cytoplasm and triangular intensely stained nuclei corresponding to Spielmeyer's "ischemic cell change." Autopsy specimen from a 75-year-old woman suffering from cardiac arrhythmia, decompensation, recurrent confusional episodes, and a progressing aphatic-agnostic-apractic syndrome. Death from ruptured myocardial infarction. Senile plaques and neurofibrillary tangles were absent in the cortex.

SYMPTOMATOLOGY OF THE ORGANIC BRAIN SYNDROME IN OLD AGE

The definition of OBS as a condition associated with impairment of brain tissue function implies that the clinical symptoms cover wide ranges of neurological and psychiatric symptomatology.

Mental Deterioration

This is the most striking feature of the syndrome, and the diagnosis is dependent on the identification of some degree of impairment of orientation, memory, cognitive function, and appropriate emotional response. There is a wide variation, from mild impairment of these functions to confusional states, either acute or chronic, and dementia. The majority of old people considered to have signs of OBS are those with mild impairment of brain function. Extrapyramidal symptoms and postapoplectic syndromes complicate the symptomatology.

There are two symptoms which are common in aged patients with OBS but which are almost completely neglected and usually mentioned only very briefly in geriatric textbooks. These symptoms are decreased alertness and disturbance of balance and posture control in old age.

Decreased Alertness

Changes in alertness, which also can be called arousal or vigilance, have been studied by means of neurophysiological and psychological methods. The concept of vigilance was first developed by Head (27), who stated that vigilance is "a high state of physiological efficiency present at all levels of the nervous system and capable of either general or local depression." A decreased alertness implies an impaired response to external stimuli and a deterioration of subject-environmental relations. It has been generally accepted that a slowing of sensorimotor performance occurs with age (28), and such a slowing down could be interpreted as a decrease in vigilance or alertness.

A decrease in alertness can be caused by disease, drug effects, or degenerative changes of brain tissue owing to the aging process. Other causes of decreased alertness in the aged are sensory deprivation, which also includes a decrease of proprioceptive perception and lack of environmental stimuli in old age. According to Welford (28,29), the old brain has more random activity or "inner noise" than the young brain. This brings about a decrease in channel capacity of perception.

Disturbance of Balance and Posture Control

In patients with OBS, deterioration of posture control and disturbance of balance are common findings and often an indication for hospital admission. Postural mechanisms depend on information from proprioceptive, visual, and labyrinthine efferents and the integration of that information with appropriate motor responses by the basal ganglia, cerebellum, and cerebral cortex. The sense of balance is dependent on the quality of the sensorimotor functions, including control of the horizontal and vertical planes, which is essential in promoting a normal gait. Typical symptoms of impaired postural control are dizzy turns, a sensation of uncertainty during walking, and "marche aux petits pas." These symptoms are pronounced in old people who have been confined to bed. Another familiar phenomenon in these patients is the tendency to attempt balance by leaning backward. The patients complain usually of dizziness, but seldom of rotatory vertigo. A primary vestibular cause is exceptional. After a stroke, the postural mechanisms are often severely impaired, and assessment and restoration of these abilities is an essential part of the rehabilitation program of stroke patients.

Urinary Incontinence

The relationships between OBS and urinary incontinence in the elderly has been extensively reviewed by Brocklehurst and Dillane (30). They studied 100 incontinent elderly women and found a disease of the central nervous system in 83 of the patients. Of these, 42 had suffered a stroke, 27 had cerebral arteriosclerosis, and 14 had other CNS diseases. The general intellectual capacity of the incontinent patients was compared with a control group of nonincontinent aged women. Tests of orientation and toy tests were used. Highly significant differences were found between the two groups in orientation in time and place and in performance. The findings indicated a considerable amount of brain damage in this series.

CARDIOVASCULAR INVOLVEMENT

The physician examining his patient with OBS may often neglect the underlying cardiovascular changes. The conditions of importance are the following: cardiac decompensation, rhythm disturbances, arterial hypertension, and orthostatic hypotension.

Cardiac Involvement

In patients with transient cerebral attacks or palpitations, Goldberg et al. (31) described dangerous arrhythmias. They used ambulatory electrocardiographic recording, which was made continuously over 24 hr, in 130 ambulant outpatients complaining of syncope, dizzy turns, or palpitations. Analysis of the tape recording showed appreciable dysrhythmias in 74% of the group. In most cases the dysrhythmias were complex mixtures of rapid supraventricular and ventricular rhythms. Bouts of ventricular tachycardia were seen in 7 patients, all of whom were women. Episodic complete heart block was seen in only 2 patients, but prolonged ventricular gaps (greater than 1.5 sec) not associated with ectopic beats were found in 26 cases. A study of 60 asymptomatic subjects in six decades from the ages of 20 upward failed to show any dysrhythmias in 95%, and important dysrhythmias such as supraventricular tachycardia occurred only in 1%.

Impaired brain function is a common finding in myocardial infarction of the aged. Rodstein (32) and Pathy (33) have studied series of patients with myocardial infarction and separated cases of brain affection without classical signs of heart disease. It is obvious that OBS is a common finding in the acute phase of myocardial infarction in the aged. The cause is decreased cardiac output and cerebral blood flow. Konu has studied the epidemiology of myocardial infarction in the aged in Turku, Finland (34). He studied 228 patients and his series comprised 241 infarcts, 108 in men and 133 in women. The mean age was 73 years in men and 74 in women. The prevalence of clinical symptoms of brain affection is shown in Table 16-1.

Functional impairment of the brain occurred in 22.1% and was two to three times more common in women than in men. In 11 men and in 15 women, hemiplegia had preceded the myocardial infarction – in 15 patients only 1 to 2 weeks before the latter occurred.

TABLE 16-1. *Incidence of symptoms due to brain involvement in 228 elderly patients*

	Men	Women	All (%)
Confusion	3	9	5
Unconsciousness	8	14	9.1
Hemiplegia	0	2	0.9
Dizziness	4	13	7.1

Myocardial infarction as a cause of acute functional brain affection is often overlooked. In acute confusional states, when acute falls and dizziness attacks occur, an EKG recording and appropriate blood enzyme estimations must be regarded as routine examinations in the elderly.

Hypertension

It is difficult to define "normal" levels for blood pressure in old age, although generally it can be stated that hypertension in advanced age is seldom of a malignant type. In consequence, hypertension in the elderly might be classified mainly as "benign essential hypertension." However, in some cases established hypertensive brain disease does occur, and in these cases, there is usually a long history of hypertension.

Orthostatic Hypotension

Orthostatism occurs in 10 to 30% of old people living at home.

In senescence, the two most important factors are drugs with a hypotensive effect and cerebrovascular disease. The relevant terminology is somewhat variable, although two main types of orthostatism are generally discerned. In postural hypotension, the systolic and especially the diastolic pressure drop on arising, indicating failing arteriolar constriction in the presence of venous pooling. The stroke volume decreases while the heart rate remains largely unchanged. There is no rise in the plasma norepinephrine content on arising. The basic cause of the disorder lies in sympathetic nervous insufficiency of diverse origin, as follows: idiopathic, secondary to diabetes, multiple sclerosis, cerebral vascular disease, and administration of tranquilizers and ganglionic or adrenergic blocking agents, including most of the antihypertensive drugs.

In orthostatic hypotension, on the other hand, the systolic pressure is lowered, reflecting decreased stroke volume, whereas the diastolic pressure usually exhibits some elevation, indicating arteriolar constriction. There is also marked cardiac acceleration, yet the cardiac output falls because of relatively greater reduction of the stroke volume. The plasma norepinephrine is increased, with consequent reflex sympathetic activation, although this is insufficient to compensate for the basic failure. The basic failure is a greatly decreased venous return resulting from pooling of blood in the dependent, often weak-walled or varicose veins.

Of these two types of orthostatism, the former asympathetic or postural hypotension occurs chiefly in persons over the age of 50. Men are affected three times more often than women.

TREATMENT AFFECTING THE CIRCULATORY SYSTEM

A number of cardiac and circulatory drugs can be used in the treatment of the OBS at various etiological stages.

Heart Failure and Rhythm Disturbances

Treatment of heart failure with digitalis and diuretics in the aged is of great importance for maintaining appropriate perfusion of the brain. However, digitalis is often poorly tolerated in the aged and toxic effects are quite common. Bradycardia due to digitalis treatment decreases the CVR. The most common rhythm disturbance of significance is atrial fibrillation. Electroconversion is usually not indicated in the elderly. Beta blockers are indicated and tolerated even in very old age, and patients with a combination of rhythm disturbances, coronary artery disease, and hypertension are often beneficially treated with these drugs. The patients must be observed carefully, at least during the first 2 weeks of treatment, for early detection of heart decompensation and bradycardia, with impairment of CVR.

In cases with Adam-Stokes syndrome, an artificial pacemaker is indicated even in the very old. Lagergren and Olsson (35) demonstrated a highly significant improvement in mental efficiency in a group of 12 patients with artificial pacemakers. They showed an increase in their heart rate from an average of 46 beats/min to 72 beats/min. Mental efficiency was measured by psychomotor and perceptual tests, including simple and choice reaction time, critical flickerfusion rate, visual acuity, and digit symbol.

Hypertension

Treatment of hypertension in the aged is usually not indicated, as such treatment must be started earlier in life, before established hypertensive brain disease occurs. Furthermore, vigorous treatment of patients with hypertensive brain disease, diffuse cerebral symptoms, and dementia, with antihypertensive drugs, is contraindicated (36). There is an urgent need to screen for hypertension in the younger age groups, but not in old age. Newly detected arterial hypertension in aged patients is only an indication for treatment when a lowering of the arterial blood pressure is necessary to prevent cardiac decompensation.

Orthostatic Hypotension

There are two drugs commonly used in the treatment of orthostatic hypotension: ethylnorphenylephrine (Effortil®) and dihydroergotamine.

Lund et al. (37) studied the effect of ethylnorphenylephrine on orthostatic hypotension in 15 severely disabled geriatric patients. The investigation was carried out as an intraindividual crossover study with placebo control. There was a statistically significant difference in favor of ethylnorphenylephrine. Nordenfelt and Mellander (38) studied the central hemodynamic effects of dihydroergotamine on 10 female patients with orthostatic hypotension. Dihydroergotamine increased the cardiac stroke volume in the standing position, decreased the pulse rate, and increased the central blood volume. This effect is obviously beneficial in patients with orthostatic hypotension.

PERIPHERAL VASODILATORS

The clinical studies of the effects of vasodilators on OBS in aged subjects are beset by great difficulties. The results must be interpreted critically with the following objections in mind. Methods of observing the patients and measuring the changes of the observed parameters are poor. This criticism concerns both rating scales and global assessment of the patients especially. Many studies have included patients with ill-defined clinical conditions, such as "geriatric" or "disabled" patients.

The degree of alertness can change in a few hours and can be considerable during a few days. Diseases can change the alertness of the patients during a follow-up period and the subjects can show either a decrease or increase in the observed parameters which has nothing to do with the effect of the drug. Double-blind controlled studies have been reported which, in contrast to what should be expected, have shown significant improvement in most of the parameters observed. It is a well-known fact, however, that there are numerous well-designed clinical studies which have failed to show any effect of the drug in question. These studies have usually remained unpublished and have been forgotten. This means that the selection of published papers favors the successful ones.

The effect of vasodilating drugs in the treatment of patients with cerebrovascular disease has been widely discussed, but opinions as to the benefit of this kind of treatment are divergent. An often expressed opinion stresses that vasodilation can be possible only in intact or nearly intact vessels of the brain. Vasodilation of these vessels changes the blood flow in the brain so that the perfusion of those areas where the vessels are rigid and narrow decreases. Thus, the effect of the vasodilation, in spite of increasing the total blood flow of the brain, might decrease the regional blood flow of the more heavily affected areas. In 75% of cases, a cerebrovascular accident is a thrombosis and causes an infarction of the affected area of the brain. The total blood flow of the brain decreases, but in the neighboring area of the infarction, there is a maximal vasodilation which sometimes can be demonstrated angiographically and is called laxory perfusion. Obviously the carbon dioxide (CO_2) released from the infarcted tissue causes the vasodilation. There then ensues development of collateral circulation, on which the survival and function of the neighboring areas of the infarction are dependent. After a period of some weeks, up to 2 months, this acute phase is over and the situation becomes more stable.

Nevertheless, it has been shown that with some agents, in some patients, cerebral circulation can be improved, even in ischemic regions. Generally it can be said that the value of cerebral blood flow measurements is questionable and that there are great difficulties in promoting controlled clinical studies of vasodilator effects, especially in old patients. CO_2 is the most potent vasodilator of the cerebral vessels, but because of toxicity it has no place in the treatment of patients. In 1952, Jayne et al. (39), using the Kety-Schmidt method, demonstrated that intravenous administration of 200 mg papaverine increased mean cerebral blood flow 13%, or from 56.6 to 63.9 ml/100 g/min in 18 patients. The authors thought that the mechanism whereby papaverine increases cerebral blood flow and decreases cerebral vascular resistance is its direct vasodilating effect on cerebral vessels. These findings were confirmed by Aizawa et al. in 1961 (40) and Gottstein (41). Meyer et al. (42) first produced evidence to suggest that papaverine would increase oxygen availability. Other vasodilating agents which have been reported beneficial in the treatment of stroke patients are hexobendine, dihydroergotamine, cyclandelate, nylidrin, and the carbonic anhydrase inhibitor, acetazolamide.

The ergot alkaloid preparation, dihydroergotamine, has been studied extensively. It has been claimed that it improves the brain metabolism and blood supply of the brain. Although it is not strictly a vasodilator, controlled clinical studies have shown significant improvement of performance and mental ability of the observed subjects (43–48).

Cyclandelate (Cyclospasmol®) was given on a double-blind basis to 11 patients with cerebrovascular disease by O'Brien and Veall (49), and CBF measurements were performed by the xenon inhalation method, after both placebo and drug. The patients receiving cyclandelate had 6.51 ± 1.55 ml/100 g/min increase in CBF, which was significant. Several clinical trials have suggested that patients treated with cyclandelate may show improvement in their mental and neurological state. Ball and Taylor (50) reported a double-blind trial with cyclandelate and placebo and showed a significant improvement in the results of mental function tests in the group of patients treated with cyclandelate. Young et al. (51) studied 21 patients suffering from cerebral arteriosclerosis, diagnosed on defined clinical criteria and treated with cyclandelate in a double-blind, controlled crossover trial lasting

12 months. They found that the usual decline in various psychiatric, neurological, behavioral, and psychometric parameters did not occur during the cyclandelate-treated phase.

CLINICAL TRIAL OF CYCLANDELATE

A study was performed by one of the authors (L.S.), with the aim of observing the effect of cyclandelate on sensorimotor performance in aged patients. This involved comparing two groups, one consisting of patients with a past history of cerebrovascular accident (CVA) and another, patients without evidence of past CVA.

The study was carried out as a double-blind trial, comparing cyclandelate with a placebo in groups of patients who either had or had not suffered a CVA. Forty patients, whose mean age was 74 years, completed the trial; 18 patients (Group I) had suffered a CVA not less than 2 months previously, and 22 patients (Group II) had no clinical signs of cerebrovascular disease but a comparable history of hospitalization for a variety of physical disorders. Half of the patients in Groups I and II were treated with cyclandelate (1,600 mg/day) for a period of 6 weeks, whereas the remainder received a placebo for a similar period. Prior to commencing treatment, and again after the 6 weeks of treatment, all patients were tested by a number of psychological methods assessing perceptual factors. These methods have been described by Sourander et al. (52). A total of 14 variables were assessed by these techniques, of which four measured sense of balance, four measured kinesthetic perception. and six measured visual perception.

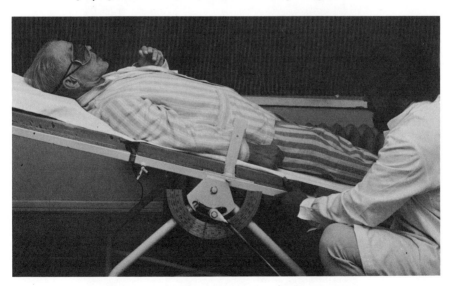

FIG. 16-5. Test for sense of balance: horizontal tilting. [Figs. 16-5 and 16-6 reproduced from *Geriatrics* © 1970 by Harcourt Brace Jovanovich, Inc. (52)].

Test for sense of balance. The purpose of this test was to measure the subject's sense of balance in the vertical and the horizontal position with vision excluded. In variables 1 and 2, the subject lay blindfolded on a bed which could be tilted like a seesaw, and in variables 3 and 4 the subject sat blindfolded in a chair which could be tilted sideways.

The subject was asked to state when he thought himself to be in the horizontal or vertical position, and this data was then recorded by four different maneuvers as follows.

Variable 1: Head lifted 20° and then lowered toward the horizontal.
Variable 2: Head lowered 20° and then lifted toward the horizontal.
Variable 3: Patient tilted 20° to the right followed by gradual decrease of tilt.
Variable 4: Patient tilted 20° to the left followed by gradual decrease of tilt.

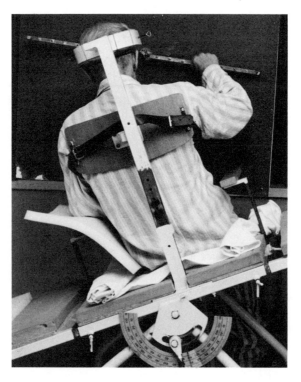

FIG. 16-6. Test for sense of balance: sideways tilting.

Test for kinesthetic perception. The purpose here was to measure the subject's perception of the horizontal. The subject sat in the chair with body and head supported. At a distance of 40 cm from the blindfolded subject's face was a rod 70 cm long and 2 cm wide, pivoted from its midpoint. The subject was instructed to feel the rod and to adjust it until it was horizontal (see Fig. 16-2). The experimenter then recorded the deviation, in degrees, of the subject's projection of the horizontal from the true horizontal. As before, four variable maneuvers were employed as follows.

Variable 5: Rod moved down with chair upright.
Variable 6: Rod moved up with chair upright.
Variable 7: Rod moved down with chair tilted 20° to the left.
Variable 8: Rod moved up with chair tilted 20° to the left.

Test for visual perception. This experiment was performed in a dark room, with only the rod, painted with luminous paint, being visible. The rod was 2.5 meters in front of the subject at the height of his eyes. The experimenter changed the tilt of the rod slowly, clockwise and counterclockwise in turn, and the subject was asked to give a signal when it was vertical and a second signal when it was horizontal. In this test, six variables were used as follows.

Variable 9: Rod moved down with chair upright.
Variable 10: Rod moved up with chair upright.
Variable 11: Rod moved down with chair tilted 20° to the left.
Variable 12: Rod moved up with chair tilted 20° to the left.
Variable 13: Rod moved down with chair tilted 20° to the right.
Variable 14: Rod moved up with chair tilted 20° to the right.

RESULTS

The data obtained from these 14 variables were statistically analyzed by analysis of variance, comparisons being made between Groups I and II in terms of the differences observed before and after treatment with cyclandelate and placebo. These results are shown in Tables 16-2 and 16-3.

For the four variables assessing sense of balance, there were highly significant differences ($p < 0.01$) in favor of cyclandelate for the CVA (Group I) group of patients. Next, considering the four variables assessing kinesthetic perception, there were also differences in favor of cyclandelate in the CVA group (Group I), although these just failed to achieve an acceptable level of statistical significance. Finally, the six variables assessing visual perception showed no significant overall difference between the CVA (Group I) and the non-CVA group (Group II).

The mean changes in the four variables measuring sense of balance, for Groups I and II, are shown in Table 16-4.

The results of the study suggest that treatment with cyclandelate benefits

TABLE 16-2. *Effect of cyclandelate (Cyclospasmol®) on sensorimotor abilities in 18 patients with past cerebrovascular accidents (Group I) ($\bar{\chi}$ degrees)*

| Test | Variable | Cyclandelate treated | | | | Placebo treated | | | |
| | | Before | | After | | Before | | After | |
		$\bar{\chi}$	SD	$\bar{\chi}$	SD	$\bar{\chi}$	SD	$\bar{\chi}$	SD
Sense of balance	1	16.0	19.6	11.3	7.4	6.8	4.9	6.2	6.3
	2	13.5	20.9	5.1	4.9	10.3	5.7	6.8	4.7
	3	7.0	3.6	5.8	4.4	6.2	6.0	4.8	3.6
	4	9.8	9.9	2.8	2.7	5.6	4.7	3.8	3.0
Kinesthetic perception	5	20.5	19.9	5.3	3.5	16.5	13.0	17.2	11.2
	6	16.6	23.3	3.5	2.6	20.2	13.5	19.5	11.9
	7	23.3	18.6	10.6	6.6	24.6	11.5	14.3	7.7
	8	21.6	22.4	9.6	8.9	19.0	8.3	20.3	14.2
Visual perception	9	12.1	11.9	9.3	5.0	10.3	4.6	11.3	6.4
	10	9.8	4.8	7.1	4.5	10.0	6.3	12.0	7.2
	11	22.0	12.3	13.1	7.9	16.2	6.2	15.6	9.7
	12	13.1	7.6	12.3	10.1	12.1	3.9	16.5	7.8
	13	24.0	21.4	16.3	16.9	14.0	7.7	23.2	13.5
	14	8.6	7.0	13.0	8.5	14.8	9.5	16.2	10.9

TABLE 16-3. *Effect of cyclandelate (Cyclospasmol®) on sensorimotor abilities in 22 patients without signs of clinical cerebrovascular disease (Group II) ($\bar{\chi}$ degrees)*

| Test | Variable | Cyclandelate treated | | | | Placebo treated | | | |
| | | Before | | After | | Before | | After | |
		$\bar{\chi}$	SD	$\bar{\chi}$	SD	$\bar{\chi}$	SD	$\bar{\chi}$	SD
Sense of balance	1	9.0	8.7	8.0	4.9	10.6	12.2	9.5	8.5
	2	10.3	10.7	11.2	7.8	7.0	4.4	9.4	12.7
	3	9.6	9.9	4.5	3.3	7.2	4.5	6.2	9.0
	4	7.4	8.4	7.0	6.4	7.0	5.6	6.0	8.7
Kinesthetic perception	5	17.6	19.4	10.9	8.0	13.8	9.4	12.3	9.4
	6	20.4	20.5	8.6	4.2	12.7	7.9	13.2	11.5
	7	23.4	24.9	13.9	9.1	15.2	6.2	13.6	11.2
	8	20.3	17.1	12.0	8.3	20.7	13.5	15.6	12.5
Visual perception	9	9.2	7.8	10.0	7.0	9.8	6.4	14.9	7.8
	10	9.7	10.8	9.0	4.2	8.9	5.8	12.5	7.6
	11	14.0	7.4	13.7	10.8	15.4	9.2	16.4	7.9
	12	11.4	8.7	11.9	7.0	11.1	5.0	17.2	11.5
	13	11.8	6.7	13.8	8.6	12.1	7.4	18.0	8.3
	14	7.6	4.9	9.1	5.3	10.1	4.6	15.5	9.1

TABLE 16-4. *Mean changes* (± SD) in sense of balance variables before versus after treatment, of patients receiving cyclandelate and placebo

	CVA (Group I); $n = 18$		Non-CVA (Group II); $n = 22$	
	Cyclandelate	Placebo	Cyclandelate	Placebo
Variable 1	−4.7 ± 2.4	−0.6 ± 1.1	−1.0 ± 0.7	−1.1 ± 0.6
Variable 2	−8.4 ± 3.1	−3.5 ± 2.0	+0.9 ± 0.3	+2.4 ± 1.7
Variable 3	−1.2 ± 0.9	−1.4 ± 0.7	−5.1 ± 3.2	−1.0 ± 1.4
Variable 4	−7.0 ± 3.4	−1.8 ± 1.3	−0.4 ± 0.5	−1.0 ± 1.1

aged patients with past cerebrovascular accidents, in that there is an improvement in spatial orientation and control of the horizontal plane.

OTHER FORMS OF DRUG THERAPY

Anticoagulants

Anticoagulants may protect some arteriosclerotic patients against recurrent small cerebral infarcts, thrombotic episodes, and ensuing cerebral ischemia. However, their use is still controversial; some authors are enthusiastic about them (53), but others doubt the general effectiveness of anticoagulants in the management of patients with early OBS due to arteriosclerosis (54). The most obvious indication for anticoagulant treatment in the aged is atrial fibrillation and the prevention of embolism. Another indication is recurrent transient ischemic attacks in the elderly.

Naftidrofuryl

Naftidrofuryl (Praxiline®) has been claimed to increase the respiration rate of brain tissue and increase the glucose metabolism of the brain in animal experiments (55). Some improvement in intellectual performance has been registered, in controlled clinical trials, in geriatric patients suffering from OBS (56,57).

Piracetam

Perhaps the most interesting new drug claimed to act beneficially on brain function is piracetam. It belongs to a group of psychotropic drugs which have been called nootropic substances by Giurgea (58). Lagergren and Levander (59) studied whether, and to what extent, piracetam is protective against the effects of a decreased cerebral circulation (i.e., assumedly against hypoxia). They investigated the effects of piracetam at varied heart rates in patients with artificial pacemakers. Four psychometric tests were used, measuring vigilance, and the results suggested that piracetam indeed had certain effects on performance. Furthermore, the drug ameliorates the decrement in performance induced by a decrease in heart rate, and thereby, presumedly, a reduction in cerebral blood flow. In another study, Mindus et al. (60) found that piracetam produced improvement in mental tasks demanding acuity and vigilance, in elderly persons with slight symptoms of OBS.

The most striking results in elderly patients with OBS are achieved by a well-planned rehabilitation program which includes physiotherapy, activation, resocialization, and remotivation of the patient. It cannot be denied, however, that some benefit with vasodilating and psychotropic drugs has been recorded in numerous controlled clinical studies. It is obvious that a critical but not nihilistic attitude toward drug therapy in aged patients with OBS is highly indicated.

CONCLUSIONS

1. Organic brain syndromes (OBS) in old age are often caused by or related to cerebrovascular insufficiency (CVI). Careful observation of the patient with OBS provides a good opportunity for the clinician to distinguish between circulatory disorders and' primary neurodegenerative diseases affecting the aged brain. There is, however, still a widespread misunderstanding among clinicians of the basic hemodynamic and neuropathologic changes in OBS.

2. Cerebrovascular insufficiency is often a result of extracranial changes of the circulatory system and not merely the result of cerebrovascular arteriosclerosis. Cardiovascular diseases and impaired autoregulation are of utmost importance. Cerebrovascular blood flow (CBF) is diminished because of a decreased cardiac output, increased cerebrovascular resistance (CVR), or hypotensive episodes. The result is ischemic lesions and multiple infarcts of the brain. Therefore, in patients with OBS a review of their cardiovascular status is important.

3. Treatment must be adequate and based on clinical findings. Appropriate treatment of heart failure and rhythm disturbances is crucial in the prevention of ischemic brain lesions in the aged. The uncritical use of drugs which are considered to "improve brain function" should be abandoned. Treatment of hypertension must start early in life, not in senescence. Therefore, early screening for hypertension may be of importance, while the hypotensive effect of many drugs must be kept in mind.

4. Some common symptoms related to a mild degree of OBS, such as diminished alertness and disturbance of the sense of balance and postural control, obviously can be improved by pharmacotherapy.

5. The effect of vasodilating agents, such as cyclandelate, on the integrative cerebral functions maintaining postural control may be of im-

portance. Such treatment beneficially assists rehabilitation in aged patients with past CVA. The effect of vasodilating agents, however, is still dubious, and such agents should not be considered routine therapy in patients with OBS. Some new drugs such as piracetam are interesting, but it is still not possible to assess their final value.

REFERENCES

1. Fazekas, J. F., Kleh, J., and Witkin, L. Cerebral haemodynamics and metabolism in subjects over 90 years of age. *J. Am. Geriatr. Soc.*, 1953, 1, 836.
2. Corday, E., Rothenberg, S. F., and Putnam, T. J. Cerebrovascular insufficiency. An explanation of some types of localized cerebral encephalopathy. *Arch. Neurol. Psychiatry*, 1953, 69, 551.
3. Sokoloff, L. Circulation and metabolism of brain in relation to the process of aging. In: *The Process of Aging in the Nervous System*, edited by J. E. Birren, H. A. Imus, and W. F. Windle. Charles C Thomas, Springfield, Ill., 1959, p. 113.
4. Sokoloff, L. Aspects of cerebral circulatory physiology of relevance to cerebrovascular disease. *Neurology*, 1961, 11, 34.
4a. Sokoloff, L. Cerebral circulation and metabolism in the aged. In:*Aging*, Vol. 2, edited by S. Gershon and A. Raskin. Raven Press, New York, 1975, p. 45.
5. Gellerstedt, N. Zur Kenntnis der Hirnveränderungen bei der normalen Altersinvolution. *Upsala Läkarefören*. N.F. Vol. 38, 1933.
6. Hassler, O. Vascular changes in senile brains. A micro-angiographic study. *Acta Neuropathol.*, 1965, 5, 40.
7. Hassler, O. Arterial deformities in senile brains. *Acta Neuropathol.*, 1967, 8, 219.
8. Fisher, C. M. Dementia in cerebral vascular disease. In: *Cerebral Vascular Diseases. Sixth Conference*, edited by J. F. Toole, R. G. Siekert, and J. P. Whisnant. Grune and Stratton, New York, London, 1968.
9. Tomlinson, B. E., Blessed, G., and Roth, M. Observations on the brains of non-demented old people. *J. Neurol. Sci.*, 1968, 7, 331.
10. Worm-Petersen, Y., and Pakkenberg, H. Atherosclerosis of cerebral arteries, pathological and clinical correlation.*J. Gerontol.*, 1968, 23, 445.
11. Hachinski, V. C., Lassen, N. A., Marshall, J. Multiple-infarct dementia. A cause of mental deterioration in the elderly. *Lancet*, 1974, 2, 207.
12. Torvik, A., and Jorgensen, L. Thrombotic and embolic occlusions of the carotid arteries in an autopsy material. Part 1. Prevalence, location and associated diseases. *J. Neurol. Sci.*, 1964, 1, 24.
13. Ingvar, D. H., and Lassen, N. A. (Eds.). Brain work. The coupling of function, metabolism and blood flow in the brain. *Alfred Benzon Symposium. Series VIII*, Munksgaard, Copenhagen, 1976.
14. Corday, E., and Rothenberg, S. F. The clinical aspects of cerebral vascular insufficiency. *Ann. Intern. Med.*, 1957, 47, 626.
15. Corday, E., and Irving, D. W. Effect of cardiac arrhythmias on the cerebral circulation. *Am. J. Cardiol.*, 1960, 6, 803.
16. Brierley, J. B. Pathology of cerebral ischaemia. In: *Cerebral Vascular Diseases. Eighth Conference*, edited by F. H. McDowell and R. W. Brennan. Grune and Stratton, New York, London, 1973, p. 59.
17. Zülch, K. J., and Behrend, R. C. H. The pathogenesis and topography of anoxia hypoxia and ischaemia of the brain in man. In: *Cerebral Anoxia and the Electroencephalogram*, edited by H. Gastaut and J. S. Meyer. Charles C Thomas, Springfield, Ill., 1961.
18. Riishede, J. Cerebral apoplexy. *Acta Psychiatr. Neurol. Scand.* (Suppl. 118), 1957, Vol. 32.
19. Lassen, N. A. Cerebral blood flow and oxygen consumption in man determined by the inert gas diffusion method. A review. Christtreus Bogtrykkeri, Kobenhavn, 1958.
20. Paulsson, G. W., and Perrine, G., Jr. Cerebral vascular disease in mental hospitals. In:

Cerebral Vascular Diseases. Sixth Conference, edited by J. F. Toole, R. G. Siekert, and J. P. Whisnant. Grune and Stratton, New York, London, 1968, 232.

21. Dalessio, D. J., Benchimol, A., and Dimond, E. G. Chronic encephalopathy related to heart block. *Neurology,* 1965, 15, 499.

22. Abdon, N.-J., and Malmcrona, R. Symptomatic patients with bradyarrhythmias hidden in the population. *Lancet,* 1973, 2, 607.

23. Abdon, N.-J., and Heister, B. Intermittenta hjärtarytmier hos senildementa. *Sv. Läkartidning,* 1974, 71, 1296.

24. Matthew, N. T., and Meyer, J. S. Pathogenesis and natural history of transient global amnesia. *Stroke,* 1974, 5, 303.

25. Perez, F. I., Rivera, V. M., Meyer, J. S., Gay, A., Taylor, R. L., and Matthew, N. T. Analysis of intellectual and cognitive performance in patients with multi-infarct dementia, vertebrobasilar insufficiency with dementia and Alzheimer's disease. *J. Neurol. Neurosurg. Psychiatry,* 1975, 38, 533.

26. Sjögren, H., and Sourander, P. Senil demens – en eller flera sjukdomar. *Läkartidningen,* 1974, 71, 1293.

27. Head, H. The conception of nervous and mental energy II. Vigilance: A physiological state of nervous system. *Br. J. Psychol.,* 1923, 14, 126.

28. Welford, A. T. On changes of performance with age. *Lancet,* 1962, 1, 335.

29. Welford, A. T. Performance, biological mechanisms and age: A theoretical sketch. In: *Behaviour, Aging and the Nervous System,* edited by A. T. Welford and J. E. Birren. Charles C Thomas, Springfield, Ill., 1965, p. 3.

30. Brocklehurst, J. C., and Dillane, J. B. Studies of the female bladder in old age II. Cystometrograms in 100 incontinent women. *Gerontol. Clin.,* 1966, 8, 306.

31. Goldberg, A. D., Raftery, E. B., and Cashman, P. M. M. Ambulatory electrocardiographic records in patients with transient cerebral attacks or palpitation. *Br. Med. J.,* 1975, 4, 569.

32. Rodstein, M. The characteristics of non-fatal myocardial infarction in the aged. *Arch. Intern. Med.,* 1956, 98, 84.

33. Pathy, M. S. Clinical presentation of myocardial infarction in the elderly. *Br. Heart J.,* 1967, 29, 190.

34. Konu, V. Myocardial infarction in the elderly. A clinical and epidemiological one year follow-up study in the coronary register of Turku. *(To be published.)*

35. Lagergren, K., and Olsson, J. E. The effect of exogenous changes in heart rate upon mental performance in patients treated with artificial pacemakers for complete heart block. Karolinska Sjukhuset, Stockholm, 1973.

36. Hughes, W., Dodgson, M. C. H., and McLennan, D. C. Chronic hypertensive cerebral disease. *Lancet,* 1954, 2, 770.

37. Lund, V., Scherwin, J., and Wirenfeldt Asmussen, N. Treatment of orthostatic hypotension in severely disabled geriatric patients. *Curr. Ther. Res.,* 1972, 14, 252.

38. Nordenfelt, I., and Mellander, S. Central haemodynamic effects of dihydroergotamine in patients with orthostatic hypotension. *Acta Med. Scand.,* 1972, 191, 115.

39. Jayne, H. W., Scheinberg, P., Rich, M. et al. The effect of intravenous papaverine *hydrochloride* on the cerebral circulation. *J. Clin. Invest.,* 1952, 31, 111.

40. Aizawa, T., Tazaki, Y., and Gotoh, F. Cerebral circulation in cerebrovascular disease. *World Neurol.,* 1961, 2, 635.

41. Gottstein, U. Pharmacological studies of total cerebral blood flow in man with comments on the possibility of improving regional cerebral blood flow by drugs. *Acta Neurol. Scand.* (Suppl. 14), 1965, 136.

42. Meyer, J. S., Gotoh, F., Gilroy, J. et al. Improvement on brain oxygenation and clinical improvement in patients with strokes treated with papaverine hydrochloride. *J.A.M.A.,* 1965, 194, 957.

43. Emmenegger, H., and Meier-Ruge, W. The actions of Hydergine on the brain. A histochemical circulatory and neurophysiological study. *Pharmacology,* 1968, 1, 65.

44. Gerin, J. Symptomatic treatment of cerebrovascular insufficiency with Hydergine. *Clin. Ther. Res.,* 1969, 11, 539.

45. Jennings, W. G. An ergot alkaloid preparation (Hydergine) versus placebo for treatment

of symptoms of cerebrovascular insufficiency: A double-blind study. *J. Am. Geriatr. Soc.,* 1972, 20, 407.

46. Bazo, A. J. An ergot alkaloid preparation (Hydergine) versus papaverine in treating common complaints of the aged: Double-blind study. *J. Am. Geriatr. Soc.,* 1973, 21, 63.
47. Cerletti, A., Emmenegger, H., Meier-Ruge, W. et al. Experimental cerebral insufficiency. Models for the quantification of dihydrogenated ergot effects on brain metabolism and functions. Scientific Exhibit. Federation of Amer. Societies for Exp. Biol., 57th Annual Meeting, Atlantic City. N.J., April 15–20, 1973.
48. Mongeau, B. The effect of hydergine on cerebral blood perfusion in diffuse cerebral insufficiency. *Eur. J. Clin. Pharmacol.* (accepted for publication).
49. O'Brien, M. D., and Veall, N. Effect of cyclandelate on cerebral cortex perfusion-rates in cerebrovascular disease. *Lancet,* 1966, 2, 729.
50. Ball, J. A. C., and Taylor, A. R. Effect of cyclandelate on mental function and cerebral blood flow in elderly patients. *Br. Med. J.,* 1967, 3, 525.
51. Young, J., Hall, P., and Blakemore, C. Treatment of cerebral manifestations of arteriosclerosis with cyclandelate. *Br. J. Psychiatry,* 1974, 124, 177.
52. Sourander, L., Ruikka, I., and Rautakorpi, J. Psychological methods applied to evaluate symptomatic geriatric treatment. *Geriatrics,* 1970, 6, 41.
53. Walsh, A. C., and Walsh, B. H. Senile and presenile dementia: Further observations on the benefits of a dicumarol-psychotherapy regime. *J. Am. Geriatr. Soc.,* 1972, 20, 127.
54. Baker, R. N., Millikan, C. H., Siekert, R. G., and Schick, R. M. Anticoagulant therapy of cerebral infarction: Report of a National Co-operative Study. In: *Cerebrovascular Disease,* Chapter XX, edited by C. H. Millikan. Proc. Assoc. Nerv. and Ment. Dis., New York City, Dec. 8–9, 1961. Williams and Wilkins, 1966, p. 287.
55. Meynaud, A., Grand, M., and Fontaine, L. Effect of naftidrofuryl upon energy metabolism of the brain. *Arzneim Forsch.,* 1973, 23, 1431.
56. Judge, T. G., and Urquhart, A. Naftidrofuryl – a double-blind crossover study in the elderly. *Curr. Med. Res. Opinion,* 1972, 1, 166.
57. Bouvier, J. B., Passeron, O., and Chupin, M. P. Psychometric study of praxilene. *J. Int. Med. Res.,* 1974, 2, 59.
58. Giurgea, C. The "nootropic" approach to the integrative activity of the brain. *Cond. Reflex,* 8, 1973, 108.
59. Lagergren, K., and Levander, S. A double-blind study on the effects of piracetam upon perceptual and psychomotor performance at varied heart rates in patients treated with artificial pacemakers. *Psychopharmacologie* (Berl.), 1974, 39, 97.
60. Mindus, P., Cronholm, B., Levander, S. E., and Schalling, D. Piracetam and mental performance in aging people. Presented at the APA Annual Meeting, May 5–9, 1975, Anaheim, Calif.

ACKNOWLEDGMENT

The authors are indebted to Dr. Hakon Sjögren for clinical examinations (clinical pathological investigations), to Timo Laes, M. A. for psychometric testing, and to Dr. Colin Blakemore for statistical analysis (clinical trial of cyclandelates).

Stress and the Heart, edited by D. Wheatley,
Raven Press, New York © 1981.

Nootropic Drugs and Human Brain Function

Bernd Saletu

Geriatric psychopharmacology has long been a neglected area in psychopharmacologic research. This is surprising, as the geriatric population is growing rapidly in all developed countries. In fact, the elderly in need of drug therapy for somatic and psychic complaints outnumber any other diagnostic group in neuropsychiatry (1). The state of the art is best characterized by the large number of synonyms for substances of this class of drugs. As some of these drugs lack usual pharmacologic activities and selectively improve efficiency of higher telencephalic and integrative activities, Giurgea (2) proposed the term "nootropics." These substances have one property in common: they combat hypoxia. Hypoxia, according to Strughold (3), is an impairment of the "cerebral biological oxidation," which may be due to an hypoxic, nutritive, histotoxic, ischemic, metabolic, or hypochreotic cause. Unfortunately, the problem of assessing objectively and quantitatively the therapeutic efficiency of such drugs on the central nervous system (CNS) is intrinsically complex.

One of the few techniques proved to be of value in obtaining objective and quantitative data concerning pharmacodynamics of encephalotropic drugs in man is the quantitative pharmaco-EEG method (4–6). Utilizing digital computer period analysis or power spectral density analyses of the human electroencephalogram (EEG), along with some statistical procedures, it is possible to determine drug effects at the target organ: the human brain. By means of this rather simple and noninvasive technique, some conclusions can be made: (a) whether or not a drug is active on the CNS as compared with placebo, (b) to which psychotropic class it eventually belongs, (c) its duration of action, and (d) the effective dosage.

The aim of this chapter is to survey the growing body of neurophysiologic data (collected primarily in our own laboratory) of the main representatives of this new drug class. It should be understood, however, that treatment of underlying disorders, such as heart failure and rhythm disturbances, when present, is of utmost importance in the therapy of the organic brain syndrome, as outlined in the preceding chapter. This aspect of the problem is not discussed in this chapter.

METHODOLOGIC ASPECTS

In our own investigations, all neurophysiologic data were obtained utilizing the double-blind, placebo-controlled, crossover study design. Usually, groups of eight to 10 geriatric subjects over the age of 60 were studied; healthy younger volunteers in the age range of 20 to 45 years were also included.

In the single dose trials, the subjects received, randomized and at weekly intervals, single oral doses of the test substance (usually three different dosages), placebo, and a control substance. They were not allowed to take any psychoactive drugs 3 weeks before and/or during the study. To prevent the well-known decrease of vigilance after heavy meals, the subjects received snacks every other 2 hr.

A 3-min vigilance-controlled EEG (V-EEG) and a 3-min resting EEG (R-EEG) were recorded before and 1, 2, 4, 6, and 8 hr after oral administration of one single dose on an 8-channel Beckmann R611 polygraph or an SLE electroencephalograph. During the V-EEG recordings, the technician attempts to keep the vigilance of the subject constant; as soon as drowsiness patterns appear, the subject is aroused by the technician. The subject lies with eyes closed in a relaxed position on a bed located in an electrically shielded room. Scalp electrodes are placed according to the international 10/20 system. The 02-CZ lead plus three other leads (01-CZ, P3-CZ, P4-CZ) are recorded on a Hewlett-Packard 3968 tape recorder and analyzed offline primarily on an Intertechnique Plurimat S computer system utilizing power spectral density programs. The latter permit analysis of the dominant frequency, the relative and absolute power in the dominant frequency, and the total power, as well as the absolute and relative power in nine different frequency bands. Each 10- or 20-sec epoch with muscle movement or eye artifacts was excluded from the analysis.

ERGOT ALKALOID PREPARATIONS

Codergocrine Mesylate

Single doses of 5 mg hydergine®, a dihydrogenated ergot alkaloid containing dihydroergocornine, dihydroergocristine, and dihydroergokryptine in equal proportions, produced in the spectral analyzed V-EEG of geriatric subjects a statistically significant ($p < 0.05$, ANOVA) decrease of delta and theta activities, as well as an increase in alpha and slow beta activities (Fig. 17.1). In contrast, placebo did not induce any significant changes (with the exception of a decrease in the beta activity in the sixth hr). Hydergine-induced changes reached the level of statistical significance from the fourth hr on and increased thereafter until the eighth hr. In the R-EEG, similar alterations were observed, which reached the level of statistical significance in the second and sixth hr (7).

In the second study (8), almost identical alterations could be obtained (Fig. 17.2); in a third study, the changes did not reach the level of statistical significance.

Nicergoline

Nicergoline (Sermion®) is a 1,6-dimethyl-8 beta (5-bromonicotinoylooxy-methyl)-10 alpha-methoxyergoline (8). After single oral doses of 15, 30, and 60

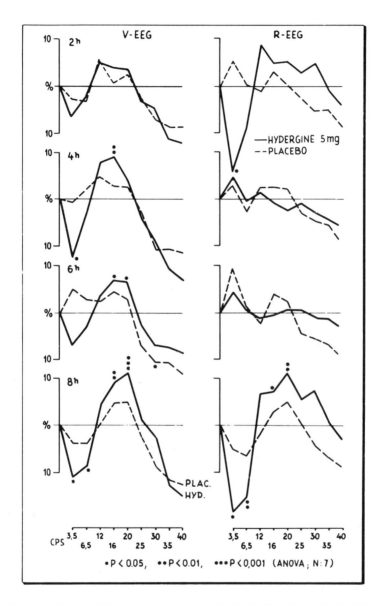

FIG. 17.1. Quantitative EEG changes after 5 mg hydergine® and placebo (relative power; 02-CZ; *N* = 7). Nine frequency bands are shown in the abscissae; drug-induced changes (in percentage of the pretreatment value) are represented in the ordinates. **Left:** Changes in the V-EEG. **Right:** Alterations in the R-EEG. While placebo does not induce statistically significant changes, hydergine attenuates delta and theta waves and augments alpha and slow beta activities. The peak effect is in the eighth hr.

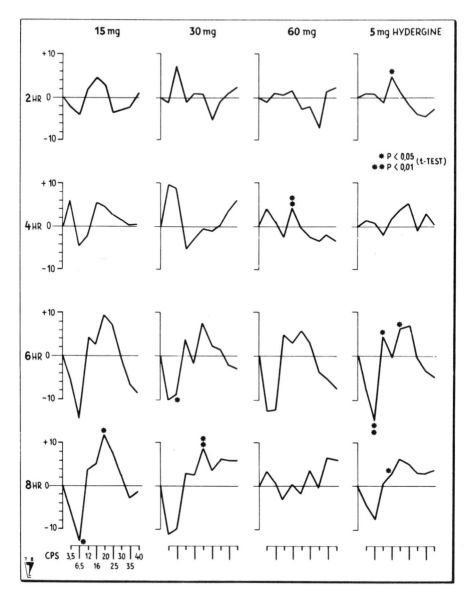

FIG. 17.2. Quantitative EEG changes in the V-EEG after nicergoline (15, 30, and 60 mg) and hydergine® (5 mg) as compared with placebo (3 min; V-EEG; 02-CZ; relative power; $N =$ 10). Nine frequency bands are shown in the abscissae; differences between drug-induced changes and placebo-induced alterations are shown in the ordinate. Placebo is represented by the zero-line. Both ergot alkaloids produce a decrease of delta and theta activities and an increase of alpha and slow beta activities, which are most pronounced at 6 to 8 hr (later recordings were not obtained).

mg, geriatric subjects showed significant changes in the spectral analyzed EEG as compared with placebo, which were characterized by a decrease of delta and theta activities and increases in alpha and (predominantly slow) beta activities (Fig. 17.2).

The described changes in brain activity were already observed with the lowest dosage of 15 mg, while an increase to 30 and 60 mg resulted in no increase of the CNS effect. Pharmacodynamic investigations regarding time-efficacy relationships demonstrated that the CNS effect-increase over time was maximally pronounced between the sixth and eighth hr. The control substance (5 mg hydergine®) induced similar changes, which were also most pronounced between the sixth and eighth hr. The equipotent dosage of nicergoline as compared to 5 mg hydergine® is between 15 and 30 mg. Psychometric investigations showed a significant improvement in the nonsense syllable learning test as compared with placebo and 5 mg hydergine®.

In a subsequent study, chronic CNS effects of nicergoline were observed in geriatric subjects (9). Using a double-blind crossover design, they received 30 mg nicergoline daily for 2 weeks, as well as placebo for an additional 2 weeks (with a drug-free interval of 1 week). Statistical analyses of the power spectrum data after one oral single dose confirmed our previous results, since the same pharmaco-EEG profile was obtained (Fig. 17.3) as in the earlier studies (Fig. 17.2). While delta and theta activities decreased, alpha and beta activities and the dominant frequency (Fig. 17.4) increased as compared with placebo, suggesting an improvement of vigilance. In both the neurophysiologic and psychometric data, the chronic effect was less pronounced than the acute one (Fig. 17.3).

Clinical Implications

Both of the ergot alkaloid preparations described above (codergocrine and nicergoline) induced the same type of changes, characterized by a decrease of delta and theta activities and an increase of alpha and slow beta activities. Such alterations are indicative of an increase in vigilance.

The term vigilance was proposed by Head (10) and stands for the adaptive ability of the CNS, which again is determined by the dynamic state of the total neuronal network. Indeed, a diminutive adaptive ability of the vigilance regulating systems in old age has been suggested by Kanowski (11). Several authors (12–15) could demonstrate that with increasing age, an increase in delta and theta activities, a decrease in alpha and slow beta activities, a trend toward an increase in fast beta activities above 30 cps, and a slowing of the dominant frequency occur (Fig. 17.5). Ergot alkaloid preparations induce alterations in the EEG which are opposite to the aforementioned alterations (Fig. 17.5) as demonstrated by Matejcek and Devos (12), Bente et al. (16), and our group (7–9). Matejcek and Devos (12) showed that the quantitative EEG changes during treatment of geriatric patients were associated with clinical improvement.

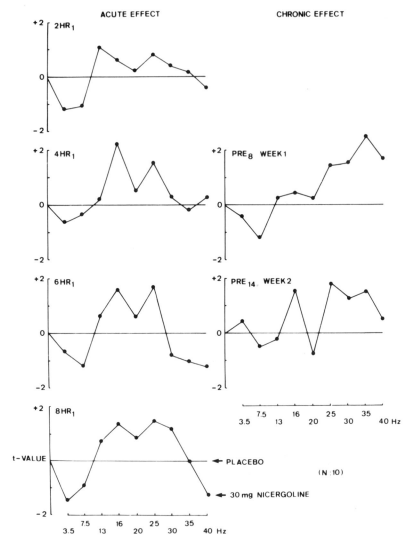

FIG. 17.3. V-EEG changes (relative power) after acute **(left)** and chronic **(right)** administration of nicergoline (30 mg daily) in the elderly as compared with placebo. Nine frequency bands are shown in the abscissae; differences between nicergoline- and placebo-induced alterations are shown in the ordinate. Placebo is represented by the zero-line. Single doses of nicergoline induce a decrease of slow activities and an increase of alpha and slow beta activities. After 1 and 2 weeks of treatment, the changes are similar; theta activity decreases and beta activities increase. The chronic effect seems less pronounced than the acute one.

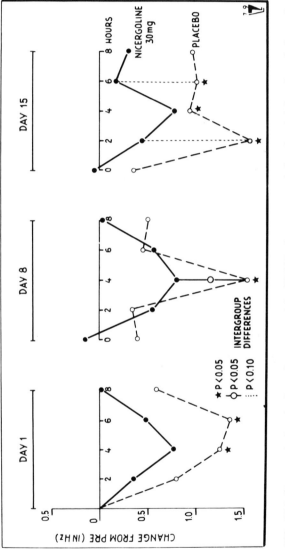

FIG. 17.4. Changes in the dominant frequency of the V-EEG after acute and chronic administration of nicergoline and placebo in the elderly (N = 10). Time is shown in the abscissae; changes from the predrug baseline (in cps) are indicated in the ordinate. Nicergoline attenuates the decrease of dominant frequency which occurs in the placebo condition.

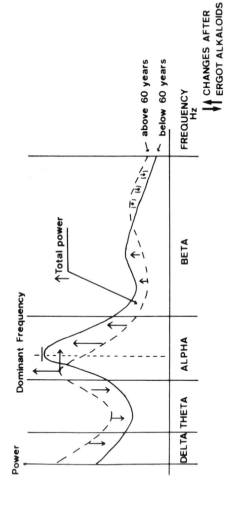

FIG. 17.5. Changes in the EEG power spectrum with advancing age and after ergot alkaloid preparations. Frequencies are shown in the abscissae, power in the ordinate. With advancing age, there is an increase in delta and theta activities, a decrease in the dominant frequency, and an attenuation of alpha and slow beta activity. Ergot alkaloid preparations induce the opposite effects (12).

Indeed, clinical evidence is mounting that ergot alkaloids are of value in the treatment of geriatric disorders. There are numerous double-blind clinical studies in which the therapeutic effects of hydergine were significantly superior to placebo (17,18). Regarding nicergoline, two double-blind studies have demonstrated a significant superiority of this natural rye ergot alkaloid over placebo. Michelangeli et al. (19) noted a significant improvement in the Wechsler memory test after long-term treatment with nicergoline, while Grel and Normand (20) observed a superiority of nicergoline as compared with placebo with respect to general activities and intellectual functions. Two studies involved the double-blind comparison of the activity of nicergoline and hydergine in elderly patients (21,22).

The therapeutic changes after hydergine reveal great variances. For instance, Geraud et al. (23) described improvements in physical impairment and activities of daily living but no changes in psychologic (mental) status; Triboletti and Ferri (24), however, noted improvement in attitude and mood but no alterations in physical manifestations and activities of daily living.

In two of our pharmaco-EEG studies with hydergine, we saw statistically significant changes but no significant changes in the third investigation. Thus the baseline is an important factor, as is the evaluation technique in clinical studies. One must be cautious in utilizing global rating scales and evaluation methods and should focus on well-defined smaller sections of mental performance and psychopathology. The principle mechanism of action of ergot alkaloids is probably a metabolic effect rather than the direct regulation of the cerebral circulation (25), although the latter has been demonstrated by some authors (26–28).

HEXOBENDINE, ETHOPHYLLINE, ETHAMIVAN, AND COMBINATIONS

In an early study, Instenon forte®, a fixed combination of 60 mg hexobendine + 60 mg ethophylline + 100 mg ethamivan, was investigated in healthy volunteers aged 23 to 32 years (29). Power spectrum analysis demonstrated a decrease of delta activity as well as an increase of alpha and beta activities, as compared with placebo (Fig. 17.6). The changes were dose-dependent and statistically significant until the second hr after 1 and 2 dragees and up to the sixth hr after 4 dragees. The effect was most pronounced in the first 2 hr. One ampule of Instenon induced significant changes (theta decrease, beta increase) in the first 2 hr after the injection, the equipotent dose being between 1 and 2 dragees.

As we were interested in which component of the combination Instenon forte is responsible for the above-described changes, we carried out a double-blind, placebo-controlled, pharmaco-EEG study involving 120 mg hexobendine, 120 mg ethophylline, 200 mg ethamivan, and combinations of 120 mg hexobendine + 120 mg ethophylline, 120 mg hexobendine + 200 mg ethamivan, and 120

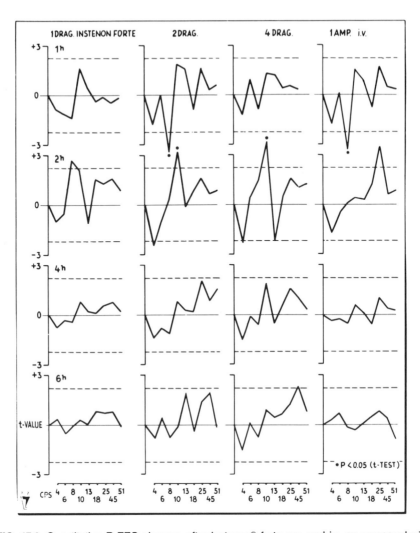

FIG. 17.6. Quantitative R-EEG changes after Instenon® forte p.o. and i.v. as compared with placebo (relative power; 02-CZ; $N = 10$). Nine frequency bands are shown in the abscissae; drug-induced changes as compared with placebo are expressed in t-values and are indicated in the ordinates. *Dotted lines,* significance at the p 0.05 level. Placebo is represented by the zero-line. Instenon forte induces a dose-dependent decrease in delta activity as well as an increase in alpha and beta activity as compared with placebo. The peak effect is within the first 2 hr.

mg ethophylline + 200 mg ethamivan in a similar population including 10 normal healthy volunteers aged 21 to 33 years (mean, 27 years). Power spectral density analysis of 3-min V-EEG and 4-min R-EEG periods at 0, 1, 2, 4, and 6 hr after oral administration demonstrated that the peak CNS effect occurred within the first hour after drug ingestion for all preparations.

Single Components of the Combination

The most effective single component of Instenon forte was 120 mg hexoben-dine, followed by 120 mg ethophylline and 200 mg ethamivan (Fig. 17.7). The significant attenuation of slow activities, augmentation of alpha activity, and the increase in the dominant frequency after 120 mg hexobendine indicate im-provement of vigilance (Fig. 17.7). Similar although less pronounced alterations were produced by 120 mg ethophylline, while 200 mg ethamivan induced only a decrease of fast activities (Fig. 17.7). If one combines 120 mg hexobendine with 120 mg ethophylline, an additive interaction may be observed, as the effect of hexobendine is potentiated by ethophylline (Fig. 17.7). In fact, this combina-tion was the most CNS active preparation at the time of the peak effect (first hr). Moreover, any combination of two components of Instenon forte produced more EEG changes than the single components alone. On the other hand, combi-nation of all three substances induced less neurophysiologic alterations than the hexobendine + ethophylline and hexobendine + ethamivan combination.

Our neurophysiologic findings with Instenon forte were accompanied by an increase in psychomotor activity and critical flicker frequency (CFF), by im-provement in quantitative and deterioration in qualitative aspects of attention, and by an improvement in mood and affectivity. Several clinicians have described significant improvements of creativity, memory, mood, and energy in geriatric patients. This has been more fully discussed by Saletu and Grünberger (29). An increase in CFF had already been described by Ambrosi and Neumayer (30) after intravenous injection of single doses of Instenon, as well as after the injection if its components ethophylline and ethamivan, but not after hexo-bendine.

On the other hand, our own investigations with orally administered single components of Instenon forte did not reveal any significant change in CFF, as compared with placebo, nor in attention, attention variability, tapping, com-plex reaction, and mnestic function ($p < 0.05$, Newman Keuls test). However, 120 mg hexobendine produced activation (prolongation of the aftereffect of the Archimedean spiral) in the second hr, and improvement in affectivity (fourth hr); 120 mg ethophylline decreased concentration (second hr) and improved reaction time (sixth hr) and mood (fourth hr); 200 mg ethamivan improved psychomotor activity. The combination hexobendine + ethophylline improved mood (second and fourth hr) and affectivity (fourth and sixth hr). As in the EEG, there were no significant changes after the hexobendine + ethamivan combination; while after the ethamivan + ethophylline combination, psychomo-tor activity (fourth hr) and reaction time (sixth hr) improved. Time- and dose-efficacy studies based on changes in 13 psychometric variables demonstrated that after hexobendine and the hexobendine + ethophylline combination, the maximal psychotropic effect occurred as early as the second hr (earlier psycho-metric tests could not be carried out), while the other preparations did not show any relevant time course from the second to the sixth hr. As in the EEG, the

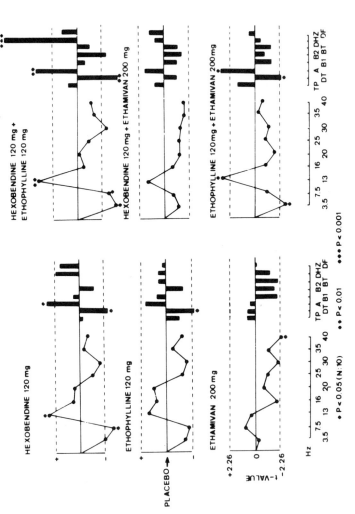

FIG. 17.7. Pharmaco-EEG profiles of hexobendine, ethophyline, ethamivan, and their combinations are compared with placebo (V-EEG; 1 hr post; relative power). Quantitative EEG measurements are shown in the abscissae; drug-induced changes as compared with placebo are indicated in the ordinates. Placebo is represented in the zero-line. Hexobendine (120 mg), ethophyline (120 mg), and the three different combinations attenuate delta and theta waves, increase alpha waves, and decrease fast beta activities. The hexobendine-ethophyline combination induces the most pronounced changes.

most effective preparation was the hexobendine + ethophylline combination.

Concerning the mode of action of these three substances, hexobendine is known to produce a selective vasodilation of cerebral and coronary vessels by increasing the uptake of glucose and free fatty acids. As the cerebral oxygen consumption remains virtually unchanged by hexobendine, citrate, malate, and possible other C_4 acids accumulate, leading to a metabolic acidosis with release of H^+ and CO_2, which in turn attenuates the effect of Ca^{2+} on the contractile system of the smooth muscle of precapillary vessels. This results in a decrease of muscular resistance, and the cerebral blood flow increases. The latter was demonstrated by means of the Xenon 133 injection method, H_2 clearance method, cerebral radiocirculography, rheoencephalography, and ophthalmodynamometry. [This is more fully described by Saletu and Grünberger (29).] Ethamivan induces cortical stimulation through the midbrain reticular formation, as well as stimulation of the respiratory and vascular centers. Ethophylline is a CNS stimulatory drug and has, in addition, a positive inotropic effect on the heart and an ability to relax smooth muscles of the bronchi, which results in an increase in vital capacity.

TINOFEDRINE

Tinofedrine (D8955), the hydrochloride of a basic thiophene derivative, is chemically a [1,1-dithienyl-(3)-propen-(1)-yl-(3)]-[1-phenyl-1-hydroxypropyl-(2)]-amine-hydrochloride. In animal experiments and clinicopharmacologic studies, a dose-dependent increase in cerebral blood flow was found after both intravenous and oral administration of the substance (absorption, 78%). The cerebrocirculatory time is reduced. The influence on the cerebral metabolism in the dog and rat is characterized by an enhanced glucose uptake and an increased formation of high energy phosphates. Learning in healthy volunteers, as well as on the avoidance test in rats, is promoted. Tinofedrine has been shown to be a cerebral protector against impairment in learning as produced by electroshock in the rat. Because of its positive inotropic effect, tinofedrine leads to an increase in stroke volume and cardiac output. Mean arterial pressure and heart rate are only slightly increased, while peripheral and pulmonary vascular resistances are lowered. These cardio- and circulatory-dynamic alterations, as well as the decrease in blood viscosity, fibrinogen, triglycerides, beta-lipoproteins, and the inhibition of platelet aggregation, are individual effects contributing to the effect of tinofedrine in enhancing cerebral blood flow.

In an early pharmaco-EEG study in 10 healthy young adults (mean age, 26 years) involving orally administered doses of 20, 30, and 40 mg tinofedrine and 6 mg i.v. tinofedrine, as compared with placebo and 1,600 mg pirazetam, we observed an attenuation of delta, increase of alpha and slow beta, and decrease of fast beta activities (31). Vigilance-improving qualities of the drug were suggested by the V-EEG changes in relative power after 20 mg, which were rather small, but those after 30 and 40 mg were better, with pronounced peaking in the fourth hr. The attenuation of delta activity after the highest dosage (40 mg) reached the level of statistical significance as early as the first hr; this was still significant at the sixth hr.

After placebo, an increase in theta activity was observed in the first hr, and of beta activity in the sixth hr. In contrast to the 20 and 30 mg doses, 6 mg i.v. tinofedrine produced a significant delta attenuation and alpha augmentation in the first hr, which could still be observed by the sixth hr at a significant level.

In the R-EEG, a significant increase in theta and decrease of alpha and beta activities were observed after placebo and significantly so in the fourth hr, indicating a decrease in vigilance. The latter was markedly attenuated by 40 mg tinofedrine.

Recently, we could replicate the vigilance-promoting effect of tinofedrine in geriatric patients (mean age, 65 years; mean SCAG-score, 56.2) (32). In a cross-over study, they received in randomized order either placebo or 8 mg i.v. tinofedrine. A 10-min R-EEG was recorded at 2, 30, 60, 120, 180 min. Spectral analysis demonstrated an acceleration of the dominant frequency, a decrease in delta and theta activities, and an increase in alpha and beta activities, as compared with placebo (Fig. 17.8). These tinofedrine-induced alterations reached the level of statistical significance by 7 min after administration and were still detectable 3 hr after (Fig. 17.9).

Chronospectrographic investigations immediately after intravenous injection showed a marked attenuation of the spontaneously occuring increase in the delta + theta/alpha quotient (Fig. 17.10). Our findings confirm those of Spehr (33), who described almost identical changes after 4 mg i.v. tinofedrine in 10 normal volunteers; they indicate that tinofedrine is indeed an antihypoxidotic drug.

CINNARIZINE

Cinnarizine (Stugeron®), a piperidine derivative, in a dose of 150 mg, produced a decrease in delta activity, an increase in alpha activity, and a decrease in fast beta activities in the V-EEG of geriatric subjects (6) (Fig. 7.11). From all alterations, only the alpha augmentation reached the level of statistical significance; placebo showed similar changes. Different changes were observed in the R-EEG, characterized by an increase of delta and theta waves and a decrease of alpha and slow beta activities, which was significant by 4 hr after drug administration. While the above mentioned V-EEG changes indicate an improvement in vigilance, the augmentation of slow waves observed in the R-EEG suggests the opposite. In this connection, it is of interest that cinnarizine is chemically related to antihistaminics (cyclizine), some antiparkinsonian drugs (hexyphenidyl), and certain parasympathicolytics. Cinnarizine shows a long-lasting antihistaminic effect, as well as a sedative effect, and it also inhibits labyrinthal excitation (34). It has a positive effect on cerebral dysfunctions and

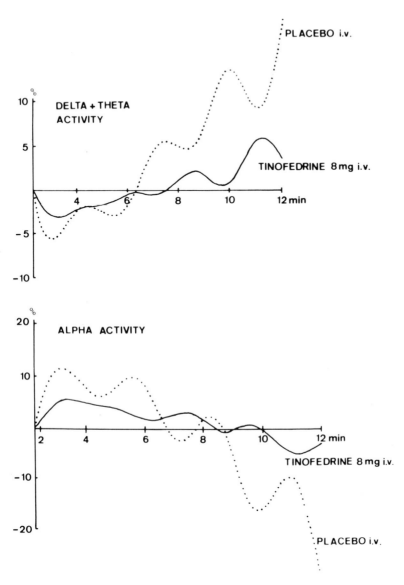

FIG. 17.8. Time-response relationship in relative power of slow waves (delta + theta band) and alpha band (R-EEG) of geriatric patients 2 to 12 min after 8 mg tinofedrine and placebo i.v. Time after the injection is shown in the abscissae, changes in the ordinate. Tinofedrine attenuates the increase in slow activities and decrease of alpha activity occurring after placebo, thus improving the vigilance of the geriatric patients.

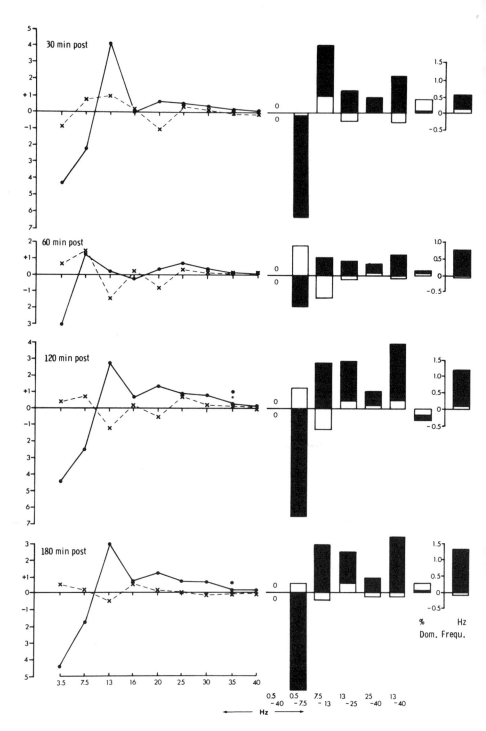

FIG. 17.9. Changes in relative power 30, 60, 120, and 180 min after 8 mg tinofedrine and placebo i.v. given to geriatric patients. Quantitative EEG measurements are shown in the abscissae; changes (as compared with baseline) are indicated in the ordinates. In contrast to placebo, tinofedrine induces a decrease in delta and theta activities and an increase of alpha and beta activities. The dominant frequency increases with tinofedrine but not with placebo.

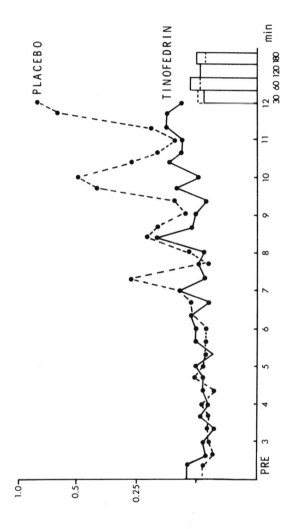

FIG. 17.10. Time course in the delta + theta/alpha quotient (absolute power R-EEG) of geriatric patients 2 to 12 min after 8 mg tinofedrine and placebo i.v. With placebo, an increase in the delta + theta/alpha quotient occurs over time, reflecting a decrease in vigilance. In contrast, after 8 mg i.v. tinofedrine, only minimal changes can be seen, mirroring a stabilization of vigilance.

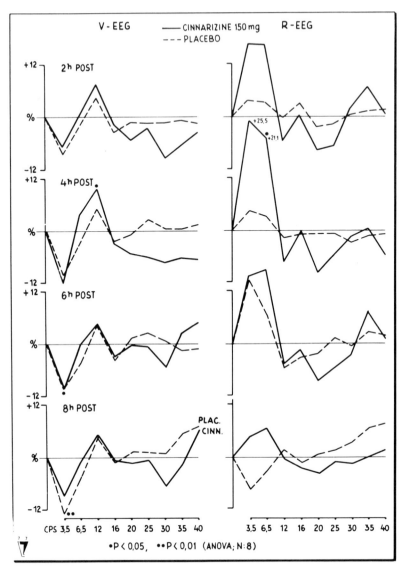

FIG. 17.11. Quantitative EEG changes after 150 mg cinnarizine and placebo (spectral analysis; relative power; 02-CZ; $N = 8$). For description of the axes, see Fig. 1. While in the vigilance-controlled state, 150 mg cinnarizine produces a decrease of delta and a significant increase of alpha activity; an increase of slow waves can be seen in the resting state.

impairment of mental performance in the higher age groups (35,36), which seems to be due to a direct musculotropic vasoactivity, as it inhibits the influx of Ca^{2+} into the depolarized cell, thus attenuating the availability of free calcium ions for the maintenance of muscular contraction (37).

ISOXSUPRINE

Isoxsuprine is a beta-sympathicomimetic and alpha-sympatholytic drug, which has been marketed for some time as a vasodilator. While there is some evidence that isoxsuprine fulfills the criteria of cerebral vasodilators (6), Heiss (38) failed to show any increase in cerebral blood flow with the drug by means of the Xenon method. In our own investigations, we were more concerned with encephalotropic, psychotropic, and pharmacodynamic properties of the drug. In an early single-blind, placebo-controlled, nonrandomized, crossover study, 5-min R-EEGs were recorded in healthy geriatric subjects at 0, 2, 4, 6, and 8 hr after the injection of 40 and 80 mg isoxsuprine retard (Xuprin®), a sustained release preparation of the drug, in order to investigate the "retardation effect" of this new formulation of the substance (6). We were able to document that the CNS effect did not commence before 4 hr but thereafter increased during the sixth hr and was maximal by the eighth hr postdrug (later recordings were not scheduled). There were no clear differences between the 40 and 80 mg dosage; but there were no significant changes after placebo. Surprisingly, the isoxsuprine-induced changes were characterized by an increase in delta, theta, and alpha activities, as well as by a decrease in beta activity, dominant frequency, and total power, indicating some centrally inhibitory properties (alpha-sympaticolytic?) of the substance. As sedation effects have not been found in other experiments, and as the acute effect might differ from the chronic one, we recently carried out a double-blind, placebo-controlled, crossover study in 10 geriatric subjects aged 58 to 73 years (mean; 64 years), who were treated for 15 days with 40 mg isoxsuprine retard and placebo twice daily. A treatment-free interval of 1 week was introduced between both treatment periods to allow for washout.

The two-way analysis of variance demonstrated significant changes over time in three EEG variables after the active drug, as compared with no significant changes after placebo in the V-EEG. In the R-EEG, isoxsuprine induced significant changes in nine variables, as compared with two after placebo. Evaluation of the acute effect of 80 mg isoxsuprine confirmed our previous observations. On all three recording days (0, 8, and 15), the augmentation of slow waves was the most consistent finding compared to placebo (Fig. 17.12). There was an additional decrease of alpha activity and an inconsistent trend toward an increase of fast beta activity (Fig. 17.12). Based on Friedman's ANOVA of placebo-corrected, sign-free changes in 11 variables of the spectral analyzed V- and R-EEG power, the peak effect of the drug was found to occur 10 hr after oral administration of a single dose, thus confirming the "retardation effect"

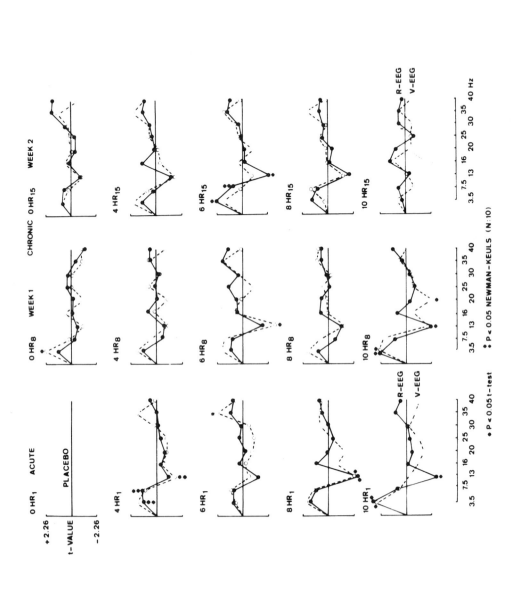

of the new formulation of isoxsuprine, as described earlier (6). While similar in type, the chronic effect was weaker than the acute effect; also, the effect of an additional single dose of isoxsuprine on day 15 was smaller than on day 0 of the chronic administration.

Psychometric analyses demonstrated inconsistent changes in the acute experiment, with the exception of mood, which was found significantly improved, as rated by the von Zerrsen scale. Chronic treatment resulted in a clear trend toward improvement of attention, deterioration of concentration and attention variability, improvement in psychomotor activity and tapping, increase in CFF, shortening of reaction time, activation as evaluated on the Archemedian spiral, improvement in affectivity based on a semantic differential polarity profile, a trend toward widening of the pupil size, and a significant improvement in mood (von Zerrsen scale), all compared with placebo.

Mnestic functioning based on a nonsense syllable learning test was significantly improved after 1 week of treatment with isoxsuprine; there were no statistically significant differences from placebo. Similarly, verbal memory improved significantly after 2 weeks of treatment with the active compound and even more so after an additional single dose, but the latter was observed also during the eighth hr after placebo, and the drug-placebo comparison yielded no significant differences regarding these variables. Generally, the trend toward improvement in psychometric testing observed in our study supports previous observations of other investigators. In a double-blind, placebo-controlled study, Affleck et al. (39) could show that isoxsuprine significantly improved intellectual functioning, while there was no improvement in the adaptation of the patient to hospitalization.

Dhrymiotis and Whittier (40) demonstrated the superiority of isoxsuprine over placebo in patients with cerebral ischemic episodes. Our psychometric findings (especially the improved mood) are of interest in light of the fact that the pharmaco-EEG profile of isoxsuprine retard (increase of slow, decrease of alpha, and increase of fast beta activities) somewhat resembles the quantitative EEG changes observed after some antidepressants. Unfortunately, the observed isoxsuprine-induced changes were generally small and especially inconsistent in the fast beta band. There is some evidence that beta-adrenergic stimulants, such as salbutamol, may have antidepressant properties (41–43).

FIG. 17.12. Placebo-corrected quantitative EEG changes after acute and chronic administration of 80 mg isoxsuprine in the elderly (relative power). Quantitative EEG measurements are shown in the adscissae; drug-induced changes as compared with placebo are indicated in the ordinates. The zero-line represents placebo. After one single dose (acute effect), an increase in delta and theta activities and a decrease in alpha activity can be seen. Beta activity shows inconsistent changes, although in the sixth hr a significant increase of fast beta activity in the V-EEG occurs. Chronic changes (after 1 and 2 weeks at baseline) are less pronounced than acute changes. On the 8th and 15th day, the effect of an additional single dose was recorded up to 10 hr. The same type of changes can be observed as on day 1.

METHYLTHIOMETHYLPYRIDINE

In connection with the slow wave-inducing properties of cinnarizine and isoxsuprine, an observation on a patient population with yet another nootropic substance—methylthiomethylpyridine (EMD-21657)—is of interest (44).

This drug is a derivative of a pyritinol metabolite and was found to be significantly superior to placebo in the treatment of organic brain syndrome in the alcoholic patient, both from a clinical and a psychometric point of view. Quantitative EEG analysis demonstrated similar changes in both the drug- and the placebo-treated patients, which were characterized by a decrease of average frequency, attenuation of the average frequency of the alpha activity, attenuation of delta, fast alpha, and beta waves, and an increase of theta and slow alpha waves; a spontaneous improvement of organic brain syndrome inevitably occurs under the condition of strict abstinence of hospitalized patients.

There was one statistically significant intergroup difference. EMD-treated patients showed more theta increase than placebo-treated patients. The question arises whether the theta augmentation was a drug-specific effect or the neurophysiologic correlate of psychopathologic improvement of the alcoholic patient. An increase of slow activity and a decrease of fast activity have been described frequently as indicative of reduction of psychopathology in psychiatric populations during psychopharmacotherapy (6,45). On the other hand, augmentation of theta activity by EMD-21657 was seen also by two other research teams investigating quantitatively analyzed EEG changes in normal subjects. Administering oral doses between 700 mg and 1 g EMD-21657, Hopes et al. (46) described an increase in power of the theta frequencies as the most dominant EEG alteration. Fink (47) also noted an increase in theta activity in the form of sporadic bursts in about 30% of normal subjects receiving 1 g EMD-21657. Dolce (48) described other EEG changes characterized by a decrease in amplitude variability and an increased intensity in spectral segments of the alpha region (which was significant in one subject but nonsignificant in the others), while Hinrichs et al. (49) observed EEG changes which differed from region to region and which were also dependent on the personality of the subject.

Thus the question as to whether the observed quantitative EEG changes are neurophysiologic correlates of clinical improvement or indicate a drug-specific effect, or actually reflect both, cannot be answered at this time. From our own and others' experiences, the class of agents with nootropic qualities is a heterogenous one, since different quantitative EEG changes occur with different representatives of this class. The mode of action of these substances (as far as is known) also differs.

PIRACETAM AND ANALOGS

Piracetam (Nootropil®, Normabrain®, Nootrop®,) a 2-oxo-1-pyrrolidine-acetamine and cyclic γ-aminobutyric acid derivative, in single oral doses of 1,600 mg, produced highly statistically significant augmentation of beta activity in the 20 to 25, 25 to 30, 30 to 35, and 35 to 40 cps bands in both the V-EEG and R-EEG (Fig. 17.13). These changes increased until the fourth hr, at which time they reached the level of statistical significance and were maximally pronounced in the sixth hr after drug administration (31). In the R-EEG, an additional attenuation of alpha activity was observed at that time (as was seen after placebo), while the augmentation of theta waves (seen after the placebo administration due to a spontaneous decrease in vigilance over time) was less pronounced after piracetam (Fig. 17.13).

Piracetam was shown to improve significantly the noopsyche in patients with senile involutional syndromes (50,51) and acute and chronic brain syndrome (52), in alcoholics (53), and in normal students (54) and aging individuals (55).

The neurophysiologic basis for this clinical therapeutic efficacy seems to be an improvement in vigilance, which was documented in patients by Bente et al. (56) in terms of an increase in beta activity (predominantly in the 18 to 25 cps range), by a decrease in slow waves, and by an acceleration and increase of alpha activity. In the latter study, the patients received 4.8 g piracetam daily over 8 to 13 months.

In our own investigations involving the CNS effect of single oral doses of 1,600 mg piracetam in healthy young subjects, we also saw an increase in beta activity, which was by far the most pronounced EEG change. In the resting condition, the theta augmentation was less pronounced than after placebo, while delta augmentation showed the opposite trend. According to Giurgea (2), piracetam has a selective effect on the telencephalon without involvement of the reticular and limbic structures, although the detailed mechanism of such selectivity is still obscure. Nicholson and Wolthuis (57,58) proposed that piracetam on the one hand protects against hypoxia, via stimulation of adenylatkinase, catalyzing the conversion of ADP into ATP, and on the other hand facilitates noetic functions via the inhibition of protein breakdown. Investigating the effect of piracetam on the neuronal respiratory chain, Woelk and Peiler-Ichikawa (59) found that it enhances the formation of ethanolamine plasmalogen by an increased synthesis or turnover of cytochrome b_5.

Etirazetam

We had the opportunity recently to investigate the encephalotropic, psychotropic, and pharmacodynamic properties of a new piracetam analog etirazetam (UCB-6474).

The neurophysiologic activities of etirazetam are of a nootropic nature, as it exerts a facilitating effect on memory and learning (spinal fixation and watermaze test), facilitates cortical integrative functions (as demonstrated by transcallosal evoked potentials), increases cortical control over the lower centers of

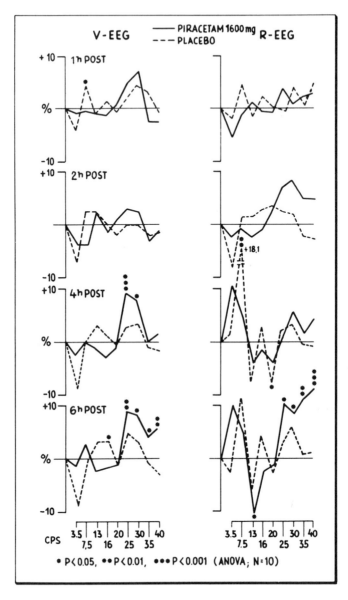

FIG. 17.13. Quantitative EEG changes in the V-EEG and R-EEG after 1,600 mg piracetam and placebo (spectral analysis; relative power; 02-CZ; *N* = 10). For description of axes, see Fig. 1. In contrast to placebo, 1,600 mg piracetam produces a significant increase in beta activities in both the resting and the vigilance-controlled state. In the R-EEG, there is an additional decrease in alpha activity (as after placebo) and a trend toward an increase in slow activity, which is less pronounced than after placebo. The peak effect is in the sixth hr postdrug.

the CNS (facilitation of fixation of an experience on the spine, inhibition of central nystagmus), and protects against certain adverse effects on the CNS, such as those produced by hypoxia, cerebral ischemia, and severe barbiturate intoxication.

Etirazetam is characterized, as is its precursor piracetam, by a lack of activity in most standard tests. In higher doses, however, it produces slight hypotony and sedation, potentiates barbiturate sleep, and induces temporary ataxia. Etirazetam does not potentiate or inhibit stereotypic behavior induced by dexamphetamine but protects animals against audiogenic epilepsy and has no effect on the cortical EEG of rabbits. Toxicologic experiments have demonstrated a very low toxicity with the drug. The absorption of orally given etirazetam is rapid, and peak levels are reached in less than 1 hr, while the half-life is approximately 9 hr. The drug is not metabolized (60).

In an acute and subacute pharmaco-EEG and psychometric study, 10 healthy, normal volunteers (five males and five females), aged 20 to 28 years (mean, 24.3 years), received single oral doses of placebo and 250, 500, and 1,000 mg doses of etirazetam. Recordings were carried out at 0, 1, 2, 4, and 6 hr postdrug. Thereafter, the subjects were treated with the drug (same dosages per day) for a period of 1 week. The neurophysiologic and psychometric investigations were repeated at the same intervals after an additional single dose.

After the single doses of 250, 500, and 1,000 mg, etirazetam induced a statistically significant CNS effect as compared to placebo, which in the spectral analyzed EEG was demonstrated predominantly by an increase in beta activity, especially in the 16 to 20 cps range but also in the 30 to 35 cps band (Fig. 17.14). There was an additional trend toward an alpha attenuation. Theta waves decreased initially after 250 mg, while after 500 mg, a trend toward an increase was observed.

Chronic administration over 1 week resulted in an augmentation of theta activity, which was significant after the 500 and 1,000 mg doses, as well as in a trend toward an increase in beta activity (Fig. 17.15). Alpha activity tended to increase after the low dosage and to decrease after the middle and high dosage, while delta activity was significantly decreased with the low doses and tended to increase with the higher doses.

An additional single dose to the chronic administration of the drug induced an additional augmentation of beta and attenuation of alpha activity after the 500 and 1,000 mg doses and alpha augmentation after the low doses. Considering quantitative EEG changes after single dose administration, there is a definite resemblance between the pharmaco-EEG profile of piracetam and etirazetam. Pharmacodynamic investigations were undertaken by means of the Friedman's rank ANOVA, based on changes in all EEG parameters. In relation to the time-efficacy relationship (Fig. 17.16), the peak effect occurred in the fourth hr (with the sixth, second, and first hr ranking behind); in relation to dose-efficacy (Fig. 17.17), most changes were observed after 500 mg etirazetam (with 1 g and 250 mg etirazetam and placebo ranking behind).

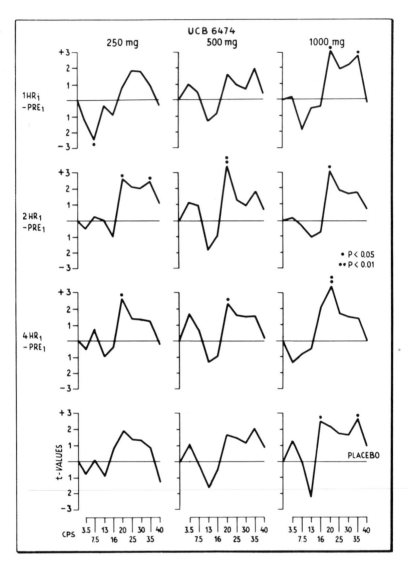

FIG. 17.14. Quantitative V-EEG changes after single doses of etirazetam as compared with placebo (3 min V-EEG; 02-CZ; relative power; $N = 10$). Nine frequency bands are shown in the abscissae; differences between drug-induced changes and placebo-induced changes at different times are indicated in the ordinate (in terms of t-values). The zero-line represents placebo. All three doses of etirazetam are CNS effective. The most characteristic change is the augmentation of slow beta activity, which statistically is significant after 250 and 500 mg at 2 and 4 hr and after 1 g at all times. There is a trend toward a decrease of alpha and increase of slow activities after the middle and high dosage.

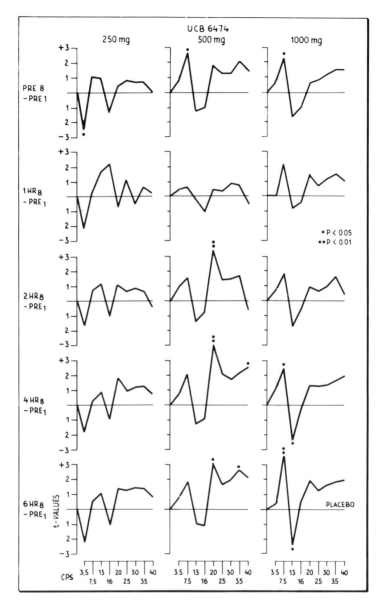

FIG. 17.15. Quantitative V-EEG changes after 1 week on etirazetam and after one additional single dose, as compared with placebo (3 min EEG; 02-CZ; relative power; $N = 10$). For description of the axes, see Fig. 7. Chronic administration of etirazetam results in a decrease of delta activity at 250 mg/day and in an increase of theta activity at 500 to 1,000 mg/day. An additional single dose to chronic administration produces significant changes only with 500 and 1,000 mg, which are characterized again by an increase of (mostly slow) beta activity. The highest dosage produced a significant increase in theta activity and a decrease in alpha activity.

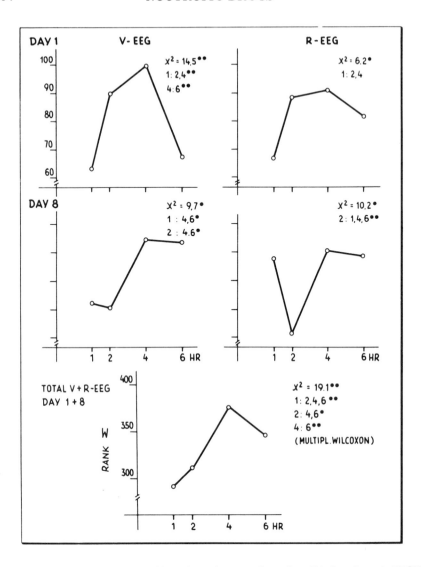

FIG. 17.16. Time-efficacy relationships after etirazetam (based on Friedman's rank ANOVA of sign-free changes in 11 EEG variables). Time is shown in the abscissae; rank sums in the V-EEG or R-EEG on day 1 and day 8, as well as on both days together, are indicated in the ordinate. There is a slight increase in CNS effect from 1 to 2 hr, and a marked increase from the 2 to 4 hr ($p < 0.01$, multiple Wilcoxon). The peak effect is at 4 hr; Thereafter, the CNS effect decreases slowly.

Psychometric tests after single low doses (250 mg) of etirazetam usually showed a shortening of reaction time and time estimation, an increase in the aftereffect measured by the Archimedean spiral indicating CNS activation, a decrease in psychomotor activity, and an improvement in mood and affectivity.

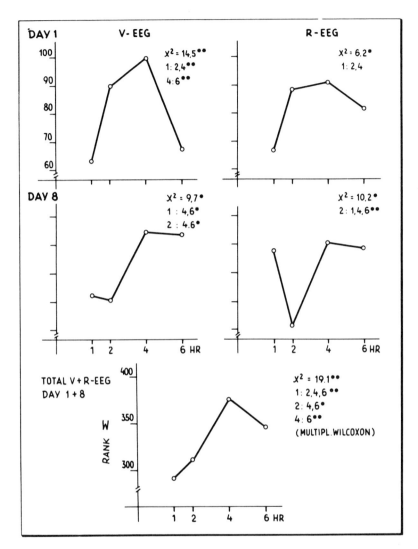

FIG. 17.17. Dose-efficacy relationship after etirazetam (based on Friedman's rank ANOVA of sign-free changes in 11 EEG variables). Doses are shown in the abscissae, rank sums in the ordinates. Etirazetam produces significantly ($p < 0.01$ multiple Wilcoxon) more changes than placebo. The most effective dosage is 500 mg, following by 1,000 and 250 mg.

After single doses of the medium dosage (500 mg), there was an improvement in attention and psychomotor activity and a lengthening of time estimation but a deterioration of affectivity, as compared with placebo. After the highest dose (1 g), attention variability but also concentration decreased, and reaction time deteriorated, while time estimation was shortened. Chronic administration resulted in a shortening of time estimation with the low dosage: with the middle dosage, a deterioration of mood and affectivity occurred; and with the high dosage, a decrease of attention variability was observed. Learning of nonsense syllables deteriorated after single doses of 250 and 500 mg but improved after chronic administration of 500 mg. There were no significant differences compared to placebo. Our results indicate an activating effect of etirazetam in low doses and some sedative properties of the drug in higher doses.

CONCLUSIONS

Since antihypoxidotic/nootropic drugs protect against impairment of cerebral biologic oxidation due to hypoxic, nutritive, histotoxic, metabolic, or hypochreotic causes, their target patient population is one of the largest in medicine. Nevertheless, there is a paucity of objective and quantitative data concerning their effectiveness on the human CNS. The quantitative pharmaco-EEG, along with psychometric tests, seems to be an outstanding tool to evaluate encephalotropic, psychotropic, and pharmacodynamic properties of these drugs. Representative substances of this class were studied by such methods and the literature reviewed.

Ergot alkaloid preparations, such as hydergine and nicergoline, the tiophene derivative tinofedrine, hexobendine, ethophylline, and the hexobendine/ethophylline/ethamivan combination Instenon forte, produced statistically significant changes in the spectral analyzed EEG as compared with placebo. The latter are characterized by an increase in alpha and slow beta activity as well as by a decrease in delta and theta activity. Interestingly, such changes are opposite to quantitative EEG changes observed with advancing age and indicate an improvement in vigilance.

Improvement in vigilance may be one of the most important principles in the pharmacotherapy of the elderly, as a diminished adaptive ability of the vigilance regulating systems in old age has been known for some time.

Piracetam and the new piracetam analog etirazetam produce a significant increase in beta activity as well, while alpha activity is augmented or attenuated according to the given dosage. After chronic administration of etirazetam and especially after high doses, an increase in theta activity may be observed. Psychometric tests also demonstrate stimulatory qualities in low doses and slight sedative properties in high doses.

Cinnarizine, isoxsuprine, and methylthiomethylpyridine, a derivative of a pyritinol metabolite, exhibited somewhat different effects. However, these drugs also may produce beneficial effects in the elderly suffering from impairment of mental functions.

REFERENCES

1. Wieck, H. H., and Blaha, L. Therapeutische Möglichkeiten bei zerebrovaskulärer Insuffizien. *Therapiewoche*, 1976, 26, 5282–5290.

2. Giurgea, C. Vers und pharmacologie de l'activité intégrative du cerveau. Tentative du concept nootrope en psychopharmacologie. *Actual. Pharmacol.,* 1972, 25, 115–156.
3. Strughold, H. Hypoxydose. *Klin. Wochenschr.,* 1944, 23, 221–222.
4. Fink, M. EEG and human psychopharmacology. *Ann. Rev. Pharmacol.,* 1969, 9, 241–258.
5. Itil, T. M. Quantitative pharmaco-electroencephalography. In: *Psychotropic Drugs and the Human EEG,* edited by T. M. Itil, pp. 43–75. Karger, Basel, 1974.
6. Saletu, B. *Psychopharmaka, Gehirntätigkeit und Schlaf.* Karger, Basel, 1976.
7. Saletu, B., Grünberger, J., and Linzmayer, L. Classification and determination of cerebral bioavailability of psychotropic drugs by quantitative "pharmaco-EEG" and psychometric investigations (studies with AX-A411-BS). *Int. J. Clin. Pharmacol.,* 1977, 15, 449–459.
8. Saletu, B., Grünberger, J., and Linzmayer, L. Bestimmung der encephalotropen, psychotropen und pharmakodynamischen Eigenschaften von Nicergolin mittels quantitativer Pharmako-EEG und psychometrischer Analysen. *Arzneim. Forsch.,* 1979, 29, 1251–1261.
9. Saletu, B., Grünberger, J., Linzmayer, L., and Anderer P. Proof of CNS efficacy and pharmacodynamics of nicergoline in the elderly by acute and chronic quantitative pharmaco-EEG and psychometric studies. In: *Drug Treatment in Chronic Cerebrovascular Disorders,* edited by G. Tognani and S. Garattini, pp. 245–272. Elsevier, Amsterdam, 1979.
10. Head, H. The conception of nervous and mental energy. II. Vigilance: A physiological state of the nervous system. *Br. J. Psychol.,* 1923, 14, 125–147.
11. Kanowski, S. The aging brain: Current theories and psychopharmacological possibilities. In: *Neuropsychopharmacology,* edited by P. Deniker, C. Radonco-Thomas, and A. Villeneuve, pp. 23–31. Pergamon Press, Oxford, 1978.
12. Matejcek, M., and Devos, J. E. Selected methods of quantitative EEG analysis and their application in psychotropic drug research. In *Quantitative Analytic Studies in Epilepsy,* edited by P. Kellaway and I. Peterson, pp. 183–205. Raven Press, New York, 1976.
13. Obrist, W. D. Electroencephalographic changes in normal aging and dementia. In: *Brain Function in Old Age,* edited by F. Hoffmeister and C. Müller, pp. 102–111. Springer, Berlin, 1979.
14. Surwillo, W. Timing of behavior in senescence and the role of the central nervous system. In: *Human Aging and Behavior,* edited by E. Talland, pp. 1–33. Academic Press, New York, 1968.
15. Van der Drift, J. H. A., Kok, N. K. D., Nidernayer, E., Naguet, R., and Vigouroux, R. A. The EEG in relation to pathology in simple cerebral ischemia. In: *Handbook of Electroencephalography and Clinical Neurophysiology,* edited by A. Remond, vol. 14A, p. 17. Elsevier, Amsterdam, 1972.
16. Bente, D., Glatthaar, G., Ulrich, G., and Lewinsky, M. Quantitative EEG-Untersuchungen zur vigilanzfördernden Wirkung von Nicergolin. Ergebnisse einer Doppleblindstudie bei gerontopsychiatrischen Patienten. *Arzneim. Forsch.,* 1979, 29, 1804–1808.
17. Lemperiere, T. Cerebral protectores in psychogeriatrics. In: *Neuro-Psychopharmacology,* edited by P. Deniker, C. Radouco-Thomas, and A. Villeneuve, pp. 59–65. Pergamon Press, Oxford, 1978.
18. Petrie, W. M., and Ban, T. A. Drugs in geropsychiatry. *Psychopharmacol. Bull.,* 1978, 14, 7–19.
19. Michelangeli, J., Sevilla, M., Lavagna, J., and Darcourt, G. Etude de l'action de la nicergoline (Sermion dans le pathologie vasculaire chronique du 3me agé. *Ann. Med. Psychol.,* 1975, 133, 499–510.
20. Grel, P., and Normand, F. Etude comparative en double insu contre placebo de l'action de la nicergoline dans 1-insuffisance circulatoire cérébrale. *Psychol. Med.,* 1975, 7, 1789–1793.
21. Memin, Y., and Majean Hueber, E. Etude à double insu selon une échelle d'appréciation quantitative d'un traitement des troubles vasculaires cérébraux chroniques. *Sem. Hop. Paris (Ther.),* 1973, 49, 605–608.
22. Baldoni, E., Serentha, P., Cuttin, S., and Galetti, G. L'Azione terapeutica della nicergolina negli anziani arteriosclerotici con insufficienze cerebrale vascolare. *Gass. Int. Chir.,* 1971, 76, 965–974.
23. Geraud, J., Bes, A., Rascol, A., et al. Mesure due débit sanguin cerebral au krypton 85. Quelques applications physiopathologiques et cliniques. *Ref. Neurol.,* 1963, 108, 542–557.
24. Triboletti, M. D., and Ferri, H. Hydergine for treatment of symptoms of cerebrovascular insufficiency. *Curr. Ther. Res.,* 1969, 11, 609–620.
25. Meier-Ruge, W., Enz, A., Gygax, P., Hunziker, O., Iwangoff, P., and Reichlmeier, K. Experimen-

tal pathology in basic research of the Aging 2: aging brain. In: *Genesis and Treatment of Psychologic Disorders in the Elderly,* edited by S. Gershon and A. Raskin, pp. 55–126. Raven Press, New York, 1975.

26. Herzfeld, U., Christian, W., Oswald, W. D., Ronge, I., and Wittgen, M. Richtgrössen für die Beurteilung der Hirnfunktion nach Langzeittherapie mit Hydergin. Eine Dokumentation mit dem Radiozirkulogramm und dem EEG. *Ärztl, Forsch.,* 1972, 26, 216–228.
27. Herzfeld, U., Christian, W., Oswald, W. D., Ronge, I., and Wittgen, M. Zur Wirkungsanalyse von Hydergin im Langzeitversuch. Eine interdisziplinäre Studie. *Med. Klin.,* (1972):67, 1116–1125.
28. Mamo, H., Seylaz, J., Rey, A., and Houndart, R. Etude pharmacodynamique du débit sanguin du cortex cérébral de l'homme par une méthode de mesure continue et focale. *Rev. Neurol.,* 1970, 123, 101–115.
29. Saletu, B., and Grünberger, J. Assessment of psychoactivity and pharmacodynamics of a cerebral vasodilating hexobendine-combination by quantitative electroencephalographic and psychometric analyses. *Prog. Neuropsychopharmacol.,* 1979, 3, 543–551.
30. Ambrosi, L., and Neumayer, E. Zerebrovasculäre Insuffizienz und Hirnleistung. *Weir Klin. Wochenschr.,* 1971, 83, 188–192.
31. Saletu, B. Quantitative EEG-Analysen bei zerbralen Antihypoxidotika. Presented at the Annual Meeting of the German Society for Medical Psychology and Psychopathometry, Erlangen, 1977.
32. Saletu, B., and Anderer, P. Doubleblind placebo-controlled quantitative pharmaco-EEG investigations after tinofednine i.v. in geriatric patients. *Curr. Ther. Res.,* 1980, 28, 1–15.
33. Spehr, W. Zur Zeitgestaltung de Elektroenzephalogramms unter Tinofedrin. *Arzneim. Forsch.,* 1978, 28, 1312–1313.
34. Philipszzon, A. J. Influence of cinnarizine on the labyrinth and on vertigo. *Clin. Pharmacol. Ther.,* 1962, 3, 184.
35. Bernard, A., and Goffart J. M. A double-blind cross-over clinical evaluation of cinnarizine. *Clin. Trials J. (Lond.),* 1968, 5, 945–948.
36. Toledo, P., and Marches, M. Clinical evaluation of cinnarizine in patients with cerebral circulatory deficiency. *Arzneim. Forsch.,* 1972, 22, 448–451.
37. Godfraid, T., and Kaba, A. Blockade or reversal of the contraction induced by calcium and adrenaline in depolarized arterial muscle. *Brit. J. Pharmacol.*
38. Heiss, W. D. Drug effect on regional cerebral blood flow in focal cerebrovascular disease. *J. Neurol. Sci.,* 1973, 19, 461–482.
39. Affleck, C. D., Treptow, K. R., and Herrick, H. D. The effects of isuxsuprine hydrochlorid (Vasodilan) on chronic cerebral arteriosclerosis. *J. Nerv. Ment. Dis.,* 1961, 132, 335–338.
40. Dhrymiotis, A. D., and Whittier, J. R. Effect of vasodilator (isoxsuprine) on cerebral ischemic episodes. *Curr. Ther. Res.,* 1962, 4, 124–129.
41. Lecrubier, Y., Jouvent, R., Puech, A. J., Simon, P., and Widlöcher, D. Effet anti-dépresseur d'un stimulant beta-adrénergique. *Nouv. Presse Méd.,* 1977, 6, 2786.
42. Francés, H., Puech, A. J., Chermat, R., and Simon, P. Are psychopharmacological effects of beta-adrenergic stimulants central or peripheral? *Pharmacol. Res. Commun.,* 1979, 11, 273–278.
43. Puech, A. J. Widlöcher, D., Lecrubier, Y., Francés, H., Jouvent, R., Allitaire, J. F., and Simon, P. Antidepressive effect of a stimulant of beta-adrenergic receptors. Read at the Second World Congress of Biological Psychiatry, Barcelona, 1978.
44. Saletu, B., Grünberger, J., Saletu, M., Mader, R., and Volavka, J. Treatment of the alcoholic organic brain syndrome with EMD 21657—a derivative of a pyritinol-metabolite: Double-blind clinical, quantitative EEG and psychometric studies. *Int. Pharmacopsychiat.,* 1978, 13, 177–192.
45. Saletu, B., Itil, T. M., Arat, M., and Akpinar, S. Long-term clinical and quantitative EEG effects of clophenthixol in schizophrenics clinical-neurophysiological correlations. *Int. Pharmacopsychiatr.,* 1973, 8, 193–207.
46. Hopes, M., Herbsleb, x., and Leopold, G. EMD 21657—Verträglichkeit in Dosen von 700 mg, 800 mg, 900 mg, 1000 mg bei oraler Verabreichung. Internal report, E. Merck, 1974.
47. Fink, M. EEG classification study of EMD 21657: Dose-finding studies. Report to E. Merck, 1975.

48. Dolce, C. Neurophysiologische Untersuchungen zur Wirkung von Pyrithioxin auf das zentrale Nervensystem der Katze. *Pharmakopsychiatrie,* 1970, 3, 335–370.
49. Hinrichs, H., Künkel, H., Luba, A., Niethardt, P., and Reinhardt, B. Der Stellenwert persönlichkeitsspezifischer Merkmale in der EEG-Analyse cerebraler Medikationswirkungen. Read at the 20th Jahrestagung der Deutschen EEG-Gesellschaft, Münster, 1975.
50. Stechnik, A. J. The clinical use of piracetam, a new nootropic drug. *Arzneim. Forsch.,* 1972, 22, 975–977.
51. Kretschmar, J. H., and Kretschmar, Chr. Zur Dosis-Wirkungs Relation bei der Behandlung mit Piracetam. *Arzneim. Forsch.,* 1976, 26, 1158–1159.
52. Lagergren, K., and Levader, St. A double-blind study on the effects of piracetam upon perceptual and psychomotor performance at varied heart rates in patients treated with artificial pacemakers. *Psychopharmacologia (Berl.),* 1974, 39, 97–104.
53. Weckroth, J., and Mikkonen, H. On the effect of UCB on certain intellectual, perceptual and psychomotor performance traits and traits of subjectively rated mental states. Communication of the 30th. Int. Congress on Alcoholism and Drug Dependence, Amsterdam, 1972.
54. Dimond, S. J., and Brouwers, E. Y. M. Increase in the power of human memory in normal man through the use of drugs. *Psychopharmacology,* 1976, 49, 307–309.
55. Mindus, P. Some clinical studies with piracetam—a "nootropic" substance. In: *Neuro-Psychopharmacology,* edited by P. Deniker, C. Radouco-Thomas, and A. Villeneuve, pp. 73–81. Pergamon Press, Oxford, 1978.
56. Bente, D., Glatthaar, G., Ulrich, G., and Lewinsky, M. Piracetam und Vigilanz: Elektroencephalographische und klinische Ergebnisse einer Langzeitmedikation bei geronto-psychiatrischen Patienten. *Arzneim. Forsch.,* 1978, 9, 1529–1530.
57. Nicholson, V. J., and Wolthhuis, O. L. Effect of the acquisition-enhancing drug pirazetam on rat cerebral energy metabolism in comparison with naftidrofuryl and methamphetamine. *Biochem. Pharmacol.,* 1976, 25.
58. Nicholson, V. J., and Wolthuis, O. L. Differential effects of the acquisition enhancing drug pyrrilidone acetamide (pirazetam) on the release of proline from visual and parietal rat cerebral cortex in vitro. *Brain Res.,* 1976, 114.
59. Woelk, H., and Peiler-Ichikawa, K. The action of piracetam on the formation of ethanolamine-plasmalogen by neuronal microsomes of the developing rat brain. *Arzneim. Forsch.,* 1978, 28, 1752–1756.
60. UCB 6474. *Summary on Drug Information.* Bruxelles, 1977.

Stress and the Heart, edited by D. Wheatley,
Raven Press, New York © 1981.

Tricyclic Antidepressants and Cerebral Blood Flow*

I. M. James

In the opening chapter to this section, Sourander and Sourander, in their comprehensive survey of organic brain syndromes, referred briefly to brain metabolism and the effects of the cerebral circulation upon it.

However, it should be clearly stated from the outset that until recently very little was known about the changes that occur in brain metabolism (cerebral oxygen and glucose utilization) in patients with psychiatric diseases, or with drugs that are used in the treatment of these disorders. This lack of information can be ascribed to two main factors. First, it was thought unlikely that such crude measurements as total cerebral blood flow, total brain oxygen, and glucose consumption would shed much light on the understanding and biochemistry of psychiatric diseases or, indeed, on the mechanisms of action of the various psychotropic drugs. Second, the various technical difficulties and ethical problems involved made it appear that the efforts would not be commensurate with the information or benefits likely to accrue. The great increase in the number of prescriptions issued in recent years for the tricyclic antidepressants, however, has caused general awareness not only of the beneficial qualities but also of the systemic effects of these drugs, particularly those occurring in the cardiovascular system. The effects of these drugs on the heart itself have been considered in an earlier section of this book, and it is apparent that the elderly are particularly at risk from cardiac complications with the tricyclic antidepressants. However, these drugs are frequently prescribed for the elderly or for those in whom there may be peripheral or cerebral circulatory insufficiency, and so a more complete knowledge of the effects of these drugs on the heart itself and on cerebral circulation is now required.

To set the subject into its proper context, it is helpful to review briefly some factors of physiological importance.

PHYSIOLOGICAL CONSIDERATIONS

The oxygen consumption of the normal human brain is 3.3 ml (or 0.13 mmoles) per 100 g of tissue per minute (1). Thus, the brain consumes ap-

---

* Reprinted with permission from *Stress and The Heart,* edited by D. Wheatley, Raven Press, 1977, first edition.

proximately a quarter of the total oxygen used by the body at rest. This high level of oxygen utilization is necessary for energy requirements supplied by the aerobic breakdown of glucose. Because cerebral glucose consumption normally proceeds at the rate of 0.027 mmoles/100 g tissue/min (1) and since six molecules of oxygen are required for the aerobic breakdown of glucose, it is possible to calculate that even under ideal circumstances some 15 to 20% of glucose used is broken down anaerobically with only low energy yield. These high demands for oxygen are met by a high rate of flow, namely 54 ml/100 g tissue/min (1) or one-sixth of the resting cardiac output. Nevertheless, it can be appreciated from these figures that since a quarter of the oxygen consumption of the body is utilized by the brain, the brain extraction of oxygen is greater than that of most other organs.

In the normal individual, the cerebral circulation copes with the changes in blood pressure and the changes in blood gas tensions in such a way that the metabolic environment of the brain is kept relatively constant. Thus, cerebral blood flow usually increases with increasing arterial CO_2 tensions or decreasing O_2 tensions and remains constant in the face of blood pressure variations over quite a wide range (2,3). Whether this still remains true after administration of psychotropic drugs is unknown. Changes in metabolism and changes in flow often proceed concomitantly, but this rule is far from invariable. Also, in many circumstances it is possible to determine whether a change in flow causes a change in metabolism, or vice versa, or, indeed, if they are both influenced by a third variable (4).

Increased mental activity is associated with an overall increase in flow of some 20% (5), but whether this increase is associated with increased metabolism is unknown. Certain substances which are known to produce alerting, i.e., catecholamines, cause large increases in cerebral blood flow, oxygen, and glucose consumption (6–8). In coma (9–11) and following the administration of sedatives (12–14), there is a fall in both flow and metabolism. A fall in cerebral blood flow secondary to a decrease in metabolic demands would presumably matter little, but a fall in flow with increased or unchanged metabolic requirements could precipitate relative ischemia. The cerebral vasculature, in contrast with that in other beds, was considered, until fairly recently, to be almost entirely regulated by local chemical changes (15). Evidence has recently been obtained which suggests that cerebral blood vessels are reflexly controlled and that the carotid body chemoreceptors and carotid sinus baroreceptors initiate many of the cerebrovascular responses to hypoxia, hypercapnia, and hypotension (4,16). There is a great deal of morphological evidence to show that in most species there is an adrenergic pathway originating in the superior cervical ganglion which is constrictor in nature (17). Norepinephrine infused into the internal carotid artery of the dog constricts the blood vessels of the cerebral cortex, this being mediated by the action on alpha-adrenoceptors of the cerebral arteries (8). There is also morphological evidence of a dilator pathway which may be cholinergic that is carried by the seventh cranial nerve (18).

Mchedlishvili and Nikolaishvili (19) have shown that atropine attenuates the vasodilator response of the cerebral vessels to hypotension. On the other hand, Carpi and Virno (20) claim that atropine does not inhibit cerebral vasodilation due to hypercapnia, but does inhibit the concomitant electroencephalographic arousal.

PHARMACOLOGICAL CONSIDERATIONS

Thymoleptics of the imipramine type are generally assumed to owe their antidepressant activity to a blockade of that mechanism by which biogenic amines released from nerve endings are taken up again into the nerve terminals. Although it is now established that this blockade of the membrane pump applies particularly to cerebral norepinephrine and 5HT neurons (21), it was, in fact, first described for peripheral sympathetic nerves (22). This peripheral effect explains the findings of Sigg and co-workers in 1959 that imipramine and related drugs potentiate the effects of sympathetic nerve stimulation and of administered norepinephrine (23,24). In addition to these effects upon the membrane pump, most of the tricyclic antidepressants possess distinct cholinergic blocking properties, particularly against the muscarinic action of acetylcholine. Many of the side effects seen clinically, such as blurred vision, dryness of the mouth, constipation, and urinary retention, can be attributed to this atropine-like effect (25). Thus, a potentiation of sympathetic nervous system effects, or effects due to cholinergic blockade, might well be expected following administration of tricyclic antidepressants.

Some years ago we decided to investigate this further, for several reasons. First, a more complete knowledge of the relationship between flow changes and oxygen utilization was necessary, and, second, if a characteristic biochemical response was observed, then such a response might be useful for screening compounds for antidepressant activity.

ANTIDEPRESSANT DRUGS IN DOGS

We investigated the effect of antidepressant drugs on canine cerebral blood flow and metabolism, the latter experiment being performed in the following manner. Mongrel dogs of about 15 kg were anesthetized with sodium pentobarbital, 25 mg/kg body weight. Tracheostomy was carried out and adequate ventilation assured throughout the experiment. The left femoral artery was cannulated with a polyethylene catheter and blood pressure continuously recorded with a Bell and Howell transducer Type 4–372.L221 and a servoscribe potentiometric recorder. Arterial blood samples were obtained from the same source. A branch of the left femoral vein was cathetarized so that the drug could be infused at the appropriate time.

Cerebral (cortical) blood flow was measured by the method of Ingvar and Lassen (26), using the intracarotid injection of krypton. A fine catheter was placed in the superior saggital sinus in such a way as not to impede flow, but which allowed samples of cortical venous blood to be obtained. Blood samples for oxygen content, glucose content, pH, and PCO_2 were taken from the superior saggital sinus and from the femoral artery, thus enabling cortical oxygen and cortical glucose consumption to be calculated. (Levels for cortical oxygen and glucose consumption are, incidentally, much higher than the levels for total brain oxygen and glucose utilization rates.) Oxygen content was measured directly by the method of Linden et al. (27) and glucose by a glucose oxidase method (28). The blood pH and PCO_2 were measured with the appropriate radiometer electrodes. Three sets of control measurements taken at 15-min intervals were first obtained. These were followed by several experimental periods and by at least three recovery periods. All periods were of 15-min duration.

RESULTS

The effect of the infusion of the tricyclic drug clomipramine is shown in the first figure. Similar responses were obtained in 5 other dogs.

The administration of the tricyclic drug in a total dose of 0.7 mg/kg over a 30-min period led to an increase in cerebral blood flow and in oxygen and glucose consumption. From the figure, it can be seen that the effect came fairly quickly, within 15 min of commencing the infusion, and usually lasted between 1 and 2 hr. When progressively larger doses were given, progressively greater increases in oxygen and glucose consumption were seen.

The increases in glucose utilization in percentage terms were greater than the increases in oxygen consumption. Responses similar to those outlined above were also obtained with imipramine.

The next question that needed answering was how specific was this type of response to tricyclic compounds or, indeed, to other types of antidepressants. Certainly, very similar responses have been demonstrated following isoprenaline infusion (6) and following intravenous norepinephrine (7,8). Similarly, when the monoamine oxidase inhibitor iproniazide was given, we observed a similar response.

However, in this case the effect was less marked and was delayed in onset. The administration of L-DOPA intravenously also caused a similar pattern (Fig. 18-4), although nikethamide and other analeptic drugs do not have this effect.

Interestingly enough, the effect of intravenous catecholamines can be blocked by inhalation of 5% CO_2 or by the prior administration of pro-

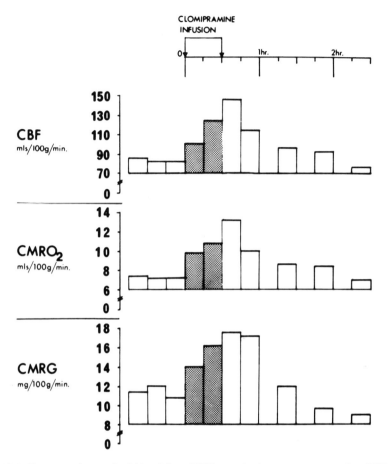

FIG. 18-1. Response by cerebral blood flow (CBF), cerebral oxygen consumption (CMRO₂), and cerebral glucose consumption (CMRG) to an intravenous infusion of clomipramine (0.7 mg/kg over 30 min) in an experiment in a single dog. Reproduced from the *Journal of International Medical Research* by kind permission of the Editor.

pranolol. High CO_2 levels and propranolol also attenuate the response of brain blood flow and metabolism to the tricyclic drugs. Evidence has been obtained recently (8) suggesting that the cerebrovasodilation observed following intravenous norepinephrine is reflex and, at least in the dog, triggered by chemoreceptor activity. To evaluate whether the increase in brain oxygen and glucose consumption could be mediated, in part, via increased chemoreceptor activity, the following experiment was performed.

Brain metabolism was measured in dogs whose chemoreceptor regions were vascularly isolated and perfused by the blood of second animals. The full experimental details of the procedure have recently been described (8). If clomipramine in a dose of 1.4 mg/kg was given to the second dog over a

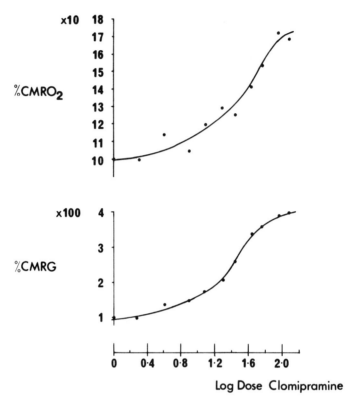

FIG. 18-2. Dose-response relation of cerebral oxygen and cerebral glucose consumption to intravenous infusions of increasing doses of clomipramine in the dog. The log of the cumulative dose in mg is shown. Reproduced from the *Journal of International Medical Research* by kind permission of the Editor.

30-min period, an increase in cerebral oxygen and glucose consumption occurred in the first dog.

Experiments were also performed where clomipramine was administered to the first dog. In these circumstances some increase in flow and metabolism was seen, but the increases were smaller than those seen in the intact animal. Thus, although some of the changes are mediated indirectly via the chemoreceptors, there would seem to be a direct effect as well.

From the animal experiments there appeared to be a fairly clear-cut response to tricyclic antidepressants. The response was dose dependent but perhaps not entirely specific in that catecholamines and monoamine oxidase inhibitors caused the same changes. Thus encouraged, we felt that it was important to extend the study to man and particularly to ascertain whether there was any relationship between the metabolic changes and the psychotropic effects caused.

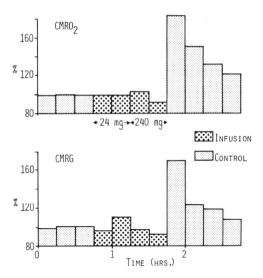

FIG. 18-3. Response by cerebral oxygen consumption (CMRO₂) and cerebral glucose consumption (CMRG) to intravenous infusion of iproniazid.

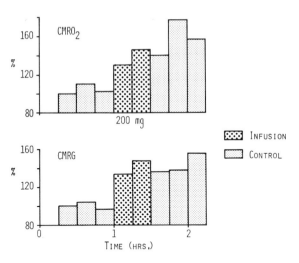

FIG. 18-4. Response by cerebral oxygen consumption (CMRO₂) and cerebral glucose consumption (CMRG) to intravenous infusion of L-DOPA.

METABOLIC AND PSYCHOTROPIC RESPONSES IN MAN

These responses were studied in patients suffering from depression, the severity of the illness being rated on the Hamilton Rating Scale. The rating was always carried out within a period of 36 hr prior to the biochemical studies.

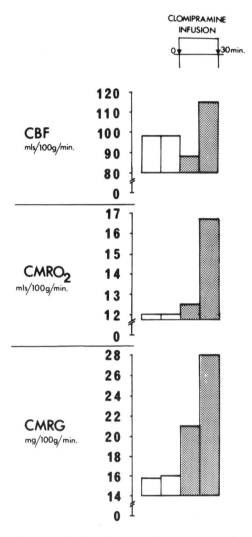

FIG. 18-5. Response by cerebral blood flow, cerebral oxygen, and cerebral glucose consumption in the first dog whose chemoreceptors had been vascularly isolated and perfused with blood from a second dog when clomipramine (1.4 mg/kg over 30 min) was infused intravenously into the second dog. Reproduced from the *Journal of International Medical Research* by kind permission of the Editor.

Cerebral blood flow was measured using a slight modification of the McHenry technique (29). Small needles of 21 gauge with special catheters attached were inserted into the jugular bulb, as described by Gibbs et al. in 1945 (30), and into a femoral artery. Ethyl chloride was sprayed liberally onto the skin at the appropriate site and then a small "bleb" of 2% procaine was raised. The needle, with catheter attached and filled with 2% procaine, was then slowly advanced by small increments, while further procaine was injected, until finally the correct position was reached. It was possible to place the needles in position in this manner without causing discomfort to the patient; once the needles and attached catheters were in position, the patient breathed for 15 min from a spirometer containing radioactive krypton.

At the end of this time the patient again breathed room air, and timed samples were taken both from the femoral artery and the jugular bulb for subsequent krypton analysis. The conventional height-over-area formula was used to derive cerebral blood flow. Arterial and venous blood samples were also taken so that the cerebral consumption of oxygen and glucose could be calculated.

Patients admitted to Friern and Halliwick Hospitals suffering from depression were studied. These were mainly patients whose symptomatology was of the so-called endogenous type, but because of the uncertain status of the various depressive syndromes, they were considered as one group. They were studied as soon after admission as was possible, whereas no patient was investigated who had received any medication in the preceding 10 days. Cerebral blood flow and metabolism were measured before and immediately after a 30-min infusion of clomipramine; the total dose given by infusion was 0.7 mg/kg in all cases. The patients were then treated with tricyclic antidepressants for a period of at least 3 weeks before they were studied again. The dose and route of administration were decided upon by the psychiatrist in charge of the patient, and so it was not possible to standardize the dose.

In this way, the effect of intravenous clomipramine was determined in three situations: 1. depressed patients before receiving drug treatment; 2. depressed patients following 3 weeks therapy with tricyclic drugs; and 3. control volunteer subjects.

ETHICS

The project was approved by two local Ethics Committees and one national committee, subject to the following conditions:

1. Only patients admitted informally should be studied.
2. The patient should be able to give informed consent, this ability being judged by an independent psychiatrist.
3. No patient should be studied whose participation could adversely affect his psychiatric state. This also was judged by an independent psychiatrist.
4. Consent by patient could be withdrawn at any stage during the study.

RESULTS IN MAN

The average values for cerebral blood flow, oxygen, and glucose consumption found in the 6 depressed patients were: 42 ml/100 g/min, 2.3 ml/100 g/min, and 3.4 mg/100 g/min, respectively. These results are shown graphically in Figs. 18-6, 18-7, and 18-8.

These values appear to be lower than normal and certainly the values for cerebral oxygen consumption are lower than values obtained in the 4 normal volunteers. Because the patients and controls were not strictly age-matched, this finding has to be interpreted with some reserve. However, it can be seen that the infusion of 0.7 mg/kg clomipramine in the depressed patients caused variable changes in cerebral blood flow and little, if any, changes in brain oxygen or glucose consumption. In 3 cases, cerebral blood flow increased and in 3 there was a fall in flow (Fig. 18-6). In those cases where there was a fall in cerebral blood flow, there was also a fall in $PaCO_2$.

Most of the depressed patients felt drowsy following the infusion, and one in particular was kept awake only with some difficulty. However, in the control group of patients the infusion caused some minor feelings of anxiety which was coupled with nausea in two out of four studies. In these patients, there was some increase in the oxygen consumption but a marked increase in brain glucose utilization (Figs. 18-7 and 18-8). It is also possible to calculate that the fraction of glucose metabolized anaerobically must have been increased. Changes in cerebral blood flow were again variable, but in

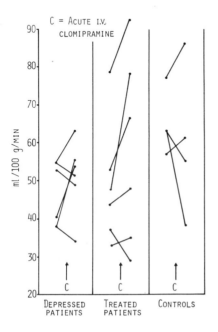

FIG. 18-6. Cerebral blood flow (CBF), before and after an acute intravenous injection of clomipramine in three experimental groups.

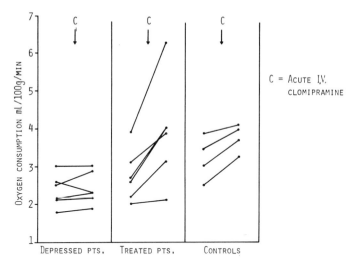

FIG. 18-7. Cerebral oxygen consumption (CMRO₂), before and after an acute intravenous injection of clomipramine in three experimental groups.

those patients where there was a fall, there was also a fall in arterial $PaCO_2$. Thus, although an equivalent dose of clomipramine was given to the depressed patients and also to the volunteers, the acute response to the drug in the two circumstances was completely different, that of the volunteers being similar to the response in dogs already described.

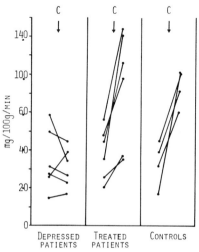

FIG. 18-8. Cerebral glucose consumption (CMRG), before and after an acute intravenous injection of clomipramine in three experimental groups.

Effects of Treatment

Following the 3-week treatment period, there was a tendency for the resting values for oxygen consumption to be higher, but no very obvious variation in resting cerebral blood flow or glucose consumption. When 50 mg of clomipramine was given, large increases in both cerebral oxygen consumption and glucose consumption occurred, which were not dissimilar to those occurring in the volunteer group. As the "treated" patients had been receiving therapy for at least 3 weeks prior to the second study, the difference in acute response on the second occasion could be due to different initial tissue levels of tricyclic drug. However, this is not an entirely adequate explanation. For example, one particular patient failed to improve, as judged by his Hamilton Rating score (i.e., 49 to 42), over the period of chronic treatment despite large doses of the drug. His cerebral oxygen and glucose response to the second acute infusion was very similar to his initial response. Fortunately, it was possible to study this patient subsequently when he had recovered and had not been on any therapy for 3 weeks. On this occasion, the response was similar to the control subjects.

The final figures show the relationship between the Hamilton Rating score and the change in cerebral glucose consumption following 50 mg clomipramine, expressed as a percentage of control.

From this it can be seen that as the depression improves, the metabolic response increases. There is also an obvious difference between the depressed patients (untreated) and the normal volunteers.

CONCLUSIONS

1. From this data some interesting facts emerge. Tricyclic antidepressants usually cause an unequivocal rise in oxygen and glucose utilization by the

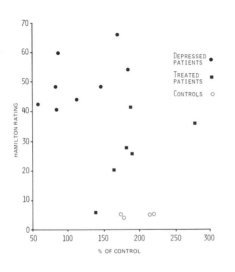

FIG. 18-9. Percent increase in cerebral glucose consumption following intravenous injection of clomipramine in three experimental groups.

brain. The effect may be beta-adrenomimetic and is probably partly dependent on chemoreceptor activation, as well as having a direct central effect.

2. Increasing doses cause a progressive increase in glucose utilization which eventually exceeds the oxygen supply and would seem to result in some degree of anaerobic glycolysis. In normal individuals this response is associated with some sensation of anxiety. Attempts have previously been made to relate brain lactic acid production to anxiety (31), and increased metabolic requirements could be the reason why in the elderly, where the cerebral circulation is not as adequate as in other age groups, the prescription of a tricyclic antidepressant occasionally results in confusion (32).

3. The lack of response in the depressed patient to acute intravenous clomipramine has an interesting parallel in the abnormal pressor response of such patients to infused catecholamines (33). However, although the response to infused drugs in depressed patients has previously been reported as abnormal, this is the first time, to our knowledge, that a difference in the response of the metabolism of the brain itself has been implicated.

4. Although the increases in oxygen and glucose metabolism were not found initially in depressed patients, they were found following chronic treatment. Despite a possibility that higher initial tissue levels of the drug played a role in the different response on the second occasion, it is difficult to accept this as the full explanation. Although it is not yet possible to explain how these differences in brain response occur, whether or not they are due to changes in brain amines (34–37) or to intracellular cyclic AMP (38–41), it would appear that they are associated with changes in the patient's psychiatric state.

ACKNOWLEDGMENTS

This research was supported by a grant from the Medical Research Council of Great Britain. The following colleagues have contributed at some stage: D. R. Pitcher, Dept. of Psychiatry, Royal Free Hospital Medical School; Lindsay MacDonell, Dept. of Pharmacology, Dalhousie University, Canada; P. C. Brant, Dept. of Medicine, University of Brasilia, Brasil; and S. Hall, Max Planck Institute, Berlin.

REFERENCES

1. Kety, S. S., and Schmidt, C. F. The nitrous oxide method for the quantitative determination of cerebral blood flow in man: Theory, procedure and normal values. *J. Clin. Invest.,* 1948, 27, 476–483.
2. Purves, M. J. Regulation of cerebral vessels by carbon dioxide. In: *The Physiology of the Cerebral Circulation.* Monographs of the Physiological Society, Cambridge University Press, 1972, pp. 173–199.
3. Harper, A. M. Regulation of cerebral circulation. *Sci. Basis Med.* (Annual Review), 1969, 60–81.
4. Purves, M. J. Cerebral blood flow and metabolism. In: *The Physiology of the Cerebral*

Circulation. Monographs of the Physiological Society. Cambridge University Press, 1972, pp. 282–333.

5. Ingvar, D. H., and Risberg, J. Increase of regional cerebral blood flow during mental effort in normals and in patients with local brain disorders. *Exp. Brain Res.*, 1967, 3, 195–211.

6. Xanalatos, C., and James, I. M. Effect of arterial CO_2 pressure on the response of cerebral and hind limb blood flow and metabolism to isoprenaline infusion in the dog. *Clin. Sci.*, 1972, 42, 63–68.

7. MacDonell, L., Xanalatos, C., Hall, S., and James, I. M. Factors affecting the response of cerebral metabolism and blood flow to a noradrenaline infusion in the dog. *Eur. Neurol.*, 1971–1972, 6, 208–212.

8. James, I. M., and MacDonell, L. Factors affecting the cerebrovascular response to noradrenaline in the dog. *Br. J. Pharmacol.*, 1975, 54, 129–143.

9. Kety, S. S., Woodford, R. B., Harmel, M. H., Freyhan, F. A., Appel, K. A., and Schmidt, C. F. Effects of barbiturate semi-narcosis, insulin coma and electroshock. *Am. J. Psychiatry*, 1948, 104, 765–770.

10. Kety, S. S., Polis, B. D., Nalder, C. S., and Schmidt, C. F. The blood flow and oxygen consumption of the human brain in diabetic acidosis and coma. *J. Clin. Invest.*, 1948, 27, 500–510.

11. James, I. M., Nashat S., Sampson, D., Williams, H. S., and Garassini, M. Effect of induced metabolic alkalosis in hepatic encephalopathy. *Lancet*, 1969, 2, 1106–1108.

12. Schmidt, C. F., Kety, S. S., and Pennes, H. H. The gaseous metabolism of the brain of the monkey. *Am. J. Physiol.*, 1945, 143, 33–52.

13. Bernsmeier A., and Gottstein, U. Die Sauerstoffaufnahme des menschlicher Gehirus unter Phenothiazinen, Barbituraten und in des Ischamie. *Pfluegers Arch.*, 1956, 263, 102–108.

14. Birzis, L., and Tachibana, S. The action of stimulant and depressant agents on local cerebral impedance and circulation. *Psychopharmacologia*, 1964, 6, 256–266.

15. Kety, S. S. The cerebral circulation. In: *Handbook of Physiology, 1: Neurophysiology*, Vol. 3, edited by J. Field. American Physiol. Society, Washington, D.C., 1964, pp. 1751–1760.

16. Ponte, J., and Purves, M. J. The role of the carotid body chemoreceptors and carotid sinus baroreceptors in the control of cerebral blood vessels. *J. Physiol.*, 1974, 237, 315–340.

17. Kajikawa, H. Mode of the sympathetic innervation of the cerebral vessels demonstrated by the histochemical technique in rats and cats. *Arch. Jap. Chir.*, 1969, 38, 227–235.

18. Lavrentieva, N. B., Mchedlishvili, G. I., and Plechkova, E. K. Distribution and activity of cholinesterase in the nervous structures of the pial arteries (a histochemical study). *Bull. Biol. Med. Exp. U. R. S. S.*, 1968, 64, 110–113.

19. Mchedlishvili, G. I., and Nikolaishvili, L. S. Evidence of a cholinergic mechanism in mediating the autoregulatory dilation of the cerebral blood vessels. *Pfluegers Arch.*, 1970, 315, 27–37.

20. Carpi, A., and Virno, M. Interaction between the electrical activity and the circulation of the brain and significance of metabolic and humeral factors under the various conditions of functional activity. In: *Cerebral Anoxia and the Electroencephalogram*, edited by J. S. Meyer and H. Gastaut. Charles C Thomas, Springfield, Ill., 1961, pp. 112–117.

21. Andén, N.-E., Carlsson, A., and Haggendal, J. Adrenergic mechanisms. *Annu. Rev. Pharmacol.* (9), 1969, 119–134.

22. Axelrod, J., Whitby, L. G., and Hertting, G. Effect of psychotropic drugs on the uptake of ³H norepinephrine by tissues. *Science*, 1961, 133, 383–384.

23. Sigg, E. B. Pharmacological studies with Tofranil®. *Can. Psychiatr. Assoc. J.*, 1959, 45, 75–85.

24. Sigg, E. B., Soffer, L., and Gyermeck, L. Influence of imipramine and related psychoactive agents on the effect of 5 hydroxytryptamine and catecholamines on the cat nictitating membrane. *J. Pharmacol. Exp. Ther.*, 1963, 142, 13–20.

25. Thursfield, D. Anticholinergic effect of clomipramine. *J. Inst. Med. Res.*, 1973, 1, No. 5, 456–459.

26. Ingvar, D. H., and Lassen, N. A. Regional blood flow of the cerebral cortex determined by krypton⁸⁵. *Acta Physiol. Scand.*, 1962, 54, 325–338.

27. Linden, R. J., Ledsome, J. R., and Norman, J. Simple methods for the determination of the concentrations of carbon dioxide and oxygen in blood. *Br. J. Anaesth.,* 1965, 37, 77–85.
28. Trinder, P. Determination of blood glucose using glucose oxidase. *Ann. Clin. Biochem.* (Proc. Assoc. Clin. Biochem.), B, 1969, 24–25.
29. McHenry, L. C., Jr. Quantitative cerebral blood flow determination: Application of krypton[85] desaturation technique in man. *Neurology* (Minneap.), 1964, 14, 785–793.
30. Gibbs, E. L., Lennox, W. G., and Gibbs, F. A. Bilateral internal jugular blood. Comparison of A-V differences, oxygen-dextrose ratios and respiratory quotients. *Am. J. Psychiatry,* 1945, 102, 184–190.
31. Pitts, F. M., and McClure, J. N. Lactate metabolism in anxiety neurosis. *N. Engl. J. Med.,* 1967, 277, 1329–1333.
32. Hamilton, M., and Mahopatra, S. B. Anti-depressive drugs. Chapter in *Side Effects of Drugs,* edited by L. Meyler and A. Herxheimer. 1972. Excerpta Medica, Amsterdam, 17–37.
33. Prange, A. J., Jr. McCurdy, R. L., and Cochrane, C. M. The systolic blood pressure response of depressed patients to infused norepinephrine. *J. Psychiatr. Res.,* 1967, 5, 1–13.
34. Schildkraut, J. J. The catecholamine hypothesis of affective disorders: A review of supporting evidence. *Am. J. Psychiatry,* 1965, 122, 509–522.
35. Schildkraut, J. J., Gordon, E. K., and Durell, J. Catecholamine metabolism in affective disorders: 1, normetanephrine and VMA excretion in depressed patients treated with imipramine. *J. Psychiatr. Res.,* 1965, 3, 213.
36. Carlsson, A., Corrodi, H., Fuxe, K., and Hokfelt, T. Effect of anti-depressant drugs on the depletion of intraneuronal brain 5-hydroxytryptamine stores caused by 4-methyl-alpha-ethyl-meta-tyramine. *Eur. J. Pharmacol.,* 1969a, 5, 357–366.
37. Carlsson, A., Corrodi, H., Fuxe, K., and Hokfelt, T. Effects of some anti-depressant drugs on the depletion of intraneuronal brain catecholamine stores caused by 4, alpha-dimethyl-meta-tyramine. *Eur. J. Pharmacol.,* 1969b, 5, 367–373.
38. Abdulla, Y. H., and Hamadah, K. 3',5' Cyclic adenosine monophosphate in depression and mania. *Lancet,* 1970, 2, 378–381.
39. Paul, M. I., Cramer, H., and Goodwin, F. K. Urinary cyclic AMP in affective illness. *Lancet,* 1970, 1, 996.
40. Paul, M. I., Ditzion, B. R., and Janowsky, D. S. Affective illness and cyclic AMP excretion. *Lancet,* 1970, 1, 88.
41. Paul, M. I., Pauk, G. L., and Janowsky, D. S. Urinary adenosine 3',5'-monophosphate excretion in affective disorders. *Am. J. Psychiatry,* 1970, 126, 1493–1497.

Stress and the Heart, edited by D. Wheatley,
Raven Press, New York © 1981.

Psychotropic Drugs in the Elderly

Anthony Hordern and David Wheatley

As indicated in the preceding chapters, geriatric psychopharmacology is destined to increase in importance, if only by reason of the continuation of the population explosion that has characterized the last 50 years. As an increasing number of individuals attain old age, the cost of providing them with health care will inexorably rise, and many will inevitably develop psychiatric disorders requiring effective, economical treatment. As people age, disabilities become increasingly common, and drug usage increases; prescribing for elderly patients merits special care in view of age-linked changes in pharmacokinetics. The major psychotropic agents currently employed include: (a) hypnotics, sedatives, and minor tranquilizers, (b) antidepressants and lithium, and (c) major tranquilizers and miscellaneous drugs.

PSYCHOGERIATRIC IMPLICATIONS OF POPULATION GROWTH

Despite the attainment of zero population growth by a number of Western nations in the 1970s, a 1978 report issued by the world bank estimated that the world population, then 4,000 million, was likely to reach 5,900 million by the year 2000. An earlier report published in 1971 by the United Nations predicted that the number of people in the world over the age of 60, then numbering 290 million, would double by the end of the century. People over 65 are already numerous in the developed nations, constituting 10% of the population of the United States, 8.5% of Australia, and 15% of England and Wales (1,2). In 1977, the director-general of the World Health Organization calculated that the majority of Western nations were spending about one half their health budgets on the elderly. Carlson (3), assuming a yearly inflation rate of only 6.2% and a rise in the number of over-65s in the United States from 20 million in 1974 to 35 million (35%) in 2000, computed that the cost of their medical care could by the latter year amount to $2,047,000 million, i.e., over $2 trillion.

Because of the rapidity and extent of psychosocial change during the last 20 years, the aged of both sexes have tended to feel increasingly unwanted. This applies to women especially; they are more numerous and in years past, few have had access to education or could enjoy a satisfying career (apart from or in addition to motherhood and rearing a family). More women over the age of 65 than men are unmarried (less than 40% versus almost 80% in the United States) and more and more women live on into widowhood. Indeed 60% of American women over 65 now live without a spouse, and although the majority reside with their children or with other family members, 41% live alone or with people to whom they are unrelated (4). Loneliness is thus common, and although social benefits and welfare services have helped, the problem is serious and worsening.

As Francis (5) has observed, three myths concerning the elderly are as follows: (a) all old people "go potty as they get older"; (b) all old people are the same; and (c) 20th-century children do not care about their parents and do not want to be bothered with them. In fact, the intelligence of most old people does not decline with age; the elderly, like their younger counterparts, have a variety of different interests, aptitudes, and accomplishments. Although most young people do care about their older relatives, society has failed to provide the environments in which care can be given. It is clear, nevertheless, as Butler (6) has emphasized, that the elderly in Western societies comprise two main groups: those who remain healthy and vigorous, i.e., those essentially enjoying an extended middle age, and the "old-old," handicapped by disease and disability.

As age increases, defects in hearing, vision, and locomotion become more common, so that there is a tendency for the aged to become increasingly isolated. In addition, as Butler has observed, the elderly are disproportionately subject to emotional and mental difficulties. With increasing age, there is an increase not only in everyday emotional problems but also in functional mental illnesses, notably depression and paranoid states, in chronic brain disease (dementia), and in suicide (in the United States, although 25% of all known suicides occur in those over 65, this segment constitutes only 10% of the population). Among men and women followed up to the age of 80 in a rural Swedish community by Essen-Moller and Hagnell (7), the rates for depression were 17.7 and 8.5% respectively; but these percentages would probably have been much higher had the study included patients whose depressions were masked or presented via physical complaints, hypochondriasis, paranoid states, alcoholism, and so forth. Roth (8) estimated that about 50% of older patients admitted to psychiatric hospitals were depressed, and many psychiatrists would put the percentage even higher (9). Furthermore, about 10% of people over the age of 65 suffer from dementia, and its incidence rises to 22% among those aged 80 and over (10). Pitt (11) has estimated that in about one-half of these patients, the dementia is at least moderately severe; yet only about one-fifth are cared for in institutions; the rest are looked after, or neglected, in their own homes.

Home is immensely important symbolically as well as practically to many old folk, representing as it does a cherished setting, providing continuous reorientation, reassuring individuals of their identities, and affording a continuous link with relatives, friends, and past experiences. Home also represents independence, safety, and predictability in social contacts, probable expenditures, commitments, and so forth. It is not surprising, therefore, that the majority of old people, even when too ill to cope and to care for themselves, strenuously resist efforts to move them out of their homes into the much more impersonal, less familiar, less predictable environment of institutions, hospitals, retirement villages, and similar places. Many of the psychotropic drugs now available facilitate home treatment and secondary developments, such as malnutrition and alcoholism, can often be controlled. Thus the elderly can be saved from designation as senile and banishment to the back wards of geriatric or psychiatric hospitals.

THE MAJOR PSYCHOGERIATRIC SYNDROMES

Neuroses presenting de novo in old age are probably extremely rare, although symptoms such as anxiety, depression, and insomnia are common. It is important to decide the severity, duration, and relationships of such complaints. Is the anxiety explicable in the light of the patient's situation? Does he or she have an organic illness which may be wholly or partly responsible for its generation? Is anxiety and depression merely part of a lifelong pattern? Or is anxiety the result of the patient's vague awareness of an early stage of dementia; i.e., is it due to "unformulated cerebral inferiority"? Is it the manifestation, as is often the case, of an agitated endogenous depression, i.e., an "involutional melancholia"? Acute organic syndromes are attributable to temporary reversible alterations of cerebral function caused by organic disease(s). The central feature is clouding of consciousness, from which all other symptoms derive.

Deliria

Characteristically lasting for days or occasionally weeks, deliria belong to the domain of general medicine and general surgery, being recognized as complications of physical illnesses, injuries, and operations. The clouding of consciousness characterizing a delirium is typically associated with three manifestations. First, there may be intellectual impairment: defects in attention and grasp, disorientation, faulty perceptions, and misidentifications of relatives, friends, and medical and nursing personnel, hallucinations and delusions, and impairment of judgment and insight. Second, emotional upsets may occur, characterized by states of fear, bewilderment, rage, or euphoria. Finally, there is disturbed behavior: noisiness, restlessness, aggressiveness, (sometimes) epileptic fits, overactivity, apathy, inability to behave rationally, to read, to write, to eat appropriately, or to control the sphincters, and, finally, exhaustion. Most delirious patients recover, especially if appropriately treated. A few—the old, the debilitated, the severely injured, and those with extremely virulent infections—die. Subsequently, a small proportion of patients pass into a subdelirious state (a subacute delirium) characterized by incoherence of thought, brief interludes of lucidity, and fluctuating levels of consciousness. Later, not uncommon sequels include the dysmnesic syndrome, i.e., a Korsakov psychosis, with prominent disturbance of recent memory, and depressions with neurasthenic features.

Dementias

Chronic organic states—dementias—are illnesses in which there is a permanent, irreversible decline in cerebral function due to organic disease(s) within the central nervous system (CNS). The central features are confusion and memory impairment, but other mental and physical symptoms are usually also present. These illnesses last, as a rule, for months or years and are dealt with medically, mainly by general practitioners, psychiatrists, geriatricians, and neurologists. Dementias may occur in youth or middle age from such causes as head injury and cerebral tumors, but they are predominantly diseases of the elderly. Of the 10% of people over 65 who are demented, 4% of the syndromes are arteriosclerotic, 4% are senile, and 2% have resulted from other causes. A mental state examination format that can provide a guide to prognosis has recently been described by Hare (12).

As in the deliria, the signs and symptoms of dementias fall into the spheres of intellectual impairment, emotional upset, and disturbance of behavior. Intellectual impairment is evident from defects in attention and grasp, disorientation (time, place, and person), defects in judgment and reasoning, memory gaps and falsifications, hallucinations and delusions, and impairment of judgment and insight. Emotional upsets are characterized by unstable, labile, or incongruous moods, with impulsivity, rage, suspicion, or apathy. Behavioral disturbances are manifested by loss of habitual restraints, i.e., undue irritability, prevarication, larceny, sexual misdemeanors, drunkenness, and a reduction in purposeful, goal-directed activities with undue rigidity in behavior and response. Furthermore, "catastrophic" reactions of anxiety, panic, or uncontrollable rage can occur when the patient is confronted with what he or she regards as an impossibly difficult task or situation. Other symptoms include deterioration of personality, disturbances of eating, sleeping, and elimination, decline in health, general slovenliness, inadequacy of personal hygiene, and incontinence (13).

Cerebral Arteriosclerosis

It is important to recognize that the dementias resulting from different causes have different courses and prognoses, and that some patients thus labeled do not have true but pseudodementias resulting from illnesses, such as depression and alcoholism. Of the true dementias, almost one-half are due to cerebral arteriosclerosis, a disease of the 60s in men, which in women usually has its onset a decade later. Arteriosclerotic dementias (ASD) usually run a jerky, intermittent course lasting 4 to 10 years, with a mean duration of 3 years. They should be differentiated from true senile dementias (SDs), which develop over the age of 75, are due to neuronal degeneration of unknown etiology, and are characterized by a smoothly progressive mental and physical decline leading to death within 2 years.

In ASD, there is often a history of hypertension with transient episodes of loss of consciousness, paralysis, inability to speak, and loss of vision, while patchy circumscribed episodes of amnesia (each corresponding to a small cerebral thrombosis) are common (in contrast to global amnesia in SD). Insight and the outward personality are preserved late (these are lost early in SD). Remissions occur early on (but not in SD), although after each episode, the patient loses more ground, so that in the long run deterioration takes place and the individual is reduced to a "vegetable" state. According to the part of the CNS affected, however, a pure "dementing" picture may be in evidence, with or without arteriosclerotic episodes, parkinsonism, or pseudobulbar palsy (dysphagia, dysarthria, and "emotional incontinence"). Headaches, dizziness, irritability, impaired concentration, and forgetfulness are common. In the early stages, the personality is well preserved, so the existence of an ASD may not be suspected. Because insight is retained, whereby the individual can compare his current state with that of the past, anxiety and depression are common, as are impulses to commit suicide. Some arteriosclerotic episodes, like ischemic coronary attacks, are probably provoked by external factors.

Clearly, it is vital for the practitioner to be able to differentiate the fair immediate, but ultimately poor, prognosis of an ASD from the adverse outlook of SD and to advise the patient and the patient's relatives accordingly. Some success in predicting outcome can be obtained from the magnitude and speed of changes in the electroencephalogram (EEG); too few data have as yet been obtained from computerized axial tomography (CAT) studies for their findings to be accorded appropriate significance. Some dementias, despite the definition of the condition, are largely reversible; thus the degree of impairment evident in many alcoholic dementias may recede dramatically when alcohol is withheld (as in the hospital), and the treatment of any associated depression may make the signs and symptoms of dementia less severe. Furthermore, not all dementias are accompanied by defects in orientation, reasoning, calculation, and memory. Thus primary or secondary tumors in the frontal lobes of the brain not uncommonly present with behavioral disturbances, characterized by inappropriate jocularity, irritability, tactlessness, and social disinhibition.

Depression

Having eliminated the presence of a significant degree of dementia, the most common psychiatric disorder in the aged is depression, usually biochemical (endogenous) to a significant extent, but often associated with personality or situational (reactive) factors. As in younger patients, evidence of functional hypothalamic shift symptoms (insomnia, anorexia, loss of weight, loss of libido, and diurnal variation in depression and drive) should be sought, and the coexistence of anxiety should not lead to doubts regarding diagnosis. Social withdrawal and a reduction in interests and fatigue are common, as is hypochondriasis, often about bowel function, leading to carcinophobia. Most of the features of depression in the elderly are not uncommon in old age per se, e.g., insomnia together with social withdrawal, concern about physical health, and similar symptoms. Alcohol is often ingested, and in women especially, the habit is often concealed. In diagnosing depression, attention should be directed to likely precipitating or aggravating factors. These may be psychologic (such as bereavement, retirement, moving house), physical (such as influenza, bronchitis, a heart attack), or pharmacologic, [such as alcohol, antihypertensives, such as reserpine, methyldopa, and propranolol, antiparkinsonian agents, barbiturates and benzodiazepines, corticosteroids and cytotoxic drugs, including immunosuppressive agents, digitalis (as a precursor or component of toxic effects), and certain neuroleptics, notably chlorpromazine, haloperidol, and depot fluphenazine].

Schizophrenia

Schizophrenic disorders presenting de novo in the elderly are often termed paraphrenias, being differentiated from schizophrenia in early adult life by the preservation of a personality which, apart from an encapsulated area of well-systematized delusions (with or without supporting hallucinations), appears normal. Not infrequently, depression is prominent in the clinical presentation, giving rise to the designation "affect-laden paraphrenia," an illness which occasions diagnostic difficulty. Impairment of hearing and sight, not uncommon disabilities in the elderly, are often present.

Alcoholism is also common in the elderly, in the range of 2 to 10% of the general population of the United States, with higher rates in widowers, medical patients, and police cases, according to Schukit et al. (14). Chronic alcoholism can be manifested in alcoholic pseudoparanoia and is frequently associated with depressive illness, with Korsakov's psychosis, and with alcoholic dementia. Because of the comparative cheapness of alcohol, its ready availability, its accepted role in social life, and its promotion by the manufacturers of alcoholic beverages, its use has been increasing steadily; with it is an increase in the problems it generates.

DISABILITIES AND DRUG USE

In the United States, 80 to 85% of those aged 65 and over have one or more chronic illnesses, in comparison to 40% of those under age 65 (15). In England, a survey by McDonnell and his colleagues (2) of those aged 65 and over living (a) in their own homes, (b) in sheltered housing, (c) in social service aged persons' hostels, and (d) in a hospital, revealed that more than 50% of those aged over 64 had some form of chronic illness, such illnesses being more common in females than in males. Nontraumatic locomotor disorders constituted the most widespread disability, being present in 19% of subjects; they were followed by disorders of eyesight, cerebrovascular disease, and respiratory infections (which were more common in men). The capacity to cope in the spheres of mobility (getting out of bed, getting about the house, getting out of the house), functional ability (feeding, toilet use, bathing, dressing), and domestic activities (shopping, cooking, cleaning) was found to be greatest in those living in their own homes, followed by those living in sheltered homes. Coping capacities were poorer in those living in social security aged persons' homes and most greatly impaired in those who were hospitalized.

17. Advocated mainly for the treatment of arteriosclerotic (multiinfarct) dementia, they can conveniently be allocated to one of three groups (a) cerebral vasodilators, (b) cerebral vasodilators that affect cerebral metabolism, and (c) drugs that have no vasodilator effect. As Saletu points out in Chapter 17, the desired property of all nootropic drugs would appear to be that they should improve hypoxia.

Cerebral Vasodilators

Cerebral vasodilators include cyclandelate (Cyclospasmol®), isoxsuprine (Duvadilon®), cinnarizine (Stugeron®), and Cosaldon. Cyclandelate in a dose of 400 to 1,600 mg daily has been claimed to improve orientation, forgetfulness, and vocabulary, but it can cause nausea, flushing, and rashes; it is contraindicated after a recent cerebrovascular accident, and many are skeptical of its value. Isoxsuprine, a cerebral vasodilator that is a beta-adrenergic stimulator, is more effective in dilating the vessels in the periphery than in the brain. In a dose of 40 to 80 mg daily, it has been claimed to reduce ischemic episodes in patients with cerebral arteriosclerosis, but it can produce flushing, dizziness, nausea, vomiting, and palpitations; it is contraindicated after arterial hemorrhage. None of the few studies performed on isoxsuprine has shown it to be of any practical value (50). Similar considerations apply to Cosaldon. This compound which is composed of nicotinic acid and 1-hexyl-3,7-dimethylxanthene, is a mixture of a vasodilator and a stimulant; it, too, is contraindicated after a recent cerebrovascular accident. In a dose of three tablets daily, Cosaldon may produce improvement in the symptoms of dementia at the price of flushing and dyspepsia, but its value is dubious.

Clinical Studies

The General Practitioner Research Group has undertaken several placebo-controlled, double-blind studies of cerebral vasodilator drugs in patients suffering from arteriosclerotic mental illness. In a study conducted over 8 weeks, cinnarizine was compared to placebo, with crossover of medications at 4 weeks and random allocation of cases to treatment (51). Results were assessed on the Crichton geriatric scale (52) initially and at the end of each 4-week treatment period. Irrespective of the order of treatment, results were similar between active and placebo medications. Thus, on combining the results from both series, the overall proportional improvement for cinnarizine was only 9%; this figure was exactly the same for placebo. Of the individual items, the best results were obtained with both compounds, in restlessness (cinnarizine, 18%; placebo, 23%) and subjective mood (cinnarizine, 24%; placebo, 19%).There were no statistical differences between the results from active and placebo drugs in relation to any of the individual symptoms.

In a more recent study, cyclandelate (Cyclospasmol®) was compared to placebo, patients being treated for 3 months with one or the other compound, according to random selection. The dose was standardized at one tablet q.d.s. (cyclandelate, 400-mg tablets); 53 patients were treated, 27 of whom received cyclandelate and 26 the placebo. A modified version of the Crichton scale was used, consisting of 12 items which could be subdivided into three groups as follows: physical (mobility, dressing, feeding, continence), mental (orientation, communication, mental alertness/confusion, memory for recent events), and psychiatric (co-operation, restlessness, anxiety, depression). In addition, the Nurses Observation Scale (NOSIE) (53) was also completed by nurses who visited the patients in their homes. The mean scores of the various assessment measures at the start and end of the trial are shown in Table 19.1

It is apparent that there were no significant changes in the mean scores on any of the assessment measures from the initial assessment to the final one. The paired t-test and Wilcoxon rank sum test were used to test for statistically significant differences between pre- and post-scores and between groups, respectively; these confirmed that no such differences existed.

Records were also made of blood pressure, pulse rate, degree of cardiac enlargement (if present), degree of cardiac failure (if present), and degree of paralysis (if present). With one exception, no significant differences were demonstrated on any of these measures in either treatment group. The one exception was an increase in mean diastolic blood pressure from 85.6 ($\pm$ 3.1) to 88.4 ($\pm$ 3.3) mm Hg ($p < 0.04$) with cyclandelate. Further analyses of the results in those patients who had not suffered a stroke, in those patients showing the best compliance in drug taking, and in the cases of shortest duration did not demonstrate any between-drug differences.

Cerebral Activators

Cerebral vasodilators, which in addition to their vascular action affect cerebral metabolism, are termed "cerebral activators." They are thought to improve cerebral utilization of oxygen and glucose. Dihydroergotoxine mesylate (Hydergine®), an alpha-adrenergic blocking drug referred to in Chapter 17, increases the activity of enzymes of intermediary metabolism in ganglion cells in animal studies. The drug produced only minimal improvement in a wide variety of indices of mental function in various clinical trials, however, and can give rise to sinus bradycardia and hypotension (50). Naftidrofuryl (Praxilene®, Nafronyl®), a second cerebral activator which inter alia increases cerebral concentrations of adenosine triphosphate and which reduces lactic acid, receives more favorable mention because clinical studies have shown that it can improve memory and behavior. Both Maclay (54) and Yesavage (55) disagree with some statements criticizing dihydroergotoxine mesylate (50), and each has separately emphasized that the drug has been shown to be effective in numerous investigations, in which it has been found to produce few side effects. Maclay (54) also stresses that the drug is indicated in the early stages of senile dementia

TABLE 19.1. Results of a clinical trial comparing cyclandelate (C) to placebo (P)[a]

| | Crichton scale | | | | | | | | NOSIE | |
| | Physical | | Mental | | Psychiatric | | Total | | | |
Dose	C	P	C	P	C	P	C	P	C	P
Initial	5.3 (±0.8)	4.4 (±0.7)	6.8 (±0.6)	6.6 (±0.7)	4.4 (±0.6)	4.0 (±0.5)	16.5 (±1.4)	14.9 (±1.4)	41.2 (±3.8)	46.4 (±4.9)
3 Months	5.3 (±0.8)	4.3 (±0.9)	6.7 (±0.7)	6.4 (±0.8)	4.7 (±0.6)	3.6 (±0.4)	16.7 (±1.6)	14.3 (±1.4)	44.3 (±3.7)	49.4 (±4.7)

[a]Mean scores ± SEM.

rather than in multiinfarct dementia. Pentifylline, a third cerebral activator, related to caffeine and conjugated with nicotinic acid, is said to increase glucose uptake in the brain, but more trials are required before its true value can be assessed.

A third group of compounds claimed to be effective in arteriosclerotic dementia affect cerebral metabolism but have no vasodilator effects. Pyritinol hydrochloride (Encephabol®) increases cerebral blood supply by improving neuronal metabolism, and, according to Flood (56), has been demonstrated to be effective in more than 20 studies on patients with organic brain disease. One double-blind trial in patients with senile dementia showed that it was significantly superior to placebo in improving physical activity, alertness, interest, and mental power. Meclofenoxate (Lucidril®) reduces cerebral need for oxygen. In a daily dose of 900 to 1,500 mg, it may improve learning capacity but can produce lassitude and irritability (49). Levodopa (Laradopa®), which alleviates dopamine deficiency in the striatum in parkinsonism, has also been tried in patients with senile dementia; one double-blind trial performed by Lewis and his colleagues (57) in female patients with an average age of 78.9 years showed that it could produce improvement in intellectual function. Procaine (Gerovitol H3®), which is a weak and reversible MAOI *in vitro,* is claimed by some to have both a physical and a mental rejuvenating effect in the elderly, but its value is controversial (13). Finally, there is recent evidence that a small daily dose of aspirin is effective, in men particularly, in preventing or reducing transient ischemic episodes in the brain (58); thus, at least in some patients, it may delay the onset and progression of arteriosclerotic dementia.

CONCLUSIONS

It is clear that, barring total war, universal famine, or an unforseen cosmic catastrophe, the proportion of old people in the population in both developed and developing countries is destined to increase, thus throwing an increasing burden on already fully extended health care resources. As age increases, defects in vision, hearing, and locomotion become more frequent, together with other organic physical illness and functional and organic psychogeriatric ailments.

The major psychogeriatric syndromes are well defined, and accurate differential diagnosis is essential for appropriate drug treatment. The increase in the number and severity of disabilities that takes place as age increases has been accompanied by an increase in the use of drugs. Prescribing drugs for the elderly is a skilled task requiring special care in view of age-linked changes in pharmacokinetics; appropriate doses and incremental increases in the elderly usually conform to the maxim, "start low and go slow."

Psychotropic drugs play an important role in the treatment of many of the disabilities and ailments of old age. Thus the benzodiazepines are invaluable in aiding elderly patients to sleep and in treating the anxiety symptoms that so commonly occur as the lifespan of the individual draws to its inevitable conclusion. The problem of dependence with these drugs is perhaps of less importance under these circumstances. The advent of the short-acting hypnotic benzodiazepines is an important advance in avoiding daytime sedation and mental confusion that can result from the use of the longer acting drugs of this type.

Depression in the elderly is an important problem which is often overlooked by the physician and can be aggravated by the overenthusiastic use of sedative drugs. Specific treatment with antidepressant drugs is of paramount importance, but many elderly patients have underlying cardiovascular abnormalities which render them susceptible to the cardiotoxic effects of the tricyclic antidepressants. Fortunately, the newer antidepressants seem to be relatively free of this disadvantage. This subject is extensively considered elsewhere in this volume.

The use of nootropic drugs, and in particular claimed cerebral vasodilators, to improve mental functioning in the elderly remains a matter of controversy. Although many of these drugs are available and there is experimental and other evidence to suggest that they may produce some effects on the aged brain, convincing proof is lacking. However, this is a hopeful field for further research in the development of cardiac and psychotropic drugs that may improve cerebral functioning in the elderly.

REFERENCES

1. Norman, T. R., Burrows, G. D., Scoggins, B. A., and Davies, B. Pharmacokinetics and plasma levels of antidepressants in the elderly. *Med. J. Aust.,* 1979, 1, 273–274.
2. McDonnell, H., Long, A. F., Harrison, B. J., and Oldman, C. A study of persons aged 65 and over in the Leeds Metropolitan District. *J. Epidemiol. Commun. Health,* 1979, 33, 203–209.
3. Carlson, R. J. *The End of Medicine.* Wiley, New York, 1975.
4. Somers, A. R. Marital status, health, and the use of health services. *JAMA,* 1979, 241, 1818–1822.
5. Francis, J. The growing problem of growing old. *The Australian,* 1 October 1979.
6. Butler, R. N. Psychiatry and the elderly: An overview. *Am. J. Psychiatry,* 1975, 132, 893–900.
7. Essen-Moller, E., and Hagnell, O. The frequency and risk of depression within a rural population in Scania. *Acta Psychiatr. Scand.,* [Suppl.], 1961, 162, 28–32.
8. Roth, M. The natural history of psychiatric disorders in old age. *J. Ment. Sci.,* 1955, 101, 281–301.
9. Raskin, A., and Sathananthan, G. Depression in the elderly. *Psychopharmacol. Bull.,* 1979, 15, 14–16.
10. Leading Article. Dementia—the quiet epidemic. *Br. Med. J.,* 1978, 1, 1–2.
11. Pitt, I. B. Dementia in old age. *Update,* February 1973, 315–319.
12. Hare, M. Clinical check list for diagnosis of dementia. *Br. Med. J.,* 1978, 2, 266–267.
13. Ban, T. A. Organic problems in the aged: Brain syndromes and alcoholism. *Geriatr. Psychiatry,* 1978, 7, 105–159.
14. Schuckit, M., Morrissey, E. R., and O'Leary, M. R. Alcohol problems in elderly men and women. *Addic. Dis.,* 1978, 3, 405–416.
15. Guttman, D. Patterns of legal drug use by older Americans. *Addict. Dis.,* 1978, 3, 337–356.
16. Cooperstock, R. Quoted in Korcok, M., 1978 ref. 21, 1978.
17. Mellinger, G. D., Batter, M. B., Manheimer, D. I. et al. Psychic distress, life crisis, and use of psychotherapeutic medications. *Arch. Gen. Psychiatry,* 1978, 35, 1045–1052.

18. Craig, T. J., and van Netta, P. A. Current medication use and symptoms of depression in a general population. *Am. J. Psychiatry,* 1978, 135, 1036–1039.
19. Green, B. The politics of psychoactive drug use in old age. *Gerontologist,* 1978, 18, 525–530.
20. Pfeiffer, E. Quoted in Korcok, M. ref. 21, 1978.
21. Korcok, M. Drugs and the elderly. *Can. Med. Assoc. J.,* 1978, 118, 1320–1326.
22. Beber, C. Quoted in Korcok, M., ref. 21, 1978.
23. Judge, T. C., and Caird, F. I. *Drug Treatment of the Elderly Patient.* Pittmann Medical, Tunbridge Wells, U.K., 1978.
24. Hartford, J. T. How to minimize side-effects of psychotropic drugs. *Geriatrics,* 1979, 34, 83–93.
25. Beattie, B. L., and Sellers, E. M. Psychoactive drug use in the elderly: The pharmacokinetics. *Psychosomatics,* 1979, 20, 474–479.
26. Shader, R. I., and Greenblatt, D. J. Pharmacokinetics and clinical drug effects in the elderly. *Psychopharmacol. Bull.,* 1979, 15, 8–14.
27. Oswald, I. The why and how of hypnotic drugs. *Br. Med. J.,* 1979, 1, 1167–1168.
28. Annotation. Benzodiazepine withdrawal. *Lancet,* 1979, 1, 196.
29. Review Article. Drugs in the elderly. Medical Letter (New York). 1979, 21, 43.
30. Lader, M. H., Makin, E. J. B., and Nicholson, A. N. (Eds.). Temazepam and related 1:4 benzodiazepines: Effects of sleep and performance. *Brit. J. Clin. Pharmacol. [Suppl.],* 1979, 8.
31. General Practitioner Research Group. Comparison of sleep patterns with flunitrazepam and nitrazepam. *J. Pharmacother.,* 1978, 1, 4, 131.
32. Magnus, R. V. A controlled trial of chlormethiazole in the management of symptoms of the organic dementias in the elderly. *Clin. Ther.,* 1968, 1, 387–396.
33. Dehlin, O., Falkheden, T., Gatzinska, R., and Nordqvist, P. The hypnotic effect of chlormethiazole during long-term treatment of geriatric patients. *Clin. Ther.,* 1978, 2, 41–46.
34. Illingworth, R. N., Stewart, M. J., and Jarvie, D. R. Severe poisoning with chlormethiazole. *Br. Med. J.,* 1979, 2, 902–903.
35. McInnes, G. T., Young, R. E., and Avery, B. S. Poisoning with chlormethiazole. *Br. Med. J.,* 1979, 2, 1218–1219.
36. Hession, M. A., Verma, S., and Bhakta, K. G. M. Dependence on clormethiazole and effects of its withdrawal. *Lancet,* 1979, 1, 953–954.
37. Glatt, M. M. Uses and abuses of chlormethiazole. *Lancet,* 1979, 1, 1093–1094.
38. Majumdar, S. K. Uses and abuses of chlormethiazole. *Lancet,* 1979, 1, 1093.
39. Exton-Smith, A. N., and McLean, A. E. M. Uses and abuses of chlormethiazole. *Lancet,* 1979, 1, 1093.
40. Scott, C. J. Uses and abuses of chlormethiazole. *Lancet,* 1979, 1, 1094.
41. Hordern, A. *Tranquility Denied.* Rigby, Adelaide, Australia, 1976.
42. Lynch, J. J. *The Broken Heart.* Basic Books, New York, 1977.
43. Hordern, A. *Depressive States.* Charles C Thomas, Springfield, Ill., 1965.
44. Nies, A., Robinson, D. S., Friedman, M. J. et al. Relationship between age and tricyclic antidepressant plasma levels. *Am. J. Psychiatry,* 1977, 134, 790–793.
45. Ravn, J. The history of thioxanthenes. In: *Discoveries in Biological Psychiatry,* edited by F. J. Ayd and B. Blackwell, Lippincott, Toronto, 1970.
46. Leading article. Drugs and male sexual function. *Br. Med. J.,* 1979, 2, 883.
47. Silverman, G. Management of the elderly agitated demented patient. *Br. Med. J.,* 1977, 2, 318–319.
48. Fine, W., and Walker, D. J. Management of the elderly agitated demented patient. *Br. Med. J.,* 1977, 2, 580.
49. Review article. Drugs for dementia. *Drug Ther. Bull. (Lond.),* 1979, 13, 85–87.
50. Leading article. Vasodilators in senile dementia. *Br. Med. J.,* 1979, 2, 511–512.
51. General Practitioner Clinical Trials. Manifestations of cerebral arteriosclerosis unaffected by a vasodilator. *Practitioner,* 1969, 203, 695.
52. Guy, W. *ECDEU Assessment Manual.* U. S. Dept. of Health, Education and Welfare, Rockville, Md., 1976.
53. Honigfeld, G., and Klett, C. The Nurses' Observation Scale for Inpatient Evaluation (NOSIE): A new scale for measuring improvement in chronic schizophrenia. *J. Clin. Psychol.,* 1965, 21, 65–71.
54. Maclay, W. P. Vasodilators in senile dementia. *Br. Med. J.,* 1979, 2, 866.

55. Yesavage, J. Vasodilators in senile dementia. *Br. Med. J.,* 1979, 2, 1223–1224.
56. Flood, M. H. Pyritinol hydrochloride (Encephabol) and senile dementia. *Br. Med. J.,* 1979, 1, 1148.
57. Lewis, C., Ballinger, B. R., and Presly, A. S. Trial of levodopa in senile dementia. *Br. Med. J.,* 1978, 1, 550.
58. Yatsu, F. M., and Carter, C. C. Drugs for the stroke-prone patient with TIAS. *Mod. Med. Aust.,* 1980, 23, 5–11.

Stress and the Heart, edited by D. Wheatley,
Raven Press, New York © 1981.

Sociopharmacologic Aspects

Anthony Hordern

Coronary heart disease in particular and cardiovascular disorders in general are now of immense importance in developed nations because the former is the principal cause of premature death in relatively young men and the latter are widespread in older people of both sexes. Coronary artery disease can result in the loss, or the enduring disablement, of the family's main breadwinner, the mother's husband, the children's father. More than one-third of all deaths in developed countries are attributable to coronary disease, which has become, as Carruthers (1) has observed, "by far the greatest peacetime killer of western man." For example, between 1950 and 1970, the incidence in England and Wales alone almost doubled in men aged 35 to 44, rose by more than one-half in those aged 45 to 54, and by one-quarter in those aged 55 to 64. In comparison, the increase was only about one-fifth in women aged 35 to 44, with no increase in the other age groups (2).

Hypertension is also very common, a diastolic pressure of 100 mm Hg or more in the sitting position being present in about one-sixth of patients in the London area; once again, the incidence is higher in males than in females (3). Cerebrovascular disease is a fairly frequent complication of advancing years, while arteriosclerotic dementias, often accompanied by depression, develop in some 5% of those over the age of 65, customarily occurring a decade or more earlier in men than in women. It is clear that, in cardiovascular terms especially, males are vastly inferior to their female counterparts, who are protected by estrogens, although this advantage, the present writer has elsewhere observed (4), is somewhat counterbalanced by the fact that women are 2.5 times more likely than men to develop endogenous depressions.

The majority of the inhabitants of the Western world currently reside in technosocieties characterized by city living, overcrowding, noise, traffic, and the "rat race," with its constant deadlines and its prevailing job insecurity. It is hardly surprising that tension, anxiety, depression, and somatic discomforts are almost universal complaints. Men in particular are often beset with multiple frustrations. A fortunate few are involved in stimulating, creative, satisfying work, but the majority are habitually employed in monotonous, boring, soul-destroying tasks which do not provide adequate psychological satisfaction. Many men are compelled to compete in the status-affluence race; and since they lack suitable outlets for their tensions, they eat too much, drink to excess, and smoke too heavily. Indeed, many aspects of contemporary Western life—the overconsumption of refined sugar and saturated fats (with resultant obesity), excessive cigarette smoking, lack of exercise, and emotional stress—are almost tailor-made to engender coronary artery disease.

Stress, as Selye (5) has observed, means different things to different people; for the present purpose, it is regarded as corresponding to the definition by Scotch (6): "any stimulus or stimuli, experienced consciously or unconsciously, which is potentially harmful or threatening to the individual." In such a sense, life for the majority of the human race, whether in developed or developing countries, has never been stress-free. Stresses have changed, however, as civilization has progressed through the successive revolutions generated by agriculture (*ca* 10,000 BC), industry (*ca* 1800 AD), and computers (from 1971 AD onward). Starvation, cold, and crude physical dangers have been largely replaced, at least in the Western democracies, by subtler psychologic pressures; and many modern inventions originally regarded as beneficial have turned out to have deleterious effects. The accelerating speed of technologic innovation has outstripped the far slower pace at which social institutions, organizations, and customs can modify themselves to adapt to new practices, new products, and new processes.

From a biologic, social, and medical standpoint, it is important to recognize that although science and technology have advanced exponentially and although society has made steady if unspectacular progress, men and women, as biologic entities, have altered hardly at all. Their bodies, evolved for the life of the hunter/gatherer, for physical exertion, for childbearing and rearing, with the free display of emotion, are not optimally suited to withstand the stresses of contemporary Western society. Such stresses are greatest in the United States, the acknowledged leader in altering lifestyles through technologic innovations introduced on a universal scale, but other Western countries have not lagged far behind.

TECHNOLOGIC INNOVATIONS: SOME ADVERSE CONSEQUENCES

The writer has elsewhere described (4) 10 technologic advances which have done much to create the shape—and the stresses—of the modern world. The 10 include advances made in (a) energy generation, (b) food manufacture, (c) transportation, (d) mass production, (e) urbanization, (f) big business, (g) communication, (h) new materials, (i) disease control, and (j) microelectronics and computers. Problems have developed in the wake of every innovation.

Energy Requirements

Energy generation from oil has become beset with political difficulties due to the higher prices and greater influence demanded by the major producer nations of the Middle East. Coal mining has become safer because of the introduction of mechanical cutters and so forth, but nuclear power carries the risk of immediate or long-term pollution, theft by terrorists, and use in nuclear war. More efficient food production is unfortunately still accompanied by inequalities in distribution, with persisting hardship and famine in poor countries. Individuals in affluent societies, in contrast, habitually consume too many calories and eat too much fat, sugar, salt, and red meat; their diets are short of roughage, and the food additives employed to aid flavor and color, as well as to act as preservatives, may be deleterious. Snacks obtained from take-out food counters or eaten in front of the TV set have reduced family cohesion by replacing formal mealtimes. Improvements in transport have literally speeded up life. The chances of dying in an accident in a commercial airliner or train are low; but roads are now made hazardous by millions of automobiles, which deplete world resources of petroleum, pollute skies, generate frustration, aggression, and (sometimes) a desire to show off in drivers, and, in company with other transport systems, discourage individuals from getting adequate exercise. Mass production has produced an oversupply of so many goods that demand has had to be artificially stimulated through advertising, and strategies such as planned obsolescence have been introduced to ensure that products break down or are discarded before the end of their useful lives. Mass production is highly efficient in turning out cornucopias of consumer durables; but work on automobile assembly lines, for example, is so tedious and boring that strikes are frequent, despite reasonable levels of pay, and there as elsewhere workers are being replaced by machines.

Influences of the Media

Urbanization has led to the overcrowding of the disadvantaged into the decaying centers of many cities where traffic densities are high and associated with noise, loss of urban amenities, ugliness, poverty, mental and physical ill health, alcoholism, prostitution, drug abuse, and crime. Big business has created wealth for the few at the expense of the many; it has also given many individuals a feeling of insignificance and powerlessness; they see themselves not as masters of their environment but as tiny cogs in an enormous machine. Such convictions do not engender confidence in personal abilities or healthy self-respect. Better communications on a person-to-person level, as provided by the telephone, have been beneficial; but on a mass basis, the avalanche of information made available by newspapers, periodicals, paperbacks, radio, and television has had mixed effects.

Television, a major transformer of modern society, may also play a significant role. It is now available in more than 90% of Western homes. Through the behavior it presents and the goods it advertises it imparts, Shulman (7) has observed, a selfish materialistic view of life. Its message often derogates widely accepted authority figures, traditional standards, and the virtues of hard work, patience, and selfless endeavor. Violence, which in real life is rather rare, is presented as routine behavior, the norm for good and bad alike. A minority of programs educate and enlighten. In Great Britain, for example, BBC2 which transmits the highest proportion of such presentations, is watched by only about 5% of viewers. The majority of programs seek to superficially entertain, but even so, a proportion arouse resentment, create envy, and provide children especially with a distorted view of society. Some presentations generate anxiety by portraying intimidating situations or by conveying information too complex for the audience to comprehend. Violence on television, moreover, like violent films, Taggart and Carruthers (8) have demonstrated, is capable of evoking responses indicative of cardiovascular stress.

Elsewhere in this volume, the same authors have shown that "active" aggressive emotions, such as the anger, determination, frustration, and anxiety experienced in emotionally stressful activities such as automobile driving, public speaking, and parachute jumping, are associated not only with tachycardia and EKG changes but also with increases in plasma norepinephrine, in free fatty acid levels, and in plasma triglycerides. This is a possible mechanism whereby intense emotion may lead to atherosclerosis, especially if the raised levels of fat in the blood are not burned away by physical exercise. It is noteworthy that oxprenolol, one of the more recently introduced beta blockers, was found to be "spectacularly effective" in abolishing the cardiac and lipid responses to intense emotion.

Of all the knowledge humanity currently possesses, 75% has been discovered within the last 20 years, and the amount is doubling every 10; ideas come and go 20 to 100 times faster than a century ago. One of the most stressful effects of this "information explosion," in combination with the increased efficiency of the media, Toffler (9) has observed, is "information-overload." Thus individuals in Western technosocieties are constantly compelled to process and to filter out a fraction of the hundreds of information-rich messages they receive daily. Difficulties have also been created by the new materials that have been developed, notably plastics, for their manufacture consumes energy and finite resources; and many, not being biodegradable, present problems in regard to disposal and pollution. Aerosol cans, for example, have been banned in the United States, lest their contents contaminate the upper atmosphere.

Therapeutic Advances

Disease control improved strikingly after 1945, although the explosive population upsurge that took place, especially in Asia, Africa, and Latin America, was probably due to improved sanitation and a better diet rather than to advances in medical treatment. Controlling the major killing diseases—cholera, typhus, typhoid, yellow fever, sleeping sickness, and plague—and treating infections with antibiotics enabled a higher proportion of infants to survive to adult life, in which they have put further pressures on food, housing, education, and health-care and, by reproducing, have added to the population problem. The introduction of oral contraceptives in the early 1960s terminated the post-Second World War baby boom and facilitated the growth of women's liberation movements, but in addition to occasional adverse physical effects (hypertension, thrombosis) the pill has produced adverse psychologic sequelae, such as depression (10). Its unprecedented popularity and efficiency in reducing the number of children born has led to profound disagreements on what the role of an adult woman should be. This last has sometimes led to reverberations on families.

Microprocessors

The microprocessor or central processing unit (CPU) introduced in 1971 and fabricated on a minute silicon chip, which was preceded by the invention of the transistor (1948), the integrated circuit (1960), and large-scale integration in the late 1960s, seems destined to exert profound effects on society. Itself a computer, the CPU's efficiency, cheapness, reliability, and ready availability will affect patterns of work, education, sociopolitical organization and scientific progress. Thus many unpleasant routine tasks, including factory and clerical duties, may be taken over by computers, leading to widespread underemployment and unemployment, with a decline in living standards and consequent dissatisfaction and resentment. The "data bank society" may generate additional bitterness because of the computer's impartial bestowal of anonymity (the individual is depersonalized to a pattern of electrical impulses stored on magnetic tape or in bubbles) and its invasion of privacy (intimate personal details, estimates of credit-worthiness, records of transgressions, and so forth will all be stored in computer memories). The computer will render education more economical and will improve it by eliminating the wasteful duplication of programs by individual teachers and by developing better teaching methods; many schools and many teachers may thus become redundant. It is likely also to produce considerable sociopolitical disruption by weakening union power and rendering valueless many hard-acquired skills, as well as the sole advantage of age, namely wisdom; the young will have immediate access to computer-stored knowledge and experience. If, as seems likely, economic growth is slowed or halted (or even curtailed), industry may be unable to generate sufficient jobs to accommodate the workforce, which in any event may be too highly educated for many of the tasks that will be available. The inability of workers to satisfy their expectations, which have risen steadily for the past 50 years and which they have been encouraged to regard as legitimate, is likely to present a severe problem. Earlier retirement, perhaps at 40, is likely, with many individuals bitterly resenting their forced leisure and reduced income. The computer will help science to progress. Its application in medicine, for example, should enable people to live longer and healthier lives, although this will add to the problem of overpopulation. Finally, it is likely to be used to create higher forms of intelligence

(11). The computer is essentially an extension of the human mind; its potential for good and evil is virtually limitless.

THE PRESENT AND THE FUTURE

The changes brought about by technologic innovation—interfering with nature—have clearly been profound and seem certain to become even more marked. In the next few decades, barring nuclear war, humans will rush into an increasingly unimaginable future in which familiar terrain will become ever more scarce. At present, society is in transition and families are under pressure. The stresses encountered by individuals include those produced by society on one hand, and on the other those experienced at different ages by the two sexes.

The goal of capital growth, so single-mindely pursued in the last quarter century by Western nations (the United States' Gross National Product rose from $400 billion in 1955 to $700 billion in 1965 and $1700 billion in 1975), while generating wealth, has also been associated with resource depletion, wastefulness, and pollution. Poverty has persisted even in the richest nations, despite the spread of affluence, and crime and violence have increased. Patriarchal institutions, such as the church and the armed services, have lost their charisma, and the social structure of society has changed as the professional and managerial classes have declined in status. On the other hand, those engaged in manual occupations—especially tradespeople engaged in skilled work—have, largely through union pressure, advanced in affluence, status, and power (henceforth, because of the computer revolution, this process is likely to be halted if not reversed). Hours of leisure have increased *pari passu* with the emergence of more permissive attitudes in regard to sexual mores, standards of work, and punishment for crime. Pornography in written material as well as in stage shows and films has become commonplace; so too has venereal disease, especially gonorrhea and nonspecific urethritis (NSU).

Interpersonal Relationships

The family has been adversely affected by these changes, particularly by the geographic and social mobility now available. The typical family in the United States moves every 3 years and is nuclear in the sense that it is no longer in continuous or frequent contact with a range of relatives of different generations. Seven out of 10 families live in urban environments and are less involved than formerly with the community. Family members have fewer extrafamilial friendships, and many tend to look to each other for their psychologic satisfactions, although separated by age, place of work, and discrepancies in recreational interests, with the possible exception of television! Marriage although still popular, has become less enduring; and more and more single-parent families, most frequently headed by a divorced or separated mother, have appeared. In 1978, the United Kingdom had 730,000 such families with 1.25 million children;

possessing about half the resources of their conventional two-parent counterparts, they now constitute a section of the "new poor" (12). Increasing numbers of young Americans in the 20–34 age group are currently postponing marriage to a later age (or indefinitely) and instead adopting alternative living arrangements (13).

The aged have become subjected to stresses they have not previously encountered. Although they are now more numerous, their position is less secure than formerly, for much of their knowledge is obsolete. Many, especially the widowed and the never-married, lead lonely, monotonous lives, often skimping on food because of low income and savings eroded by inflation. New drugs and new treatments have reduced the morbidity of some of their illnesses, but defects in sight, hearing, and locomotion make them susceptible to falls and road accidents; in cities particularly, they are subject to physical assault.

Sex Comparisons

Men center their lives for the most part round their work, which to a greater or lesser extent provides status, self-esteem, stimulus, challenge, and a chance to master the environment as well as income to support themselves and their families. The rising rate of unemployment which has characterized the Western world since the mid-1970s is thus immensely unsettling. Plenty of "dirty" jobs no one wants (garbage collecting, janitorial services, and so forth) are available, but they are frequently dull and repetitive, involving long hours of work, poor wages, inadequate safety and health protection, lack of job security, and low social status. Dissatisfaction and boredom at work, sometimes associated with increased leisure, are other sources of stress. So too are the objects and lifestyles portrayed on television which can generate unrealistically high expectations, especially when income growth—or even continuity—is not assured. The greater occupational and social mobility available in modern societies to those who succeed in the "rat race" is stressful to some, challenging to others. Relationships with women evoke more anxiety than formerly, due to the liberation movement, and male impotence has become a more widespread problem. Stress leads many adult males to employ coping mechanisms, such as overindulgence in alcohol, cigarettes, and food and inertia, which lead to the "diseases of affluence"— hepatic cirrhosis, bronchial carcinoma, obesity, and "loafer's heart." Finally, the inhibition of emotional display so highly prized by Anglo-Saxons may result in increased muscle tension and fatigue with headaches, temporomandibular joint dysfunctional discomfort, diffuse aches and pains, and so forth.

Women have been particularly affected by life in Western-type technosocieties. Because of the efficiency of modern contraceptives, the cultural warping of childbirth, the reduction of breast feeding, and the trend to small families, together with tubal ligations and hysterectomies, women's bodies evolved over millions of years to conceive, bear, nurture, and rear numbers of children, are frustrated in their biological purpose. Instead some women may suffer throughout their reproductive years with stressful menstruation. Generally, motherhood has lost its charisma and matriarchy its status. Marriage has become less secure and, despite the widespread availability of labor-saving appliances, is harder physically. This is because between one-third and one-half of married women in the Western world are engaged in paid work outside their homes; doing not one but two jobs they may become chronically overtired. Many women are deprived of emotional, physical, and financial supports because of reduced contact with parents, grandparents, and so forth; nonetheless, arranging their family and home-care tasks around their working hours, they strive to contribute toward their family's welfare. They are the prime targets of television advertising and are constantly bombarded with exhortations to purchase goods and services which are unnecessary, but which they are assured will bring greater health and happiness to themselves and their families. At work, women often receive one-third less pay than their male counterparts for performing identical duties; many women's jobs are clerical and are threatened by the computer technologies. The women's liberation movements have subjected many of their members to hostility and criticism in the harsh male-ordered materialistic society. Finally, the emphasis of recent years on sexuality and on youthful attraction has led to an increase in rape and assaults on women on one hand, and to relentless pressures to keep younger, more vital and more participant in society than nature readily permits, on the other. In consequence of these stresses more women are now developing 'male' disorders such as alcoholism, lung cancer and ischemic heart disease and many are becoming dispirited and depressed.

Problems of Child-Rearing

Children are more exposed to emotional privations at every stage now than in the past. Despite the availability of contraception and legal abortion, many illegitimate babies are born; and, with the increasing prevalence of divorce, a higher proportion of youngsters are now brought up in a broken home by a single parent, with fewer caring relatives and friends. Even when the parental home remains intact, mothers frequently decide to resume work; in the United States, one in three of the 50% of women who work are mothers with children under the age of six. Television, used as an "electronic babysitter" from the age of 2 onward, is a poor substitute for a parent's company and does not encourage children to think and to learn; its program can desensitize them to violence and render them more apprehensive in later life. When the child is old enough to go to school, the mother usually feels freer to take up employment; often she cannot reach home before her child, so that a generation of children who return to an empty house or apartment has started to appear. The computer should improve education by personalizing it and making it more interesting and efficient but may create problems by taking paid work from mothers and fathers, rendering them more frustrated and enforcing more prolonged parent-child contact in a setting of reduced income.

The lack of cohesion that has developed in Western families, with each member eating alone and "doing their own thing," has become associated with a troublesome generation gap. Parents and grandparents brought up in the depressed conditions of the 1930s, when a secure job was highly prized and work was an absolute necessity, find it difficult to sympathize with the apparently hedonistic lifestyle of Western youngsters today. The latter, growing up in a more unstable society with less acute poverty and fewer penalties for failing to work (and smaller rewards for doing so!), find the work ethic inimical to their inclinations. In consequence, they refuse to conform in dress, attitudes, or behavior to the mores of a society whose peak, they feel, has passed. Individuals in their 30s are often caught between the two worlds, getting the worst of both. The failure of many youngsters to become socially integrated is reflected in lack of discipline in schools, failure to form an identity, aimlessness, lack of goals, drug-taking, antisocial attitudes, and despair. The high rate of unemployment in schoolleavers constitutes an enormous stress for today's young people, who, deprived of meaningful work, may find it difficult to gain self-respect and to plan confidently for the future. The computer revolution is likely to make the problem worse and may lead many disaffected, dissatisfied, frustrated youngsters to turn to crime and violence for stimulus and monetary gain.

PHARMACOLOGIC IMPLICATIONS

It is paradoxical that reserpine, the oldest neuroleptic, imported into Western medicine from India as a treatment for hypertension in the early 1950s, was subsequently employed by Kline (14) to control hyperactive psychotic patients. In the process, reserpine, which depletes brain serotonin, produced depression. Observation of this phenomenon indirectly led to the introduction of the monoamine oxidase (MAO) inhibitor antidepressants in 1957. Imipramine, a clinical contribution of Kuhn (15), was made available the following year in consequence of the success of chlorpromazine, which it chemically resembles, and ushered in the era of the tricyclics. Meanwhile, in the mid 1950s, meprobamate, the first of the minor tranquilizers, had appeared, followed in the early 1960s by chlordiazepoxide and other benzodiazepines. Propranolol, the first safe beta blocker, an analog of isoprenaline, was introduced in 1964. Like other similar compounds, it not only relieves angina, reduces blood pressure, and alleviates thyrotoxicosis, hypertropic cardiomyopathy, and cardiac dysrhythmias, it also exerts psychotropic effects and, as has been described in Chapter 6, is of value in anxiety states. Beta blockers should not be prescribed in congestive failure after acute myocardial infarction, in states of impaired atrioventricular conduction, or in asthmatics (16). In other situations, they appear to be effective and reasonably safe (17).

Pharmacologically, hypertension and endogenous depressive symptoms are linked by serotonin deficiency, which is produced by reserpine, methyldopa, and other hypotensive agents. Psychodynamically, the link is anxiety and hostility which, suppressed to a greater or lesser extent, is usually found in both these conditions. Ventilating such feelings in psychotherapy, however, provides only symptomatic relief, and has little effect on the course of these diseases.

Tricyclic antidepressants in particular and psychotropic drugs in general occasionally have been shown to be associated with sudden cardiac death, as described elsewhere in this book. In view of the gloomy prediction that by the time this book is published half of Britain's total population—twice as many as when the first edition appeared in 1977—will, if present trends continue, be exposed to excessive traffic noise in their homes (18), it is of interest that Davidson (see Chapter 8) found that noise stress caused death in rats with cardiomyopathies who were receiving amitriptyline or imipramine. The risk of cardiac death with tricyclics must be balanced against that of suicide and invalidism, the mortality and morbidity of untreated melancholia. In practice, the rare instances of death associated with tricyclic administration [as Symes (19) has observed, all tricyclics are potentially cardiotoxic] are sometimes associated with the concurrent administration of other drugs, such as frusemide, so that drug interactions may play an important role. It is apparent from Chapters 10 and 11, which are concerned with the new nontricyclic antidepressants, that the latter provide an important advance in reducing the risk of cardiotoxic effects when treating depressive illness with antidepressant drugs.

The question of whether concurrent anxiety plays a significant role in the genesis of hypertension, and, if so, whether the addition of a minor tranquilizer to an antihypertensive agent might be beneficial, is described in Chapter 15. Wheatley's finding that medazepam does not increase the effectiveness of methyldopa in hypertensive patients is in agreement with clinical experience. Thus individuals with moderate degrees of hypertension do not usually develop anxiety symptoms until they learn that their blood pressures are elevated. Furthermore, in giving minor tranquilizers to hypertensives, the physician is probably treating his or her own, rather than the patient's, anxiety. One wonders what the result would have been if a phenothiazine, a tricyclic, or a MAO inhibitor, any of which might have reduced blood pressure, had been added to the hypotensive agent.

In conclusion, although the stresses of modern life have probably been reflected in an increased mortality and morbidity from ischemic heart disease, knowledge of relevant etiologic factors is steadily accumulating, and with beta blockers, psychotropics, and other compounds, more help is now available for patients with diseases of the circulatory system than at any other time in history. The pharmacologic conquest of the effects of stress on the heart is within our grasp in view of the notable advances that have been made, many of which are described in this book.

REFERENCES

1. Carruthers, M. *The Western Way of Death.* Davis-Poynter, London, 1973.
2. Darke, S. J. Diet and ischaemic heart disease. *Health Trends,* 1974, 6, 42.

3. Fry, J. Natural history of hypertension. *Lancet,* 1974, 2, 431.
4. Hordern, A. *Tranquility Denied.* Rigby, Adelaide, 1976.
5. Selye, H. *Stress in health and disease.* Butterworths, London, 1976.
6. Scotch, N. A. Sociocultural factors in the epidemiology of Zulu hypertension. *Am. J. Public Health,* 1963, 53, 1205.
7. Shulman, M. *The Ravenous Eye.* Cassell, London, 1973.
8. Carruthers, M., and Taggart, P. Vagotonicity of violence: Biochemical and cardiac responses to violent films and television programmes. *Br. Med. J.,* 1973, 3, 384.
9. Toffler, A. *Future Shock.* Pan, London, 1971.
10. Adams, P. W. Pyridoxine, the Pill and depression. *J. Pharmacother.,* 1980, 3, 20.
11. Evans, C. Computers and artificial intelligence. In: *Science Fact,* edited by F. George, pp. 11–44. Topaz, England, 1977.
12. Turner, W. One-parent families: The undeserving poor?" *New Soc.,* 45, 11, 1978.
13. United Press. More dodge marriage ties in the US. *The Australian,* August 15, 1978.
14. Kline, N. S. Use of rauwolfia serpentina benth in neuropsychiatric conditions. *Ann. NY Acad. Sci.,* 1954, 59, 107.
15. Kuhn R. Uber die behandlung depressiver zustaude mit einen iminobenzylderivat (G 22355). *Schweiz. Med. Wochenschr.,* 1957, 87, 1135.
16. Leading article. Adverse reactions to beta-adrenergic blockade. *Br. Med. J.,* 1974, 2, 3.
17. Wheatley, D. *Psychopharmacology in Family Practice.* Heinemann, London, 1973.
18. Silcock, B. Noise toll will double by 1980. *Sunday Times (Lond.),* July 21, 1974.
19. Symes, M. H. Cardiovascular effects of clomipramine (Anafranil). *J. Int. Med. Res.,* 1973, 1, 460.

Subject Index